RECOVERY AND WELL-BEING IN THE PERFORMING ARTS

Investigating the critical relationship between recovery, fatigue, working conditions, and societal pressures in the performing arts, this comprehensive text brings together international experts from psychology, medicine, and sport science. It highlights important research on recovery and its physiological and psychological implications for performing artists across music, dance, acting, and circus performance.

Divided into four parts, this book contextualises recovery challenges in performing arts while maintaining positive health and well-being levels essential for performance. Chapters examine recovery from both individual and organisational perspectives, and address how recovery and well-being can be induced and sustained, preventing overuse, and enabling creativity and self-efficacy. Contributors provide scientific state-of-the-art approaches answering crucial questions that also address societal and systemic challenges in the performing arts. They provide valuable insights for researchers, while offering practical guidance for anyone involved in supporting the physical and mental health of performing artists across diverse artistic disciplines.

This essential resource will be of interest to both academic communities and applied practice professionals concerned with human health and well-being in performing arts, including artistic directors, performing artists, coaches, conductors, composers, and healthcare teams working with performers.

Eckart Altenmüller is a Professor Emeritus of Music Physiology and Musician's Medicine at the University of Music, Drama and Media, Hannover, Germany.

Michael Kellmann is a Professor of Sport Psychology at the Faculty of Sport Science, Ruhr University Bochum, Germany. He is also an Honorary Professor in the School of Human Movement and Nutrition Sciences, The University of Queensland, Australia.

Jürgen Beckmann is a Professor of Sport Psychology and Emeritus of Excellence in the School of Medicine and Health, Technical University of Munich, Germany. He is currently a member of the Psycho-Cardiological Consultation Group at the German Heart Centre Munich. He is also an Honorary Professor in the School of Human Movement and Nutrition Sciences, The University of Queensland, Australia.

Gene M. Moyle is a Professor of Dance, Sport and Exercise Psychologist and Pro Vice-Chancellor (Academic Programs and Partnerships) at the Queensland University of Technology, Brisbane, Australia.

Advances in Recovery and Stress Research: Multi-Disciplinary Approaches Series

Series Editors

Michael Kellmann, *Ruhr University Bochum, Germany, and The University of Queensland, Australia.*

Jürgen Beckmann, *Technical University of Munich, Germany, and The University of Queensland, Australia*

Advances in Recovery and Stress Research: Multi-Disciplinary Approaches covers a broad range of areas in which recovery plays a crucial role, providing the current status of research on recovery and stress. In particular, it aims to be unique in addressing fields in which recovery and stress play an important role, but recovery has not received adequate attention, for example, in the areas of health promotion as well as performance promotion in work settings. Another feature of the series is that it contains both up-to-date theoretical and applied perspectives from multi-disciplinary approaches.

Recovery and Well-being in Sport and Exercise
Interdisciplinary Insights
Edited by Michael Kellmann and Jürgen Beckmann

The Importance of Recovery for Physical and Mental Health
Negotiating the Effects of Underrecovery
Edited by Michael Kellmann, Sarah Jakowski, and Jürgen Beckmann

Fostering Recovery and Well-being in a Healthy Lifestyle
Psychological, Somatic, and Organizational Prevention Approaches
Edited by Michael Kellmann and Jürgen Beckmann

The Recovery-Stress Questionnaires
A User Manual
Edited by Michael Kellmann and K. Wolfgang Kallus

Creating Urban and Workplace Environments for Recovery and Well-being
New Perspectives on Urban Design and Mental Health
Edited by Stephan Pauleit, Michael Kellmann, and Jürgen Beckmann

Recovery and Well-being in the Performing Arts
Edited by Eckart Altenmüller, Michael Kellmann, Jürgen Beckmann, and Gene M. Moyle

For more information about this series, please visit: www.routledge.com/Advances-in-Recovery-and-Stress-Research/book-series/ARSR

RECOVERY AND WELL-BEING IN THE PERFORMING ARTS

Edited by
Eckart Altenmüller, Michael Kellmann, Jürgen Beckmann, and Gene M. Moyle

Routledge
Taylor & Francis Group
LONDON AND NEW YORK

Designed cover image: Getty Images

First published 2026
by Routledge
4 Park Square, Milton Park, Abingdon, Oxon OX14 4RN

and by Routledge
605 Third Avenue, New York, NY 10158

Routledge is an imprint of the Taylor & Francis Group, an informa business

British Library Cataloguing-in-Publication Data
A catalogue record for this book is available from the British Library

ISBN: 9781032936444 (hbk)
ISBN: 9781032936369 (pbk)
ISBN: 9781003566885 (ebk)

DOI: 10.4324/9781003566885

Typeset in Sabon
by codeMantra

CONTENTS

CONTRIBUTORS

Ackermann, Bronwen J., The University of Sydney, Australia

Altenmüller, Eckart, The Hanover University of Music, Drama and Media Hannover, Germany

Azoury, Dimity, The Australian Ballet, Australia

Beckmann, Jürgen, Technical University of Munich, Germany, and The University of Queensland, Australia

Blevins, Peta, Edith Cowan University, Australia

Brown-Appenzeller, Derrick, University of Melbourne, Australia

Coutts, Aaron J., University of Technology Sydney, Australia

Davies, Christina, University of Western Australia, Australia

Erskine, Shona, Shona Erskine Psychology, Australia

Fraser, Chad, Performing Arts Athletic Therapist Consultant, Canada

Greenspan, Stephanie, Artletic Science, Canada

Guss-West, Clare, Bern University, Switzerland

Hopper, Luke, Edith Cowan University, Australia

Jeffrey, Erica R., Dance for Parkinson's Australia, Australia

Jeffries, Annie C., The University of New South Wales, Australia

Kellmann, Michael, Ruhr University Bochum, Germany, and The University of Queensland, Australia

Leventhal, David, Mark Morris Dance Group, USA

Mainwaring, Lynda, University of Toronto, Canada

Mayes, Susan, La Trobe University, Australia

McCrary, J. Matt, Hannover Medical School, Germany

McDonnell, Aoife, The Australian Ballet, Australia

Moisseinen, Nella, University of Helsinki, Finland

Mowers, Dave, The Mowers Group, USA

Moyle, Gene M., Queensland University of Technology, Australia

Munro, David, Swinburne University, Australia

Nicholas, Joanna, Western Australian Academy of Performing Arts, Australia

Petiot, Bernard, Ecole Nationale de Cirque, Canada

Richard, Veronique, The University of Queensland, Australia

Richter, Bernhard, University Freiburg and University of Music Freiburg, Germany

Särkämö, Teppo, University of Helsinki, Finland

Schuppert, Maria, Academy of Music 'Louis Spohr', Germany

Silverman, Michael J., University of Minnesota, USA

Stegemann, Thomas, University of Music and Performing Arts Vienna, Austria

Steiner, Dirk D., Université Côte d'Azur, France

Melanie Stuckey, Ecole Nationale de Cirque, Canada

Tallent, Jamie, University of Essex, United Kingdom

Wirdnam, Matthew, LaTrobe University, Australia

Wood, Laura L., Lesley University, USA

Wyon, Matthew, University of Wolverhampton, United Kingdom

SERIES FOREWORD

Advances in Recovery and Stress Research: Multi-Disciplinary Approaches covers a broad range of areas in which recovery plays a crucial role, providing the status of research on recovery and stress. In particular, it aims to broaden the understanding of recovery and be unique in addressing fields in which recovery and stress play an important role, but recovery has not received adequate attention. Examples are the areas of health promotion as well as performance promotion in work settings. Another feature of the series is that it contains both up-to-date theoretical and applied perspectives from multi-disciplinary approaches.

It is the idea of the series *Advances in Recovery and Stress Research: Multi-Disciplinary Approaches* to publish a volume each year. We started with *Recovery and well-being in sport and exercise* (Volume 1), followed by *The importance of recovery for physical and mental health: Negotiating the effects of underrecovery* (Volume 2), *Fostering recovery and well-being in a healthy lifestyle: Psychological, somatic, and organizational prevention approaches* (Volume 3), *The Recovery-Stress Questionnaires: A user manual* (Volume 4), *Creating urban and workplace environments for recovery and well-being: New perspectives on urban design and mental health* (Volume 5), and *Recovery and well-being in the performing arts* (Volume 6). Always current information on the series can be found at www.routledge.com/Advances-in-Recovery-and-Stress-Research/book-series/ARSR.

We thank Routledge for the flexibility and engagement for this adventure to develop the series *Advances in Recovery and Stress Research: Multi-Disciplinary Approaches.*

Michael Kellmann
Jürgen Beckmann

PREFACE

This book highlights for the first time the relationship between recovery, fatigue, working conditions, and societal pressures in performing artists. Musicians, actors, dancers, and circus artists must deal with enormous physical and psychological stressors as part of their day-to-day career pursuits. Frequently, it is challenging for performing artists to maintain positive levels of overall health and well-being such as when touring or preparing new programmes, shows or performance seasons under tight time constraints. Although robust physical and psychological well-being is typically a prerequisite for outstanding performance, many performers fear taking time off for recovery, be it due to financial reasons or perceived negative impacts upon creative processes and opportunities.

The purpose of this interdisciplinary book is to address the following questions:

- How recovery and well-being can be induced and sustained in the performing arts.
- How societal and systemic challenges in the performing arts can best be addressed.
- How overuse can be prevented in performing artists.
- How performing artists can best recover.
- What measures are necessary to maintain creativity, self-efficacy, and well-being of performing artists.

This book aims at collecting actual research on recovery and its physiological and psychological implications in performing artists. Recovery is not equated with mere regeneration, but also as a prevention measure that provides resources to assist individuals increase their resilience to future stressors. Furthermore, it strives to formulate recovery routines and aims at sensitising employers, industry professionals, and educators to improve working conditions and prevent performers from engaging in dysfunctional self-exploitation.

This book will address this often neglected aspect and connect research from different scientific disciplines to the broader perspective of creating a healthy career in the performing arts. It will demonstrate that recovery is an essential but largely neglected factor in maintaining performance in the performing arts. Additionally, several chapters explore how training and workplace environments can be optimised to enhance and promote recovery. Furthermore, one part of the book addresses how music, dance, and theatre are also excellent resources for recovery in our society.

Eckart Altenmüller
Michael Kellmann
Jürgen Beckmann
Gene M. Moyle

PART I

Conceptualising the problem

1

RECOVERY CONCEPTS AND DIVERSITY OF APPROACHES TO RECOVERY IN THE PERFORMING ARTS

A general introduction

Eckart Altenmüller, Jürgen Beckmann, Michael Kellmann, and Gene M. Moyle

Introduction

A career as a professional performing artist is highly challenging both mentally and physically. Dancing, acrobatics, making music, acting, or any of the various performing artforms are highly complex by nature. Through persistent practice, physical prerequisites like muscular strength and stamina, yet also flexibility of joints and fibrous tissues, are required to be attained and maintained. Sensorimotor, auditory, visual and cognitive and emotional skills need to be perfected and stored in memory-systems. In most performing arts, meeting temporo-spatial constraints is an integral part of any activity. For example, when playing music in an ensemble, the 'right pitch' has to be played in the 'right moment'; when dancing, the 'right step' has to be executed at the 'right time'. Similar constraints exist for most of the other performing arts, be it acrobatics, juggling, or acting. What all these activities have in common is the 'nature' of performing – that is, there is always an audience. Whether that is an external or internal 'spectator', this can result in societal or personal pressure being put on, or experienced by, the performer. Performing therefore needs to be conceptualised in a systemic manner that includes broader personal and societal goals and needs.

In the process of acquiring the necessary skills, programmes for complex and highly precise motor skill/movement sequences are developed and

Altenmüller, E., Beckmann, J., Kellmann, M., & Moyle, G. M. (2026). Recovery concepts and diversity of approaches to recovery in the performing arts: A general introduction. In E. Altenmüller, M. Kellmann, J. Beckmann, & G. M. Moyle (Eds.), *Recovery and well-being in the performing arts* (pp. 3–20). Routledge.

DOI: 10.4324/9781003566885-2

memorised, knowledge for creating an appealing performance is explicitly or intuitively acquired, and emotional expressiveness to render actions meaningful is worked towards. Learning all these skills through laborious regular practice usually starts in early childhood and undergoes different levels of increasing complexities, frequently accompanied by a transition in cognitive development and associated strategies. Whereas children tend to rely more on procedural learning through observation and imitation, older children and adolescents include cognitions and explicit strategies to achieve higher skill levels (Doyon, 1997). To attain the expertise required for a professional performer's level laborious training is demanded. Here, expertise is on one hand characterised by reliably reproducible temporal and spatial precision of highly complex movement sequences, on the other hand, expressive qualities, difficult to objectively assess are part of it. Ericsson et al. (1993) formulated the 10 years and 10,000 hours 'rule of practice', emphasising the necessity of training. More comprehensive theories suggest that in addition to training developmental factors (e.g., age of starting training), ability factors (e.g., aptitudes), non-ability factors (e.g., personality traits), and background factors (e.g., opportunity to engage in training) play an important role (Hambrick et al., 2020). The *Multifactorial Gene-Environment Interaction Model* (Ullén et al., 2016) describes elegantly how these factors relate to one another.

A further characteristic of performing arts is that all actions require sensory-motor integration in anticipation, performance and evaluation of movements. Hearing, seeing, proprioception, and the vestibulo-cochlear balancing system are prerequisites for monitoring performances. For example, musicians 'hear ahead' and 'feel ahead', dancers, acrobats and jugglers 'see ahead' and 'feel ahead' in their actions. This very precise anticipation of sound, vision, and proprioception is realised in the central nervous system as 'predictive coding' in widely distributed networks of numerous brain regions (Vuust et al., 2022). Throughout years of practice, underlying processes are automated and neuronal networks of subcortical regions, including the basal ganglia and cerebellum, gradually take over functions of the cerebral regions by creating action routines (Herholz & Zatorre, 2012). This relieves the sensorimotor areas of the cerebrum and creates capacity for the assimilation of new information (Ungerleider et al., 2002). The process of practising finally occurs as a procedural, self-organising learning process and is optimised in the best case by curious exploration of new practice styles and by sharpening self-awareness (overview in McPherson, 2005). It is important to note that not only the acquisition, but also the maintenance of performance skills requires constant practice. Performing can therefore be considered as an example of lifelong learning.

Recovery

Compared to other approaches Kellmann and Kallus (2001) have postulated a broader perspective on recovery that goes beyond regeneration or 'being cured' or 'being normal again' (Beckmann et al., 2023). This broader perspective addresses recovery as a resource that enables individuals not only to recover from stress but also to develop resilience to health-threatening stress. Kallus (2016, p. 42) defined recovery as "an inter- and intraindividual multilevel (e.g., psychological, physiological, social) process in time for the re-establishment of personal resources and their full functional capacity".

A key requirement for recovery is to take time for it. The first step is to interrupt or stop a stressful activity in order to terminate or at least reduce the stress. There are different types of stress, such as physical and mental stress. Sometimes recovery can therefore also involve switching between types of stress, for example ending or interrupting a mental activity in order to switch to a physical activity. For example, a person spending the whole day teaching students may shift to physical practice of an instrument, for example playing scales on a piano, changing from predominantly mental stress to more physical stress. The latter supports replenishing the person's mental resources. Physical activity is an active recovery approach. The music professor could alternatively get a massage, i.e., pursue a passive recovery strategy.

There are large individual differences in the type of recovery that people prefer. For successful recovery, it is crucial that the most individually appropriate recovery strategy is selected and implemented. In addition, a person can pro-actively plan or schedule self-initiated recovery strategies, including social activities that are chosen by the person themselves and tailored to their needs (Kellmann, 2002; Kellmann et al., 2018, 2023). Situational conditions play a crucial role in recovery. For example, a noisy environment can impair sleep quality. Heat can also have a negative impact on recovery, for example by hindering physical activities and negatively affecting sleep quality. Especially, in the case of physical activity as preferred recovery strategy, environmental conditions are required that make an execution of physical activity possible. Additionally, the necessary conditions for the recovery activities need to be easily accessible.

Individuals' opportunities to recover from stress may be inadequate because strenuous and excessive life activities leave little time for recovery. If the necessary conditions for recovery are not given, for example because of lack of time or opportunities, a vicious cycle can be initiated. This is specifically true for performing artists who tend to be heavily overcommitted during the 'season' followed by month-long periods of inactivity, for example during the summer break of opera-houses, ballet, or concert venues. If recovery is inadequate (underrecovery) for a longer period of time, stress can become chronic. Chronic stress can lead to a neglect of the need for recovery and also interfere with recognising what the individual optimal recovery strategy would be (Beckmann, 2023). If there is timely awareness of the need for recovery, pro-active strategies can be initiated, and the vicious circle can be broken. A central aspect of the recovery model postulated by Kellmann and Kallus (2001) is the idea of a balance between stress and recovery. Increasing stress must be accompanied by an increase in corresponding recovery in order to maintain a balance between the two and thereby avoid negative consequences of underrecovery (Beckmann et al., 2024).

While this model was initially developed for the sport context it has meanwhile become employed in different contexts such as health promotion approaches (Kellmann et al., 2023), the workplace and urban development (Pauleit et al., 2025). We believe that this will also be very beneficial in the domain of performing artists.

Figure 1.1 sketches the general principles of the '*Scissor model*' of recovery, which is applicable for performing artists. Limited opportunities for recovery, such as time constraints, can prompt the vicious circle mentioned above: if the stress cannot be compensated by adequate recovery the imbalance will increase ('scissor function'). When the stress capacity threshold is reached the system may collapse such as in 'burnout' or 'overtraining' in sports. Special recovery opportunities are then required to restore a balanced system state.

The mechanisms underlying the '*Scissor model*' can be compared with the health-oriented model of salutogenesis by Antonovsky (1979, 1987). The salutogenesis model postulates a health/illness continuum. The question is

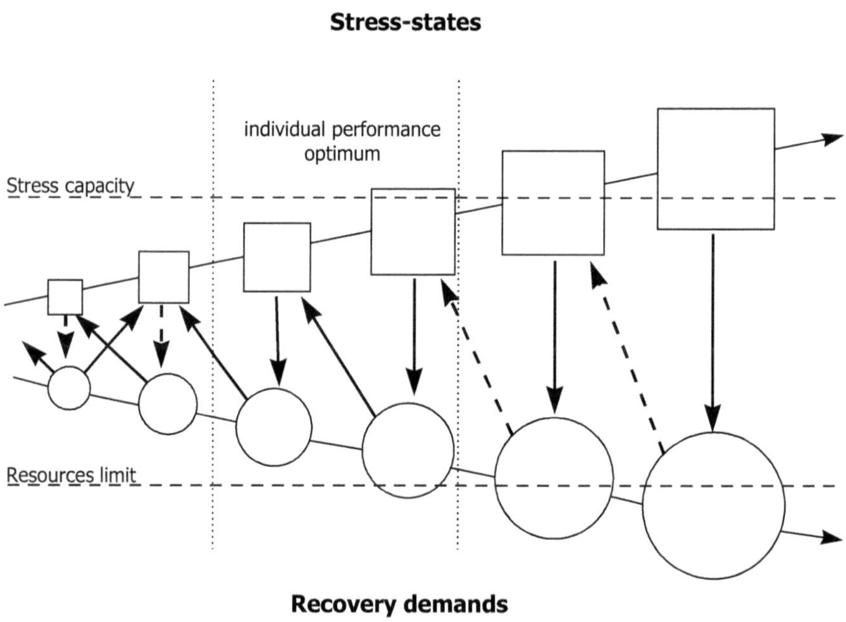

FIGURE 1.1 The '*Scissors-model*' of the interrelation of stress states and recovery demands.

Reprinted with permission from Kallus, K. W., & Kellmann, M. (2000). Burnout in athletes and coaches. In Y. Hanin (Ed.), *Emotions in sport* (pp. 209–230). Human Kinetics.

not whether someone is sick, but how far a person is from the endpoints of this continuum (i.e., healthy or sick). A person's position on the continuum depends on the person's current resilience and the availability of general resistance resources. The stress buffer created by recovery in Kellmann's (2002) model has similarities to the function of Antonovsky's general resistance resources.

In summary, Kellmann's recovery model suggests that a balance of recovery and stress prevents performance declines, illness, and reduced well-being. The model primarily states that balance is restored through appropriate recovery after a stressful experience. In addition, as a result of the recovery process, recovery can be obtained as a resource that buffers future stress. The recovery resource can raise the threshold for negative stress effects.

Specific challenges related to recovery in performing artists

Research studies have shown that consistent development and maintenance of performance at a high level requires adequate recovery (Kellmann & Beckmann, 2022). A central aspect of the Kellmann and Kallus (2001) model of recovery refers to the idea of a balance of recovery and stress. The assumption is that with increasing stress an increase in recovery must co-occur to maintain a stable balance between the two. As we understand it, recovery involves the re-establishment of individual resources but additionally involves building stress buffers (Kellmann & Kallus, 2001) or in a broader sense 'resilience' (World Health Organization, 2019). Achieving a recovery-stress balance does not simply imply recovery from stress but, in line with the World Health Organization (2019) position, promotes building up and maintaining resources that on a more general level promote a healthy state of the individual. It is essential to note that recovery is highly individuum-specific. For performing artists one of the challenges to find adequate recovery is that it requires time.

Four special features characterise the life of performing artists and have an impact on the requirements of recovery.

Beginning of professional training in childhood or youth

The decision to become a performer is often made during adolescence (Kogan, 2002; Kogan & Kangas, 2006). It is not uncommon for this decision to be influenced by parents and/or teachers, although there appears to be a lack of substantial research findings on this topic (Bright, 2006; Hague, 2018; Jaffee-Nagel, 1988). This early choice of profession leads to a self-identity and lifestyle dominated by training or performing, whereby performing is often implicitly understood as an artistic attitude. Numerous areas of life are subordinated to performance and performing. In children and adolescents, this can affect the way they organise their free time and their choice of peer group/s. Additionally, the choice of leisure sports young performing artists might participating in must not compromise their ability to perform, for example in aspiring guitarists or pianists, sports should not risk injury to hands or fingers; for aspiring dancers, sports must not put them at risk of significant injury overall (Wanke et al., 2013). Further, living as a performer impacts the consideration of nutrition and the management of body weight and composition, most obvious in dancers and acrobats. It is important to avoid alcohol as it impairs fine motor skills and memory, and also nicotine, which impairs lung function and oxygen saturation of red blood cells (Dang et al., 2020). Preparing to be a performer may influence the choice of schools, sometimes even the choice of place of residence for performer's families, particularly in highly gifted children who then relocate with their parents to attend a performing arts institution to receive optimal training and social support by an equally highly motivated peer group. Thus, numerous tasks and additional demands outside of the actual training for these children and young people start increasing, who, in addition, have to cope with bodily maturation and puberty processes, while also acquiring general social skills and participation in school education. Frequently, recovery times related to performance training are too short or incomplete due to the multiple demands these young people are confronted with.

Pleasurable, emotionally charged activity

Performing is self-rewarding and performers typically possess high intrinsic motivation. Therefore, any disruption of their ability to perform, dance, play an instrument, sing or act or any external threat to their daily training or work, such as lockdowns during the coronavirus pandemic, is met with fear (in musicians see Cohen & Ginsborg, 2022). Conversely, recovery is frequently deemed less important, since training and performing is accompanied by positive emotions and frequently of joy and flow experiences (Csikszentmihalyi, 1990; Harmat et al., 2021; Vlachopoulos et al., 2000). This is deceptive, however, because while joy and flow experiences make the concert or dance performance easier in that the effort is no longer felt and the sense of time is lost, the body still needs sufficient time for recovery.

Working at the physical and mental performance limits

Performers give their best when they are on stage, as professional success depends upon their performances, and this is evaluated by colleagues and/or audiences. For example, an orchestra member would never appear unprepared for a concert, because that would result in strong social-emotional pressure, but also disciplinary action from the company. Minimal deficits, such as those resulting from a lack of sleep, common infections (i.e., colds, influenza), hormonal changes during menstruation (or perimenopause/menopause), or a migraine, can impair performance. The fear of infection, illness or injuries that cause physical limitations can often influence the social life of professional performers. This should be a strong incentive to optimise training schedules, including appropriate recovery times. Indeed, outstanding performers frequently emphasise their time management and their reliance on sufficient recovery. However, knowledge on the role of recovery in prevention of infectious disease, headache, lack of concentration and mood fluctuations is frequently incomplete, especially in young performers (for young athletes and resilience to infections; see Beckmann & Zier, 2011).

Frequently unfavourable ergonomic conditions

While this scenario occurs regularly for musicians, it can often be experienced in dancers, actors, and acrobats depending upon their training and performing environments and/or repertoire (Chi et al., 2020). For example, orchestral instruments were developed at a time when concert life in the modern sense did not yet exist. In the Baroque era, musicians played several instruments and practised during rehearsals for the performances. Johann Sebastian Bach, for example, was proficient at playing the organ, harpsichord, viola, trumpet, conducting, composing, and was also, to his chagrin, obliged to teach Latin as the cantor of St. Thomas in Leipzig (Wolff, 2002). Systematic, hours-long study of etudes is an innovation of the Romantic period. During this time, the musicians became more professional, and – triggered by outstanding, charismatic performers such as Nicolo Paganini or Franz Liszt – the technical demands on performers increased dramatically (Lehmann, 2006). This was accompanied by specialisation in one instrument and an increase in practice and playing times, which today can be up to ten hours a day. Since many orchestral instruments were designed in the early Baroque period, when they were only played for a few hours a day, little attention was paid to ergonomic aspects. Examples are the design of the violin or viola. However, the stressful posture with holding the instruments for hours, elevation of the arm, and supination of the left forearm may lead to pain which can then become chronic (Boyette, 2005; Zamorano et al., 2023). These considerations can also be found in different genres of dance, where aesthetic aspects have often been favoured above physiological considerations. For example, in classical ballet, pointe work and grand allegro put strain on joints and muscles. Training and recovery programmes need to be adapted to these specific challenges across the performing arts disciplines.

Science in performing arts is emerging

The specific stressors which performing artists are subjected to led to publications as early as the 18th century commenting on "job-related illnesses"

(Rammazini, 1700, w.p.). Musicians' diseases were listed in detail in monographs, for example by the physicians Flesch (1925) and Singer (1926). While decades later, the first book on diseases and injuries of ballet dancers was published by Thomasen (1982). It is only since the early 1980s that professional performance has actually been considered from an occupational health perspective. Since then, the cultural taboos surrounding this issue have noticeably reduced, resulting in a gradual increase in awareness among educators and medical professionals regarding the specific healthcare needs of performers. This growing need for specialised medical care for performers is also connected to the worsening job market, with increased technical demands and the often perfectionist expectations of artists and audiences expecting the highest quality of performance.

Consequently, interdisciplinary societies like the British Performing Arts Medicine Association were founded in 1984, followed by the international Performing Arts Medicine Association in the USA in 1989. Further associations were initiated in the subsequent years, such as the International Association for Dance Medicine and Science in 1990. In these interdisciplinary associations, comprised of health professionals including medical doctors, psychologists, physiotherapists, representatives of body techniques such as Feldenkrais or Alexander technique, speech therapists, as well as music- and dance-educators, and musicians and dancers who work in the educational and medical care of performers, were brought together.

While the aims of these associations have changed over the last three decades, there is general agreement among experts that these societies have three main roles in raising awareness of the health needs of performers, prevention of performer-specific injuries, and scientific exchange in the fields of performing arts physiology and performing arts medicine.

Recovery science should be included in performing arts physiology lectures and activities. Being aware of the physical and mental processes involved in performance and having at least some basic anatomical, physiological, biomechanical and psychological knowledge of these processes is helpful for performance and for developing individual health-promoting strategies and shaped recovery plans. Therefore, it is necessary to establish curricula on the basics of performing arts physiology at conservatories, dance schools, drama schools and in acrobat and juggling training. Graduates of these institutions are then in a position to be able to share the knowledge they have gained with their own students. The early identification of individual risk factors and the observance of physiological principles in training and recovery are both essential to achieving success, while also assisting in the prevention of performance-related injuries.

Presently, the relationship between recovery and its influence and impact on performance, on injury prevention and quality of life in the performing arts is underresearched and needs to be addressed in its multilayered nature.

Concept of recovery in performing arts

In our understanding, recovery is regarded as a multifaceted restorative process in time. It includes not only physiological, but also psychological and societal aspects. If an individual's recovery is not sufficient, be it due to internal psycho-mental or muscular factors or to external conditions, for example, heavy workload in an unyielding competitive societal system such as an orchestra or a ballet or an artist company, fatigue as a condition of augmented tiredness due to physical and mental effort develops. Fatigue can be compensated with recovery, that is, the psycho-mental balance is regained by re-establishing the invested resources on a physiological and psychological level.

Recovery is an umbrella term which can be further characterised by different modalities of recovery such as regeneration or psychological recovery strategies. Regeneration as an integral part of recovery in the performing arts refers to the physiological aspect of recovery and ideally follows physical fatigue induced by training, practising or performing. Allowing regeneration is an extremely important part of injury prevention in the performing arts. Learning about regeneration and about 'when to stop training' needs to be addressed from the first training lessons, along with practice strategies and student-tailored practice schedules. Furthermore, probably more than occurs in sport, mental workload is high and requires not only memorising choreography and music scores, but also the most precise interindividual coordination (e.g., orchestras, bands, dancing, acrobatics), in addition to innumerable aesthetic decisions regarding expressivity of movement and emotional gestures. These can all produce and/or contribute to mental fatigue and require recovery approaches to be applied.

With respect to the regeneration approaches, strategies such as post-training stretches, warm relaxation baths, cold-water immersion, and rest address muscular fatigue and muscular micro-lesions. Mental fatigue and cognitive exhaustion, for example in orchestra musicians after long performances can mainly be compensated by using psychological recovery strategies such as cognitive self-regulation, resource activation, and psychological relaxation techniques. Furthermore, Kellmann (2002) distinguishes between passive, active, and pro-active approaches to recovery. Passive methods may range from the application of external methods (e.g., massage) to implementing a state of rest characterised by inactivity. Active recovery (e.g., cooldown, jogging) involves mainly physical activities aimed at compensating for the metabolic responses of physical fatigue. Pro-active recovery (e.g., social activities) implies a high level of self-determination by choosing activities customised to individual needs and preferences.

A certain degree of fatigue with 'functional overreaching' is occasionally required for performance enhancement, especially when stamina, strength and velocity need to be improved. It can be compensated through comprehensive recovery. Functional overreaching in this context describes a short-term decrement of performance without signs of maladaptation as a consequence of intensive training. In case systematic and individualised recovery is not achieved after training and functional overreaching, a continuous imbalance of inadequate recovery and excessive demands could initiate a vicious circuit, including underrecovery and 'nonfunctional overreaching' (NFO; Jeffries & Coutts, this volume, Chapter 3; Meeusen

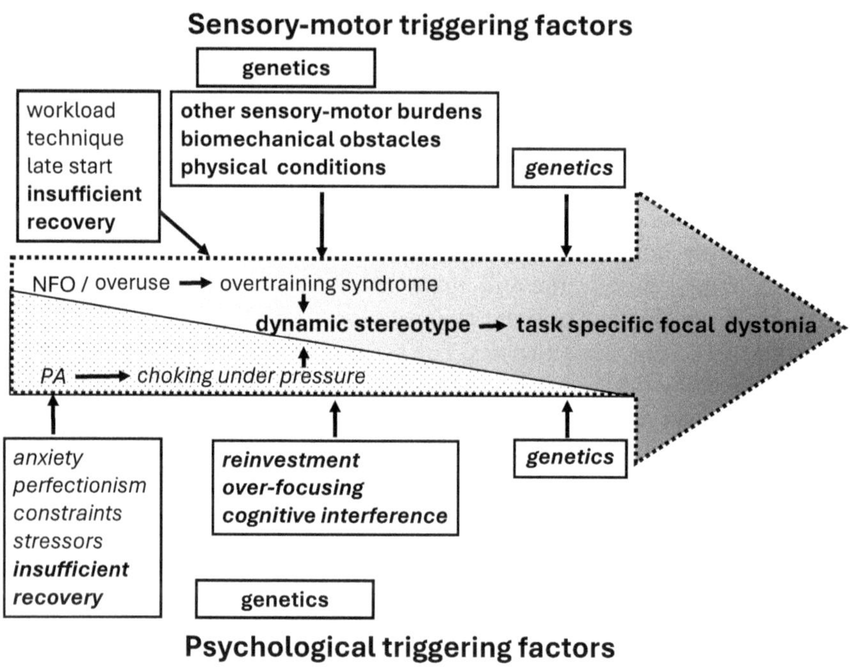

FIGURE 1.2 Heuristic model, which assumes a stepwise progression of performance failures.

Note: In the upper half of the graph, sensorimotor failures and their triggering risk factors, in the lower half psychological failures and their respective potential triggering factors are shown. Sensorimotor failures range from Nonfunctional Overreaching (NFO) or Overuse syndrome to Overtraining Syndrome, Dynamic Stereotype and finally Task-specific Dystonia. The further these problems progress, the more difficult it is to reverse the dysfunctional development. Psychological failures range from Performance Anxiety (PA) to Choking under Pressure, which may produce dysfunctional motor memories and finally Dystonia with structural memory consolidation and maladaptive brain adaptations. Potential triggering factors provoking the transition from one step to the next are categorised according to motor demands (above the arrow) and psychological contributors (below the arrow). Genetic contributions are also indicated. The increasing grey shade in the arrow symbolises the increasing deterioration of motor control. Note that the lack of sensory-motor and psychological recovery constitutes the beginning of this vicious self-augmenting development.

et al., 2013). At the end of this negative spiral, threats such as injury, loss of motivation, and, in the worst-case medical conditions like musician's dystonia (Altenmüller & Jabusch, 2010) jeopardise performers' careers (Figure 1.2).

With respect to performing arts recovery, two sports science concepts will be introduced, namely underrecovery and NFO. These represent two closely related though slightly different concepts. While according to Kellmann et al. (2018) underrecovery appears to delineate a broader condition of insufficient recovery in reaction to general stress (e.g., family, media, work demands), Meeusen et al. (2013) characterise NFO as training-specific negative psychological and hormonal alterations and subsequent decreased performance. Continuous underrecovery and NFO often serve as a precursor for overtraining syndrome (OTS). OTS is closely related to the deterioration of overtrained movements in musicians and dancers. In musicians this is termed 'dynamic stereotype' as reversible condition, and musician's dystonia as a permanent condition, needing specific retaining procedures or medical intervention, such as pharmacological treatment (Furuya & Altenmüller, 2015). This condition is relevant, since up to 2% of professional musicians suffer from it. In dancers, deterioration of motor control due to overtraining is less common; however, has been known about for a long time (Batson, 2007; Dawson, 2013).

While in sports, accumulation of underrecovery in terms of daily life demands together with long-term NFO in training and competition settings ultimately manifests in OTS, in performing arts, psychological and sensorimotor trigger factors have been identified to contribute to a deterioration of motor control (Ioannou et al., 2016). In contrast to athletes, where OTS is marked by physical symptoms such as continuous muscle soreness, pain sensations, or clinical and/or endocrinological disturbances, in performing artists, the leading symptom is lack of coordination and precision of long-term, automated skilled movements.

Underrecovery and early-stage NFO in performing artists can be compensated for by systematically applying recovery strategies and rest, along with lifestyle-related strategies like sleep, diet, and social activities. However, recovering from OTS requires a continuous restoration consisting of long rest and recovery periods lasting from weeks to months accompanied by reduced performance. For example, Ackermann and Altenmüller (2021) have established a retraining protocol for this condition in musicians.

Recovery and fatigue in performing artists can be viewed on a continuum and are jointly affected by physiological and psychological determinants. An imbalance of long-term fatigue and insufficient recovery initiates an unfavourable development, resulting in negative consequences such as underrecovery, NFO, or OTS. Ultimately, a long-term decrement of performance and well-being may manifest.

How can overuse in performing artists be prevented

There are several measures that may contribute to the prevention of the aforementioned conditions:

1. **Raising awareness regarding the health needs of performing artists.** This includes educational activities, lectures for health professionals, information in the association's magazines, and networking with educational institutions, employers of performing artists, and insurance companies for performing artists.
2. **Prevention of performing artists specific injuries and illnesses.** Preventive measures should already be implemented in the early education of performing artists. Health-promoting curricula for the training of young performing artists, the establishment of lectures or other ways of spreading information is necessary.
3. **Scientific exchange in the field of performing arts physiology and performing arts medicine.** Through an interdisciplinary approach and regularly organised symposia and conferences, performing artists can network and exchange information on the different approaches in different cultures.

It is worth mentioning why the term 'performing arts physiology' is important to reach our goal. The term physiology refers to the study of normal life processes. In our opinion, being aware of the processes in the body involved in performing and having at least some basic anatomical, physiological, biomechanical and psychological knowledge of these processes is helpful for all performers, be it singing, playing instruments, dancing, acting or performing acrobatics. Goal is a professional activity without discomfort and the development of individual health-promoting strategies including strategies for recovery. The knowledge of performing artists working in education varies greatly in this respect and is often not sufficiently imparted to students. Therefore, it is necessary to establish curricular courses on the basics of performing arts physiology at conservatories, dance, drama and acrobatic schools. Graduates of these institutions can then share the knowledge they have gained with their own students. The early identification of individual risk factors and the observance of physiological principles right from the start of training means effective prevention of illnesses and failure in performance.

Fortunately, an increasing number of performing arts students, members of orchestras, dance companies, acting and acrobatic ensembles are also requesting preventive approaches to health and well-being. In the field of music performance, this has led to the institutionalisation of music physiology and music medicine at music conservatories. In 1974, the first professorship in music physiology was established in Germany at the Hanover University of Music and Drama.

In the following four hypotheses why recovery research is needed in the performing arts are outlined:

1 **Optimal recovery will make young people resilient in a highly competitive environment**

Between 30 and 50% of young people in state youth orchestras already suffer from health complaints that can be directly linked to playing an instrument (Samsel et al., 2006). They most often manifest themselves in so-called playing-related musculoskeletal disorders. According to studies by Spahn et al. (2004), about 25% of first-semester students at the Freiburg Music Academy begin their studies with pain. In the course of their studies, 68–88% of music students in Freiburg experience illnesses that can be linked to playing an instrument. Of these, as many as 45% seek medical attention. Such percentages of stress also exist today and were replicated in Hannover (Germany) before Corona (Rosset et al., 2022).

These figures, taken from the music performance, but probably similar in other performing arts domains are disturbing, not least because they are an indication of the pressures that students can come under. Often, young artists have internalised a 'no pain, no gain' culture and want to fulfil their study obligations and assert themselves among their competitors regardless of the costs. However, many performing arts students are obviously not always able to cope with these stressors. In this case, it is the task of the educational institutions to teach students stress management strategies, including proper recovery, to help them develop insights that enable them to avoid stress, to provide them with practical exercises to help them reduce stress, and to promote an understanding of their own stress management mechanisms. The fact that over 50% of students seeking medical attention for acute or chronic pain problems are in their first or second year of university underlines the need to teach these coping mechanisms early in their studies (Ioannou et al., 2018).

2 **Performing arts medicine and physiology will help humanise a performance-related and externally determined professional environment**

Some factors that can put a strain on the performer's profession have been mentioned above. External locus of control, unrealistic performance expectations, the feeling of having to function at a high level at all times, personal tensions or dynamics within the ensemble, the orchestra, or the dance company can all detract from the joy of the profession and even result in illness. However, life stressors are often also triggers, and this was particularly evident during the coronavirus pandemic (Rosset et al., 2021). When a performer falls ill, they require the expertise of specialists, as any illness that affects their ability to perform, additionally can also impact the core of their personality. The consequences of such illnesses are far-reaching and can often lead to job-related fears, loss of self-esteem, shame, depression, social withdrawal, and anger. Performing arts health professionals must therefore be able to assess not only the triggers of physical illnesses, but also the emotional effects. For prevention and rehabilitation, it is important to address their work context and strengthen the resilience of the performers. In this sense, performing arts medicine also means active secondary prevention.

3 **Performing arts physiology and medicine will bring a culture of knowledge to the world of performers**

Performing arts medicine and science is, in the positive sense, a holistic form of medicine. The affected performing artists are not only examined and advised with regard to, for example, pain in the shoulder or anxiety in performance situations, but rather, the conditions of origin, the consequences of the illness, and a multifaceted, multidimensional therapeutic approach is addressed in a holistic way. For this reason, performing arts medicine and science are exemplary and a model for other fields. In the best case, it encompasses physiological, psychological, medical, and artist's educational aspects in an interdisciplinary manner. Performing arts medicine and science is an example of how effective healthcare can be realised for the benefit of arts, aesthetic values, and general public welfare. The prerequisites for this are an adequate time frame for the performers and the virtues of listening and appreciation.

Insights from performing arts physiology can also help students, amateurs and professionals to become more resilient and joyful. Here new applications for recovery and training may be useful tools; for example, McCrary et al. (2022) have developed an App to monitor fatigue in music students.

4 **Recovery research will help to better understand not only human performance but also human failure through interdisciplinary research**

The research areas of performing arts physiology and performing arts medicine and science are numerous. The inexhaustible field of practice and training would still be a worthwhile topic. How should one practice, when should one practice, how often should one repeat which passages/movements/text, and at what moment should one stop practicing? Where on should you focus your attention when practising? Other topics concern the resilience of performers. Why do some performers remain very healthy and well under the most severe stressful conditions, while others break down physically, psychologically and emotionally even under the most minimal challenging conditions? Why do some performers develop chronic pain, while others survive even severe physical challenges without consequences after a few days? Can changes in pain sensitivity in chronic pain be objectively measured, for example, by the reaction potentials of the sensorimotor cortex? Can the pain of performing be alleviated by modulating neuronal networks? Finally, a topic which is central to this book: How can recovery be best organised and structured? Many of these questions still require answers.

Conclusion and recommendations for practice

Improvement in the working conditions of performing artists in the next few years appears possible, and the fight against fear, self-doubt, self-deprecation and dissatisfaction will be important topics to further address. In order to provide performers with health promotion programmes tailored to their specific needs and to reduce the number of work-related complaints among performers in the long term, further prevention programmes and teaching events should be developed at performing arts training institutions. It is also important to be mindful that health-promoting behaviour and prevention begin in childhood. In-service training should be offered at schools and other primary educational institutions. The amateur sector is also far too little in the scope and focus of performing arts prevention and recovery research. Even at universities, there is a lack of obligatory basic seminars and lectures. These need to be supplemented by optional, practically oriented offers and the possibility of individual consultations with a recovery expert.

However, qualified prevention and practical performing arts medicine and science are only possible on the basis of scientifically sound principles. Regular conferences, symposia, publications, the funding of individual research projects, the awarding of scientific prizes, and the publication in empirical journals will help achieve this goal.

The social dimension is also important: the exaggerated demands of the public's expectations of performances should be queried, and care should be taken to ensure that the most important goal of performing, namely the communication of an emotional message, is given priority again.

References

Ackermann, B., & Altenmüller, E. (2021). The development and use of an anatomy-based retraining program (MusAARP) to assess and treat focal hand dystonia in musicians – A pilot study. *Journal of Hand Therapy*, *34*(2), 309–314.

Altenmüller, E., & Jabusch, H. C. (2010). Focal dystonia in musicians: Phenomenology, pathophysiology and triggering factors. *European Journal of Neurology*, *17* (Suppl. 1), 31–36.

Antonovsky, A. (1979). *Health, stress, and coping*. Jossey-Bass.

Antonovsky, A. (1987). *Unraveling the mystery of health*. Jossey-Bass.

Batson, G. (2007). Revisiting overuse injuries in dance in view of motor learning and somatic models of distributed practice. *Journal of Dance Medicine and Science*, *11*(3), 70–75.

Beckmann, J. (2023). Self-regulation of recovery. In M. Kellmann, S. Jakowski, & J. Beckmann (Eds.), *The importance of recovery for physical and mental health: Negotiating the effects of underrecovery* (pp. 53–69). Routledge.

Beckmann, J., Huber, M., & Andonian-Dierks, C. S. (2024). Chronic illness and well-being: Promoting quality of life with a broadened concept of recovery. In M. Kellmann & J. Beckmann (Eds.), *Fostering recovery and well-being in a healthy lifestyle: Psychological, somatic, and organizational prevention approaches* (pp. 3–23). Routledge.

Beckmann, J., Kellmann, M., & Jakowski, S. (2023). Recovery is more than just healing: Advocating a broader perspective on recovery in physical and mental health. In M. Kellmann, S. Jakowski, & J. Beckmann (Eds.), *The importance of recovery for physical and mental health: Negotiating the effects of underrecovery* (pp. 266–270). Routledge.

Beckmann, J., & Zier, E. (2011). Extreme Beanspruchung und ihre Folgen beim jugendlichen Leistungssportler [Extreme stress and its consequences in young competitive athletes]. *Prävention und Rehabilitation*, *23*, 2–6.

Boyette J. (2005). Splinting for adaptation of musical instruments. *Work*, *25*(2), 99–106.

Bright, J. (2006). Factors influencing outstanding band students' choice of music education as a career. *Contributions to Music Education*, *33*(2), 73–88.

Chi, J.-Y., Halaki, M., & Ackermann, B. J. (2020). Ergonomics in violin and piano playing: A systematic review. *Applied Ergonomics*, *88*, 103143. https://doi.org/10.1016/j.apergo.2020.103143

Cohen, S., & Ginsborg, J. (2022). One year on: The impact of COVID-19 on the lives of freelance orchestral musicians in the United Kingdom. *Frontiers in Psychology*, *13*, 885606. https://doi.org/10.3389/fpsyg.2022.885606

Csikszentmihalyi, M. (1990). *Flow: The psychology of optimal experience*. Harper and Row.

Dang, Y., Koutedakis, Y., & Wyon, M. (2020). Fit to dance survey: Elements of lifestyle and injury incidence in Chinese dancers. *Medical Problems of Performing Artists*, *35*(1), 10–18.

Dawson, W. J. (2013). Performing arts medicine – A bibliographic retrospective of the early literature: An historical examination of bibliographic references pre-1975. *Medical Problems of Performing Artists*, *28*(1), 47–53.

Doyon, J. (1997). Skill learning. *International Review of Neurobiology*, *41*, 273–294.

Ericsson, K. A., Krampe, R. T., & Tesch-Römer, C. (1993). The role of deliberate practice in the acquisition of expert performance. *Psychological Reviews*, *100*(3), 363–406.

Flesch, J. (1925). *Berufskrankheiten des Musikers* [Occupational diseases of the musician]. Niels Kampmann.

Furuya, S., & Altenmüller, E. (2015). Acquisition and reacquisition of motor coordination in musicians. *Annals of the New York Academy of Sciences*, *1337*(1), 118–124.

Hague, K. M. (2018). *Chasing dreams: Investigating talent identification and development in ballet.* [Masters by Research thesis, Queensland University of Technology]. QUT ePrints.

Hambrick, D. Z., Macnamara, B. N., & Oswald, F. L. (2020). Is the deliberate practice view defensible? A review of evidence and discussion of issues. *Frontiers in Psychology*, *11*, 1134. https://doi.org/10.3389/fpsyg.2020.01134

Harmat, L., de Manzano, Ö., & Ullén, F. (2021). Flow in music and arts. In C. Peifer & S. Engeser (Eds.), *Advances in flow research* (pp. 377–391). Springer.

Herholz, S. C., & Zatorre, R. J. (2012). Musical training as a framework for brain plasticity: Behavior, function, and structure. *Neuron*, *76*(3), 486–502.

Ioannou, C. I., Furuya, S., & Altenmüller, E. (2016). The impact of stress on motor performance in skilled musicians suffering from focal dystonia: Physiological and psychological characteristics. *Neuropsychologia, 85*, 226–236.
Ioannou, C. I., Hafer, J., Lee, A., & Altenmüller, E. (2018). Epidemiology, treatment efficacy, and anxiety aspects of music students affected by playing-related pain: A retrospective evaluation with follow-up. *Medical Problems of Performing Artists, 33*(1), 26–38.
Jaffee-Nagel, J. (1988). Identity and career choice in music. *Journal of Cultural Economics, 12*(2), 67–76.
Kallus, K. W. (2016). Stress and recovery: An overview. In K. W. Kallus & M. Kellmann (Eds.), *The Recovery-Stress Questionnaires: User manual* (pp. 27–48). Pearson Assessment.
Kellmann, M. (2002). Underrecovery and overtraining: Different concepts - Similar impact? In M. Kellmann (Ed.), *Enhancing recovery: Preventing underperformance in athletes* (pp. 3–24). Human Kinetics.
Kellmann, M., & Beckmann, J. (Eds.). (2022). *Recovery and well-being in sport and exercise*. Routledge.
Kellmann, M., Bertollo, M., Bosquet, L., Brink, M., Coutts, A. J., Duffield, R., Erlacher, D., Halson, S. L., Hecksteden, A., Heidari, J., Kallus, K. W., Meeusen, R., Mujika, I., Robazza, C., Skorski, S., Venter, R., & Beckmann, J. (2018). Recovery and performance in sport: Consensus statement. *International Journal of Sports Physiology and Performance, 13*(2), 240–245.
Kellmann, M., Jakowski, S., & Beckmann, J. (Eds.). (2023). *The importance of recovery for physical and mental health: Negotiating the effects of underrecovery*. Routledge.
Kellmann, M., & Kallus, K. W. (2001). *The Recovery-Stress Questionnaire for Athletes: User manual*. Human Kinetics.
Kogan, N. (2002). Careers in the performing arts: A psychological perspective. *Creativity Research Journal, 14*(1), 1–16. https://doi.org/10.1207/S15326934CRJ1401_1
Kogan, N., & Kangas, B. L. (2006). Careers in the dramatic arts: Comparing genetic and interactional perspectives. *Empirical Studies of the Arts, 24*(1), 43–54.
Lehmann, A. C. (2006). Historical increases in expert music performance skills: Optimizing instruments, playing techniques, and training. In E. Altenmüller, M. Wiesendanger, & J. Kesselring (Eds.), *Music, motor control, and the brain* (pp. 3–22). Oxford University Press.
McCrary, J. M., Ascenso, S., Savvidou, P., Schraft, S., McAllister, L., Redding, E., Bastepe-Gray, S., & Altenmüller, E. (2022). Load and fatigue monitoring in musicians using an online app: A pilot study. *Frontiers in Psychology, 13*, 1056892. https://doi.org/10.3389/fpsyg.2022.1056892
McPherson, G. E. (2005). From child to musician: Skill development during the beginning stages of learning an instrument. *Psychology of Music*, 33(1), 5–35.
Meeusen, R., Duclos, M., Foster, C., Fry, A., Gleeson, M., Nieman, D., Raglin, J., Rietjens, G., Steinacker, J., Urhausen, A., European College of Sport Science, & American College of Sports Medicine (2013). Prevention, diagnosis, and treatment of the overtraining syndrome: Joint consensus statement of the European College of Sport Science and the American College of Sports Medicine. *Medicine and Science in Sports and Exercise, 45*(1), 186–205.

Pauleit, S., Kellmann, M., & Beckmann, J. (Eds.). (2025). *Creating urban and workplace environments to promote recovery and well-being*. Routledge.
Rammazini, B. (1700). *De morbis articifium diatribia*. Modena.
Rosset, M., Baumann, E., & Altenmüller, E. (2021). Studying music during the coronavirus pandemic: Conditions of studying and health-related challenges. *Frontiers in Psychology*, *12*, 651393. https://doi.org/10.3389/fpsyg.2021.651393
Rosset, M., Baumann, E., & Altenmüller, E. (2022). A longitudinal study of physical and mental health and health-related attitudes among music students: Potentials and challenges for university health promotion programs. *Frontiers in Psychology*, *13*, 885739. https://doi.org/10.3389/fpsyg.2022.885739
Samsel, W., Möller, H., Marstedt, G., & Müller, R. (2006). Ergebnisse einer Befragung junger Musiker über Berufsperspektiven, Belastungen und Gesundheit [Results of a survey of young musicians on career prospects, stress and health]. *Musikphysiologie und Musikermedizin*, *13*(3), 86–98.
Singer, K. (1926). *Die Berufskrankheiten der Musiker* [The occupational diseases of musicians]. Max Hesse.
Spahn, C., Strukely, S., & Lehmann, A. (2004). Health conditions, attitudes toward study, and attitudes toward health at the beginning of university study: Music students in comparison with other student populations. *Medical Problems of Performing Artists*, *19*(1), 26–33.
Thomasen, E. (1982). *Diseases and injuries of ballet dancers*. Universitetsforlaget i Århus.
Ullén, F., Hambrick, D. Z., & Mosing, M. A. (2016). Rethinking expertise: A multifactorial gene-environment interaction model of expert performance. *Psychological Bulletin*, *142*(4), 427–446.
Ungerleider, L. G., Doyon, J., & Karni, A. (2002). Imaging brain plasticity during motor skill learning. *Neurobiology of Learning and Memory*, *78*(3), 553–564.
Vlachopoulos, S. P., Karageorghis, C. I., & Terry, P. C. (2000). Hierarchical confirmatory factor analysis of the Flow State Scale in exercise. *Journal of Sports Sciences*, *18*(10), 815–823.
Vuust, P., Heggli, O. A., Friston, K. J., & Kringelbach, M. L. (2022). Music in the brain. *Nature Reviews Neuroscience*, *23*(5), 287–305.
Wanke, E. M., Mill, H., Wanke, A., Davenport, J., Checcetti, F., Koch, F., & Groneberg, D. A. (2013). Dance partner or dance floor?: Exogenous factors resulting in accidents in professional dancers. *Medical Problems of Performing Artists*, *28*(3), 131–136.
Wolff, C. J. (2002). *Johann Sebastian Bach: The learned musician*. Oxford University Press.
World Health Organization. (2019). *Recovery practices for mental health and well-being: WHO Quality rights core training: Mental health and social services: Course guide*. Retrieved June 21, 2022 from https://apps.who.int/iris/handle/10665/329602
Zamorano, A. M., Kleber, B., Arguissain, F., Vuust, P., Flor, H., & Graven-Nielsen, T. (2023). Extensive sensorimotor training enhances nociceptive cortical responses in healthy individuals. *European Journal of Pain*, *27*(2), 257–277.

2

SOCIETAL, PHYSICAL, AND ORGANISATIONAL PRESSURES IN THE PERFORMING ARTS

Bronwen J. Ackermann and Dirk D. Steiner

Introduction

Becoming proficient in any of the performing arts requires a long-term dedication to training in the specific craft, typically alongside seeking out the best teachers and training institutions, while continually proving one's capacity by competing to participate and excel in public performances. Occupational demands of performing artists are diverse and yet share common features – being able to convey emotions (usually as directed), display physical mastery of skills, and communicate with their audiences – within often-challenging work environments. Job security for performing artists can be tenuous, with frequently many more applicants than available contract or permanent positions in performing arts organisations, and yet research remains scarce on the relationship between broader occupational demands and performer well-being (Willis et al., 2019). Many performing artists are freelancers and must take work opportunities when they arise or risk losing employment to others within this highly competitive workplace. Unsurprisingly perhaps, high rates of performance-related health issues (PRHI) have been consistently reported across performing arts populations in the last few decades (Hinkamp et al., 2017).

Performing arts training approaches have largely continued to follow centuries-old master-apprentice models, focussing primarily on repetition of the activities themselves and thus involving long hours of repetitive and

Ackermann, B. J., & Steiner, D. D. (2026). Societal, physical, and organisational pressures in the performing arts. In E. Altenmüller, M. Kellmann, J. Beckmann, & G. M. Moyle (Eds.), *Recovery and well-being in the performing arts* (pp. 21–40). Routledge.

DOI: 10.4324/9781003566885-3

sustained daily practice. Over the last few decades, performing arts medicine research has emerged, highlighting consistently reported high rates of PRHIs worldwide (Backiev et al., 2024; Willis et al., 2019). However, concepts such as performer well-being and adequate recovery from fatigue or increased workloads have not yet been widely recognised in performing arts domains as integral and essential components of achieving optimal performance in training or workplace environments. Without addressing performer well-being in training and workplace environments, the potential risk of performers sustaining PRHIs or burnout through factors such as muscular overuse or fatigue alongside insufficient recovery remains high.

In this chapter, a PRHI will be used to refer to the state of performing artists' health and well-being, both acute and chronic, that negatively affects their ability or capacity to perform at their desired level. Several decades of performing arts medicine research on the working conditions of performing artists undertaking creative labour, or students undertaking training, reveals that their experiences are potentially emotionally and physically damaging (Gross & Musgrave, 2020; Maxwell et al., 2015; Sun & Liu, 2024). These findings sit in stark contrast to an ever-increasing volume of research highlighting a myriad of quantifiable health benefits for those actively participating and receptively engaging in the performing arts (McCrary et al., 2021).

So why are these artists so vulnerable to these high rates of PRHIs? To become adept at their craft, performing artists across performance domains, genres and ages are exposed to a multitude of health risk factors that may be intrinsic, related to their own intrinsic capacity and functional ability, or extrinsic, related to environmental, social and organisational aspects of their work that lead to the development of these PRHIs (Shah, 2019). The quantity of performing and training hours as well as increased years of playing (older age) appears to be linked with higher frequencies of PRHIs (Greenspan, 2021), perhaps reflecting an increased exposure to potential risk factors over time. This is supported by literature highlighting the relationship between hours of playing and injury. For example, a sudden increase of playing to nine hours per day in two different youth intensive music camps in the Netherlands led to a consistent jump in injury rates from 28 to 80% (Kok et al., 2016) and in the orchestral context where full time Australian orchestral musicians who played four calls (ten hours) or more in addition to their weekly workload were three times more likely to suffer a PRHI (Ackermann et al., 2017). The variability of the work and training undertaken by performing artists, even within the same art form or genre, creates different health risks to each individual, making it extremely difficult to predict PRHIs (Shrier et al., 2022). Performing artists should receive education on recognising mental and physical signs of fatigue, understanding that a 'one size fit all' approach to duration and intensity will differ between individuals, and how to incorporate mini-breaks into practice regimes, with the understanding that work demands can vary considerably (Ackermann, 2017a). Flexibility in practice schedules, altering rehearsal schedules to incorporate breaks and acknowledging the importance of downtime and sleep need to be promoted and regarded as an integral component of performance capacity (Ackermann, 2017a). Establishing how performing artists can best implement recovery periods that are appropriate to restore regeneration and full performance capacity, not just in periods of high psychological and physical stressors but on a regular basis, requires both individual and organisational efforts.

PRHIs affecting psychological or physical well-being are globally reported to be widespread among performing artists and have been reported across the lifespan from early training years into the end of their performing careers (Maxwell et al., 2015; Munro., 2014; Ranelli et al., 2011; Shrier et al., 2009). In a national cohort of professional orchestral musicians, 50% of players were suffering injuries at the time of the survey, 25% of which had been present for more than three months (Ackermann et al., 2012). In a national survey of 782 working actors, half of the actors were suffering vocal, physical or psychological health and well-being issues at the time of the survey (Maxwell et al., 2015). Of these actors, 80% reported suffering financial stress, no doubt impacting their ability to pay for any kind of therapeutic interventions to help recovery, instead reporting high levels of alcohol and drug use to cope with problems. Similarly, dancers report high rates of injury across all forms of dance (Prakash et al., 2024), with higher injury vulnerability reported in pre-professional teenage dancers (Ekegren et al., 2014). Circus artists have been reported to suffer 9.7 injuries per 1,000 artist-exposures, a rate similar to Men's NCAA Basketball in the USA, with the highest rate of injury observed in acrobats and sudden-load (high impact) artists (Shrier et al., 2009). Alarmingly, reports of bullying have also become relatively widespread in performing arts organisations (Ackermann et al., 2017; Maxwell et al., 2015), with the 'MeToo' movement highlighting long-standing and widespread bullying and sexual harassment by famous producers and actors (Adler, 2022) that obviously has substantial adverse effects on a performer's mental health and well-being.

While the volume of data on the widespread prevalence of psychological and physical PRHIs is growing rapidly, data on the recovery from injury outcomes of performing artists is relatively sparse (Blevins et al., 2020). Nonetheless, managing the balance between stress and recovery has long been recommended to enhance performance and reduce injury risk in sport, and it is likely that the same approach would apply to performing artists (Smith, 2003). For example, the systematic organisation of training into distinct phases that vary in intensity, volume, and focus over time (periodisation) in sports domains aims to prevent overtraining and to maximise performance outcomes at specific times, such as during performances or competitions (Bompa & Buzzichelli, 2019). This often includes the use of tapering, whereby a gradual reduction of training volume, while maintaining intensity and frequency, is implemented in the lead-up to a major performance to ensure that a performer is physically rested but psychologically sharp, with the necessary energy reserves to deliver a peak performance (Bosquet et al., 2007). Despite the potential benefits of this in the performing arts, as this would appear to be a highly translatable approach, there has been little research on this topic, and in music domains in particular, little evidence of this in practice.

The implementation of progressive arts-specific rehabilitation should also be encouraged if an injury has been incurred and this should include adequate recovery periods as well as the education of the performer in how to integrate recovery periods into their future training and performance workloads. In one survey of a nationwide cohort of professional orchestral musicians, only 40% reported fully recovering from past PRHIs (Ackermann et al., 2017). Part of the difficulty in identifying recovery in the performing arts may be at least in part because individuals have markedly different experiences and perceptions throughout their recovery process. These experiences and perceptions may contrast with those of the healthcare team or performing arts administrators. Personal opinions on recovery are based on individual factors such as prior experience, level of health education, intrinsic capacity and overall state of physical and mental well-being (Hacquebord et al., 2024). For example, perceptions of physical recovery could be identified as a range of experiences from complete symptom cessation to simply being able to return to a satisfying level of functioning despite residual symptoms (Carroll et al., 2016). This quantification of recovery poses a challenge for healthcare professionals, who typically are required to quantify injury recovery using appropriate clinical outcome measures, but this may not relate to what successful recovery means to an individual, or how return to work may be impacted by anxiety and uncertainty (Middlebrook et al., 2021). Additionally, a performing artist's recovery from a PRHI and their overall well-being cannot be considered in isolation from their social and organisational environments, whether in their early days of development, during later intensive training years or as a seasoned professional. Well-being has been defined as a positive state and resource for daily life experienced by individuals and societies, encompassing quality of life and the ability of people and societies to contribute to the world with a sense of meaning and purpose (World Health Organization, 2010). It has long been known that lower levels of well-being, alongside other factors such as lack of sleep, poor diet and physical and psychological adverse health conditions, are linked to moderately negative effects on work performance (Ford et al., 2011; Sonnentag et al., 2024).

Studies of the typical working conditions of performing artists, reveal that an uncertain career looms ahead for the majority, and their career will involve them typically juggling various jobs to earn a reliable income, filled with risks, personal health challenges, insecurities, conflicts, and constraints (Kleynhans et al., 2024). Financial insecurity can create stress and reduced mental well-being, as well as decreased recovery opportunities in busy periods. Freelance performing artists in particular are often under pressure to take every gig, in the fear that refusing a gig may remove that potential source of employment in the future. Many artists also report that having limited resources prevents them being able to pay for a PRHI recovery process, such as accessing specialised healthcare providers (Maxwell et al., 2015). Similarly, musicians generally report difficulty making ends meet and report that intense financial struggles go hand in hand with increased anxiety and lower levels of psychological well-being (Gross & Musgrave, 2020). Circus artists report commonly continuing to perform with a PRHI ('pain is normal'), with their recovery pathways influenced by financial constraints, touring, and difficulty accessing suitable experienced healthcare providers (Cayrol et al., 2019; Richard et al., this volume, Chapter 12; Stuckey et al., this volume, Chapter 9). Meanwhile in a national actor's cohort, 40% of these had only earned AUD$10,000 or less in the previous financial year requiring additional varied work to supplement incomes for basic living costs (Maxwell et al., 2015).

A widespread update to educational approaches in the performing arts, incorporating information to increase resilience in managing the known physical and psychological rigours of their work, as well as other useful skills for their future careers like business management, entrepreneurship, and leadership training, is seen as an essential way to improve overall well-being of performing artists as they move into their professional careers (Clague, 2023; Wijsman & Ackermann, 2019). Furthermore, the ability to manage the stresses of a performance career by a better grounding in these organisational aspects of their career alongside understanding how to self-regulate physical and psychological demands with adequate recovery is likely to lead to enhanced well-being in performing artists (Beckmann, 2023). Systematic approaches to increasing the health literacy of performing artists have been recommended to enhance performing artists' well-being during their training and future careers and to empower them to be to optimise health and prevent or minimise the risk of PRHIs in day-to-day performance situations (Baadjou et al., 2019; Prior et al., 2015; Wijsman & Ackermann, 2019). Health literacy enhances people's knowledge and competences to access, understand, appraise, and apply health information. It has an important impact on decisions made by performing artists to prevent disease and promote health through the lifespan (Guptill et al., 2022). For this to occur, information should be context-specific, allowing them to develop personal health 'assets' accounting for the unique demands of their individual performance type within the variable environments and social situations encountered during performing arts training and work (Nutbeam & McGill, 2019).

Broader dissemination of evidence-informed health education is important not only to enhance individual well-being and health literacy but also to reduce widespread pervasive negative stigmas (devaluing and discrediting attitudes) within performing arts communities. For example, in the orchestra setting, a stigma exists that PRHIs come from poor technique, a weakness of character or lack of musicianship, with these performers deemed unreliable (Ackermann, 2017b). Dancers report a culture of injury concealment and persevere through injuries due to negative stigmas, and the fear of losing their work contracts (Vassallo et al., 2019). Inexperienced health professionals can also devalue the PRHI of the performing artist, demonstrating stigmas themselves, labelling these patients as drama queens, often telling them to just stop performing or to change profession, thus further hindering recovery and creating more stress on the suffering performing artist (Ackermann, 2017b).

Health education has the potential to empower performing artists to make better decisions regarding modifying risks to improve well-being as well as optimising recovery at university, work, and home, but information must be accessible, understandable, and applied to performing arts settings (Guptill et al., 2022; Sørensen et al., 2015). Targeted education should aim to improve resilience, a dynamic and performer-specific process that focuses on developing appropriate physiological and psychological actions to effectively recover and return to normal function following exposure to training and work stressors (Den Hartigh et al., 2024; Kellmann et al., 2018).

Societal pressures

Within the social context where people engage in daily activities, environmental, organisational, and personal characteristics can all interact to affect health and well-being (Solar & Irwin, 2010). In performing arts cultures, it is generally expected that people must train hard to succeed, and perhaps unsurprisingly many performers are reported as being perfectionistic and displaying obsessive-compulsive personality traits, which can be at times counterproductive to their creativity (Chan et al., 2022; Nordin-Bates, 2020). Regular and repetitive practice is critical to eliminating mistakes, demanding high levels of self-efficacy, control, and regulation, preparing artists to perform in exposed performance contexts where expectations are high, and feedback is both immediate and public (Jeong & Ryan, 2022). Other than repetition, relatively little effort has traditionally been placed on a well-rounded music education that enhances students' resilience and self-efficacy and creates a culture of support for optimal physical and emotional well-being as well as recovery, a concept that in contrast is relatively well-developed within dance training institutions (Kozai & Ambegaonkar, 2020; Wijsman & Ackermann, 2019). Alongside developing occupationally and culturally specific health literacy, social support plays a critical role in enhancing physical and mental recovery in training and workplaces (Ren, 2024). Including the broader community of performing artists and their administrative teams in promoting such endeavours encourages all stakeholders to be on the same page in relation to health and well-being (Eslake, 2024). Families also need to be aware of the importance of recovery and maintaining a good state of well-being for performing artists and be warned against complacency or expectations of poor health (Ackermann & Driscoll, 2013). For example, health promotion education regarding both the importance and likely better outcomes of early management of any complaints arising from performing arts participation may encourage earlier reporting or pro-active approaches by artists.

Physical pressures

To be a professional performing artist requires an exceptional set of physical and mental skills to cope with the extremely high demands of a performance career (Chan & Ackermann, 2014). They have usually trained regularly from a young age, facing challenges over their growth and development that may increase the risk of developing PRHIs, which are increased if associated with challenging psychosocial and environmental demands (Kenny & Ackermann, 2015, 2016). Too much physical (and psychological) stress with inadequate time allowed for recovery will ultimately lead to tissue breakdown and injury, such as muscle strains, ligament sprains, tendinopathies, joint inflammation and neurological dysfunctions (Hansen & Reed, 2006). While preventing such tissue damage by allowing adequate recovery in periods of high workload and fatigue is the ideal approach, early management of such injuries follows a fairly straightforward biological recovery pathway of an initial inflammation/degeneration stage, followed by regeneration of injured tissues before the final remodelling stage (Laumonier & Menetrey, 2016; Leong et al., 2020). However, without applied health education that builds performer resilience and understanding of how to best mitigate risks, performing artists often neither know how to manage physical and psychological stressors that may prevent PRHIs, now what to do if a problem arises, often ignoring symptoms and continuing to perform until symptoms are chronic and substantively affecting performance capacity (Guptill et al., 2022; Kozai & Ambegaonkar, 2020). As most performing arts students are unaware of the risks they will be exposed to during their training, they show reactive rather than pro-active attitudes to seeking health education on perceived relevant topics once a physical or psychological PRHI has emerged (Ackermann et al., 2025). Trumpeter Jonathan Vieker shares his traumatic experience with a lip injury and subsequent long and challenging road to recovery online, noting at the outset "when I was in college, it just didn't occur to me that I could seriously hurt myself playing the trumpet" (Vieker, 2013, w.p.). The training and performance schedules in performing arts institutions can easily lead to overload, such as 'doubling up' workloads if there is a shortage of certain instrumentalists or other artists to fill all roles in upcoming productions and performances, with little effort made to allow subsequent recovery by reducing the load on these individuals after the event (Wijsman & Ackermann, 2019). In some cases, education on effective active recovery interventions such as recovery massage during intensive work periods, behavioural techniques, reflective practice and strengthening programmes may help to modify the impact of physical pressures and prevent PRHIs (Blevins et al., 2020; Chan & Ackermann, 2014; Chan et al., 2014; Eslake, 2024; Hakim et al., 2020).

In a pilot study at the Australian National Academy of Music to modify physical pressures due to long orchestra rehearsals, orchestral rehearsal breaks were changed to shorter rehearsal sessions with more recovery breaks, while still maintaining the overall time spent playing, to reduce the impact of fatigue on the musicians. Additionally, students received applied health education in relation to both performance health (for example, warming-up, stretching, relative rest, relaxation strategies and so on) and general health (for example, hydration, diet, sleep, and so on). The students reported that the more frequent short rest breaks in their rehearsals were noticeable in reducing PRHIs, improving concentration and energy, and appreciated the ability to rehydrate and refuel more frequently compared to previous heavy rehearsal weeks (Ackermann, 2017a). A similar trial in Australia's premier chamber orchestra anecdotally had highly positive effects on rehearsal quality and performance outcomes. Considering flexibility with rehearsals makes sense to allow the breaks to come when needed due to the widely varying physical demands of repertoire (Ackermann, 2017a). The same approaches can apply easily to rehearsals in other performing arts domains. Leadership should recognise that regular short recovery periods are simple, practical ways to reduce muscle overuse and fatigue and reduce PRHI risk. Performing artists should incorporate broader preparation and training practices for the required highly complex physical and mental skills, including specific muscle action training, warming up, stretching, mental skills training and so on, in a way similar to the advances made in athlete preparation for optimal performance and well-being in sport (Coutts et al., 2022; Hays, 2002; Kellmann et al., 2018). Time for recovery has been scheduled into some dance environments as an injury prevention measure (Bloom, 2024), but this has not yet been reported within music or circus settings. While prospectively measuring stressors in music settings could illustrate how best to add recovery periods to reduce exposure to health risks, for example by monitoring physical and psychological workloads (Windt & Gabbett, 2017), this has to date proved difficult to measure using self-report approaches (Ackermann et al., 2014; McCrary et al., 2021).

Organisational pressures

Research from work and organisational psychology has long considered how work characteristics are important to employee health and well-being. The applicability of these findings to professional performing artists should be evident, although studies applying these concepts to such populations are few and far between. An important synthesis of the literature (Morgeson & Humphrey, 2006) on job design and a related meta-analysis (Humphrey et al., 2007) showing how work characteristics related to important health, well-being, and other outcomes of interest to individuals and their employers are instructive as we think about strategies for prevention in professional performing artists.

In reviewing the literature on job design characteristics, Morgeson and Humphrey (2006) categorised work characteristics into four major categories: task, knowledge, social, and work context characteristics. The task and knowledge characteristics include work features that are intrinsic to the nature of the work itself, things like one's autonomy in work methods, the variety of tasks to be performed, and the importance of the work. Knowledge characteristics include features such as the variety of skills needed and work complexity. The social characteristics include the degree to which one's work requires coordinating it with others, the nature of social support, and the feedback one gets from others. The work context characteristics include physical demands, working conditions, ergonomics and equipment used. Morgeson and Humphrey proposed and tested empirically a questionnaire for measuring 21 specific job design characteristics that they grouped into four categories.

The meta-analysis by Humphrey et al. (2007), in accordance with a vast literature on work design, proposed that the various design characteristics potentially contribute to psychological states such as experienced meaningfulness and responsibility as well as to various behavioural, attitudinal and well-being outcomes. A synthetic approach to presenting the meta-analytic results grouped the task and knowledge characteristics into a category called motivational characteristics and found that they collectively related to all the outcome variables, including behavioural (work performance, turnover intentions), attitudes (work-related satisfaction, organisational commitment, job involvement) and well-being (anxiety, stress, burnout/exhaustion) ones. The social characteristics explained additional variance in all these outcomes when using them as predictors in addition to the motivational characteristics. The work context characteristics proved to be useful in addition to all the others in explaining additional variance in the well-being outcomes.

Some studies have addressed aspects of work design relating to health in performing artists (Allmendinger et al., 1996; Détári et al., 2020; Holst et al., 2012; Vastamäki et al., 2023); however, the framework presented here has apparently not been applied in a complete manner. We will see that its features align easily with artistic professions. Autonomy in work methods is likely to be limited in orchestral musicians, unless they are soloists and are accorded the freedom to interpret the score as they wish. Other tasks and knowledge characteristics likely depend on the repertoire played and how varied and difficult it is over a season. Social characteristics are central to the work of performing groups such as orchestras and ballet troupes where coordinating the role of each musician or dancer is essential to the performance. On the other hand, the social support and feedback each musician or dancer receives can be highly variable depending on the relations with colleagues within the orchestra and especially with the conductor or director. Musicians easily speak of conductors who are positive, supportive, and encouraging, who recognise the quality of their contributions to the performance, and others who are authoritarian, cold, and directive and seem more focused on their personal recognition as a conductor rather than on the contributions of each member of the group. The physical demands and working conditions depend again on such things as the repertoire played, the number of rehearsals and performances, whether the musicians are on stage for a concert or in the pit for an opera or ballet, the instrument played, and so on. Thus, depending on how favourable or unfavourable these various work characteristics are for the performers, we should be able to expect positive or negative results in terms of performance quality, work-related attitudes (satisfaction, commitment), and indicators of health and well-being. For example, a nationwide series of occupational health initiatives in Australia that provided comprehensive guidelines on improving well-being in the professional orchestral environment, including training regional health providers, was highly effective in improving health and well-being (Ackermann et al., 2017). Similarly, reports from dance companies have shown that having an expert team can save money through delivering specialised healthcare assisting both recovery and enhancing well-being thereby not losing dancers to injury (Bronner et al., 2003).

Training institutions for performing artists should be responsible in their care of students and provide comprehensive and relevant skills and education to empower them to successfully complete their training and move forward into a professional career knowing how to manage potential occupational risks to their well-being (Prior et al., 2015). In line with workplace health and safety guidelines, leadership and general staff should assess and modify work or training exposures, ideally with input from appropriately specialised performance scientists, to ensure adequate recovery and reduce PRHI risks that may arise from overloading the cast or orchestra unevenly (Ackermann et al., 2017; Shrier et al., 2022). Once more rigorous performance periods are identified, interventions can be strategically implemented such as recovery massage during intensive work periods, regular injury advisory sessions, adaptive behaviour techniques, rostering arrangements and strengthening programmes – all of which have been shown to help to prevent injuries (Ackermann et al., 2014; Blevins et al., 2020; Chan & Ackermann, 2014; Chan et al., 2014; Hakim et al., 2020).

Other research in work and organisational psychology has examined the importance of organisational justice for the health and well-being of employees. Organisational justice is essentially concerned with treating employees fairly, in making decisions that concern them and in the way the decisions are made and communicated (for a general review, see Steiner, 2020, or for applications to employee health, see Steiner, 2017). When we examine organisational justice, we typically are interested in the perspective of employees and seek to discover their perceptions of whether they are treated fairly or not at work. The focus is indeed on people's perceptions of their treatment by their employer and those with whom they work, because people react to their work situations based on how they perceive them. Understanding what these perceptions are and what they are based on is key to finding ways to improve how people function at work.

Generally, we can define three major types of justice perceptions for people at work (Colquitt et al., 2023; Greenberg, 1987). Distributive justice concerns employees' evaluations of decisions made that concern them. The decisions of interest are typically ones where resources are allocated or distributed (Adams, 1965). The resources distributed can be of many kinds, including recognition, through salaries, positions, or even symbolic things such as praise and pleasant working conditions. Essentially, we find such distributions or decisions fair when they correspond to our contributions to the employer. Thus, if we are the most qualified candidate for a position, we consider that it is fair or equitable to be the one hired. Similarly, the harder we work or the better our performance, the more recognition we expect, whatever its form might be. A second type of justice, or dimension of justice, is called procedural justice. Besides evaluating whether the decision is equitable, people are interested in how the decision was made. Several principles govern whether we believe decision procedures to be fair or not. One of the most important is the opportunity to have 'voice' in a decision (Thibaut & Walker, 1975), that is, to be consulted and have the possibility to express an opinion concerning how the decision should be made. Many studies have confirmed the importance of having voice in decision making (van den Bos, 2005). Put simply, people like to be consulted or have the possibility to provide relevant information during the decision-making process. For example, a musician would likely find it fair to be asked what repertoire they would like to play, what their work schedule should be, and when a break in rehearsal is needed. Beyond having voice, other types of procedures are also associated with favourable justice perceptions: decisions that respect ethical principles, that are based on accurate information, that allow for an appeal process in the case of an unfavourable decision, or that take into consideration relevant criteria (Leventhal, 1976). Finally, the third dimension of organisational justice is interactional justice (Bies & Moag, 1986). This dimension focuses on how authorities communicate and interact with employees, especially in communicating decisions to them. People prefer warm and respectful exchanges with their superiors and colleagues, and explanations for decisions that are informative and justify the decision. They consider that such treatment constitutes fair interactions.

Numerous studies have supported the benefits of these different forms of fair treatment for employees and their employers (for example, see the meta-analyses of Colquitt et al., 2001, 2013; Whitman et al., 2012). The benefits include favourable attitudes, behaviours, performance, and health outcomes. Such benefits have been found in quite varied employment settings, and our work in progress confirms them in orchestra musicians. It is notably the benefits in terms of health that we focus on here to illustrate again how the work environment can contribute to health concerns beyond those typically studied and known for performing artists.

Robbins et al. (2012) provided a meta-analysis of how different types of fair (or unfair) treatment relate to health outcomes. They also presented a model of how unfairness results in health concerns. In the model, unfair treatment (no matter the type or dimension) affects psychological reactions including stress, rumination, and related central nervous system reactions. In turn, these reactions influence our behaviours related to health (e.g., physical activity, eating, and alcohol consumption), which have consequences for our health. In the meta-analytic results presented, different forms of unfair treatment were associated with mental and physical health, and notably with burnout, stress, and negative affect (with estimations of population-level correlations of a moderate size, i.e., approximately $r = .40$ depending on the variable).

Other research has found that being treated unfairly is notably associated with musculoskeletal disorders (MSDs), a frequent concern for professional musicians. The mechanisms for unfair treatment contributing to MSDs are similar to the ones described by Robbins et al. (2012). Unfair treatment prevents people from resting and recovering from their activity because they tend to ruminate and experience tension following unfair treatment. The link between unfair treatment and MSDs has been established in published studies (Manville et al., 2016), and we have found evidence for important contributions of unfair treatment to MSD-related pain and performance difficulties in professional orchestra musicians (Maugue & Steiner, 2023). In our research on musicians, we have controlled all the typically studied important variables that contribute to MSDs including instrument played, workload, gender, age, and other variables indicating recent instrumental work activity. Taking into account all these factors explained respectively 27% and 19% of the variance in emotional exhaustion and pain intensity at the moment of responding. Adding the various justice perceptions to the model, with a focus on how the orchestra's director and management treat the musicians, increased the variance explained to 36% and 23%, showing the importance of these considerations to musicians' health. Indeed, Liverpool Philharmonic Orchestra reported that implementing a health and well-being policy that required only 1.2% of the total orchestra wage bill has been a fantastic return on investment through musicians' sense of feeling valued, supported by employer, being able to focus on thriving artistically, and the overall orchestra culture (Garden, 2024).

Other research on organisational justice has examined how treatment by one's peers or colleagues is important in our day-to-day work experiences. In fact, many argue that in many work settings, our interactions with our peers are more frequent than those with our superiors and so their influence on our well-being is likely to be particularly strong (Estreder et al., 2024; Fortin et al., 2020). We can easily imagine that this will also be the case with musicians who work closely with their colleagues who play the same instrument and work beside them throughout the season, whereas in many orchestras, the conductor changes regularly, with many directing the same orchestra only occasionally. Training people on the principles of organisational justice, making them aware of the importance of them and guiding people through ways to apply them, has proven effective in other settings (Piasecki & Steiner, 2019; Skarlicki & Latham, 2005) and would likely produce positive benefits among performing artists. In summary, people value being treated fairly, and instilling these practices in any performing arts work group or training institution can only be beneficial for well-being.

Conclusion and recommendations for practice

Performing artists train and work in a competitive environment, where physiological and psychological capacity is frequently pushed to and above the capacity of the performer, in a culture where the show must go on. Physical and psychological PRHIs – including muscle tears, joint sprains, performance anxiety and a host of other disorders related to overload – are commonplace, and yet applied health education and injury prevention principles in their training and workplace environments are sparse. In both training institutions and work environments, applied health education should be provided regularly, focusing on key areas relevant to those performing artists, that is both practicable and understandable so that health literacy and resilience are developed. Educational initiatives should include helping performers to develop better self-efficacy and self-regulation skills, so they are able to optimise their own individual recovery approaches in response to variable stressors in their training and work environments. Creating a positive attitude towards taking the time to recover when needed by the performing artist and their peers is an essential component of well-being as well as optimising performance capacity. Like athletes, performing artists will be exposed to periods of high workload and extreme stress, and there is often little consideration to recovery periods. While it can be challenging to define an ideal work:rest ratio in the performing arts, where individual capacity and performance demands can vary widely, encouraging self-measuring of fatigue (e.g., Ratings of Perceived Exertion) may be one way to identify when recovery time is needed. Further research is needed to evaluate and develop more performing arts specific ways to measure tension, stress and fatigue, as well as appropriate ways to implement recovery into busy schedules. Building relationships with organisations and performing artists is critical to ensure that recovery can be supported within the workplace, and this may require funding and personnel to support such integral workplace health and safety initiatives. Education should also target performing arts organisation leadership to better understand the positive well-being and economic benefits that may result from strategies that allow performers to implement flexible recovery strategies prior to developing PRHIs. This may include adapting performer schedules that allow for recovery of players during busy work periods, or reducing intensity or volumes of rehearsals occurring on the same day as performances. Balancing practice, work and life for a performing artist is ultimately a lifelong learning process that should include adequate health education, access to specialised health care resources and personnel, and a culture of positive well-being within organisations that facilitate optimal performers as well as performances.

References

Ackermann, B. J. (2017a). How much training is too much? *Medical Problems of Performing Artists*, *32*(1), 61–62.

Ackermann, B. J. (2017b). The sickness of stigmas. *Medical Problems of Performing Artists*, *32*(3), 183–184.

Ackermann, B. J., & Driscoll, T. (2013). Attitudes and practices of parents of teenage musicians to health issues related to playing an instrument: A pilot study. *Medical Problems of Performing Artists*, *28*(1), 24–27.

Ackermann, B. J., Driscoll, T., & Kenny, D. T. (2012). Musculoskeletal pain and injury in professional orchestral musicians in Australia. *Medical Problems of Performing Artists*, *27*(4), 181–187.

Ackermann, B. J., Kenny, D. T., Driscoll, T., & O'Brien, I. (2017). *ARC sound practice project final report*. Australian Research Council; Australia Council for the Arts. Retrieved March 04, 2025 from https://creative.gov.au/wp-content/uploads/2021/07/Sound-Practice-final-report.pdf

Ackermann, B. J., Kenny, D. T., O'Brien, I., & Driscoll, T. R. (2014). Sound practice – Improving occupational health and safety for professional orchestral musicians in Australia. *Frontiers in Psychology*, 5, 973. https://doi.org/10.3389/fpsyg.2014.00973

Ackermann, B. J., Wijsman, S., & Halaki, M. (2025). The Australian Music Students Health Survey: Impact of past experience on student attitudes to health education. *British Journal of Music Education*, 42, 91–109.

Adams, J. S. (1965). Inequity in social exchange. In L. Berkowitz (Ed.), *Advances in experimental social psychology* (2nd ed., pp. 267–299). Academic Press.

Adler, K. W. (2022). *What #MeToo changed in Hollywood – And what it didn't*. Elle Magazine. Retrieved March 04, 2025 from https://www.elle.com/culture/a41539940/hollywood-five-years-after-harvey-weinstein-metoo/

Allmendinger, J., Hackman, J. R., & Lehman, E. V. (1996). Life and work in symphony orchestras. *The Musical Quarterly*, *80*(2), 194–219.

Baadjou, V. A., Wijsman, S. I., Ginsborg, J., Guptill, C., De Lisle, R., Rennie-Salonen, B., Visentin, P., & Ackermann, B. J. (2019). Health education literacy and accessibility for musicians: A global approach. Report from the Worldwide Universities Network Project. *Medical Problems of Performing Artists*, *34*(2), 105–107.

Backiev, L., Bastepe-Gray, S., Mueller, D., Watson, M. D., Chiang, C. C., Emam, M., & Lasner, A. N. (2024). Updates in performing arts medicine: A clinical overview for instrumental musicians and dancers. *Current Physical Medicine and Rehabilitation Reports*, *12*(2), 223–233.

Beckmann, J. (2023). Self-regulation of recovery. In M. Kellmann, S. Jakowski, & J. Beckmann (Eds.), *The importance of recovery for physical and mental health* (pp. 53–69). Routledge.

Bies, R., & Moag, J. (1986). Interactional justice: Communication criteria of fairness. In R. Lewicki, B. Sheppard, & M. Bazerman (Eds.), *Research on negotiation in organizations* (pp. 43–55). JAI Press.

Blevins, P., Erskine, S., Hopper, L., & Moyle, G. M. (2020). Finding your balance: An investigation of recovery–stress balance in vocational dance training. *Journal of Dance Education*, *20*(1), 12–22.

Bloom, H. (2024). *R&R: How rest can be the best medicine*. Retrieved March 04, 2025 from https://australianballet.com.au/blog/r-r-how-rest-can-be-the-best-medicine?srsltid=AfmBOooquU5TfOHtzLko5qwckmLc6rdUts0fQUPgVPMBMmL0oFC3rK3

Bompa, T. O., & Buzzichelli, C. (Eds). (2019). *Periodization: Theory and methodology of training*. Human Kinetics.

Bosquet, L., Montpetit, J., Arvisais, D., & Mujika, I. (2007). Effects of tapering on performance: A meta-analysis. *Medicine & Science in Sports & Exercise*, *39*(8), 1358–1365.

Bronner, S., Ojofeitimi, S., & Rose, D. (2003). Injuries in a modern dance company: Effect of comprehensive management on injury incidence and time loss. *The American Journal of Sports Medicine*, *31*(3), 365–373.

Carroll, L. J., Lis, A., Weiser, S., & Torti, J. (2016). How well do you expect to recover, and what does recovery mean, anyway? Qualitative study of expectations after a musculoskeletal injury. *Physical Therapy*, *96*(6), 797–807.

Cayrol, T., Godfrey, E., Draper-Rodi, J., & Bearne, L. (2019). Exploring professional circus artists' experience of performance-related injury and management: A qualitative study. *Medical Problems of Performing Artists*, *34*(1), 14–24.

Chan, C., & Ackermann, B. J. (2014). Evidence-informed physical therapy management of performance-related musculoskeletal disorders in musicians. *Frontiers in Psychology*, *5*, 706. https://doi.org/10.3389/fpsyg.2014.00706

Chan, C., Driscoll, T., & Ackermann, B. J. (2014). Effect of a musicians' exercise intervention on performance-related musculoskeletal disorders. *Medical Problems of Performing Artists*, *29*(4), 181–188.

Chan, P. H., Howard, J., Eva, N., & Herman, H. M. (2022). A systematic review of at-work recovery and a framework for future research. *Journal of Vocational Behavior*, *137*, 103747. https://doi.org/10.1016/j.jvb.2022.103747

Clague, M. (2023). From portfolio to platform career: Navigating the promise and pitfalls of a sustainable and meaningful life in the performing arts. *Artivate: A Journal of Entrepreneurship in the Arts*, *12*(1), 1–22. https://doi.org/10.34053/artivate.12.1.203

Colquitt, J. A., Conlon, D. E., Wesson, M. J., Porter, C. O. L. H., & Ng, K. Y. (2001). Justice at the millenium: A meta-analytic review of 25 years of organizational justice research. *Journal of Applied Psychology*, *86*, 425–445.

Colquitt, J. A., Hill, E. T., & De Cremer, D. (2023). Forever focused on fairness: 75 years of organizational justice in *Personnel Psychology*. *Personnel Psychology*, *76*, 413–435.

Colquitt, J. A., Scott, B. A., Rodell, J. B., Long, D. M., Zapata, C. P., Conlon, D. E., & Wesson, M. J. (2013). Justice at the millennium, a decade later: A meta-analytic test of social exchange and affect-based perspectives. *Journal of Applied Psychology*, *98*(2), 199–236.

Coutts, A. J., Crowcroft, S., & Kempton, T. (2022). Developing athlete monitoring systems: Theoretical basis and practical applications. In M. Kellmann & J. Beckmann (Eds.), *Recovery and well-being in sport and exercise* (pp. 17–31). Routledge.

Den Hartigh, R. J., Meerhoff, L. R. A., van Yperen, N. W., Neumann, N. D., Brauers, J. J., Frencken, W. G., Emerencia, A., Hill, Y., Platvoet, S., Atzmueller, M., Lemmink, K. A., & Brink, M. S. (2024). Resilience in sports: A multidisciplinary, dynamic, and personalized perspective. *International Review of Sport and Exercise Psychology*, *17*(1), 564–586.

Détári, A., Egermann, H., Bjerkeset, O., & Vaag, J. (2020). Psychosocial work environment among musicians and in the general workforce in Norway. *Frontiers in Psychology*, *11*, 1315. https://doi.org/10.3389/fpsyg.2020.01315

Ekegren, C. L., Quested, R., & Brodrick, A. (2014). Injuries in pre-professional ballet dancers: Incidence, characteristics and consequences. *Journal of Science and Medicine in Sport*, *17*(3), 271–275.

Eslake, S. (2024). *This health and well-being program is putting musicians' needs first*. Cut Common. Retrieved March 04, 2025 from https://www.cutcommonmag.com/this-health-and-well-being-program-is-putting-musicians-needs-first/

Estreder, Y., Álvarez, P., Martínez-Tur, V., Cropanzano, R., & Tomás, I. (2024). Peer justice and the individual. *Journal of Business and Psychology*, *39*(1), 233–248.

Ford, M. T., Cerasoli, C. P., Higgins, J. A., & Decesare, A. L. (2011). Relationships between psychological, physical, and behavioural health and work performance: A review and meta-analysis. *Work & Stress*, *25*(3), 185–204.

Fortin, M., Cropanzano, R., Cugueró-Escofet, N., Nadisic, T., & Van Wagoner, H. (2020). How do people judge fairness in supervisor and peer relationships? Another assessment of the dimensions of justice. *Human Relations*, *73*(12), 1632–1663.

Garden, P. (2024). *Musicians' performance and well-being – Creating conditions for musicians to thrive*. Conference presentation and personal communication from the launch and inaugural conference of the Association Française pour la Santé des Artistes de Performance, 10th February, Paris, France.

Greenberg, J. (1987). A taxonomy of organizational justice theories. *Academy of Management Review*, *12*, 9–22.
Greenspan, S. (2021). Injury frequency and characteristics in adolescent and adult circus artists: A pilot prospective cohort study. *Medical Problems of Performing Artists*, *36*(2), 103–107.
Gross, S. A., & Musgrave, G. (2020). *Can music make you sick? Measuring the price of musical ambition*. University of Westminster Press.
Guptill, C., Slade, T., Baadjou, V., Roduta Roberts, M., de Lisle, R., Ginsborg, J., Rennie-Salonen, B., Ackermann, B. J., Visentin, P., & Wijsman, S. (2022). Validity and reliability of the Musicians' Health Literacy Questionnaire, MHL–Q19. *Frontiers in Psychology*, *13*, 886815. https://doi.org/10.3389/fpsyg.2022.886815
Hacquebord, S., Kiers, H., van der Wees, P., & Hoogeboom, T. J. (2024). Towards a better understanding of our patients. A qualitative study about how patients and their physiotherapists perceive the recovery of shoulder problems. *Musculoskeletal Science and Practice*, *71*, 102931. https://doi.org/10.1016/j.msksp.2024.102931
Hakim, H., Puel, F., & Bertucci, W. (2020). Injury assessment in circus student-artists population; preliminary study. *Science & Sports*, *35*(3), 154–160.
Hansen, P. A., & Reed, K. (2006). Common musculoskeletal problems in the performing artist. *Physical Medicine and Rehabilitation Clinics*, *17*(4), 789–801.
Hays, K. F. (2002). The enhancement of performance excellence among performing artists. *Journal of Applied Sport Psychology*, *14*(4), 299–312.
Hinkamp, D., Morton, J., Krasnow, D. H., Wilmerding, M. V., Dawson, W. J., Stewart, M. G., Sims, H. S., Reed, J. P., Duvall, K., & McCann, M. (2017). Occupational health and the performing arts: An introduction. *Journal of Occupational and Environmental Medicine*, *59*(9), 843–858.
Holst, G. J., Paarup, H. M., & Baelum, J. (2012). A cross-sectional study of psychosocial work environment and stress in the Danish symphony orchestras. *International Archives of Occupational and Environmental Health*, *85*(6), 639–649.
Humphrey, S. E., Nahrgang, J. D., & Morgeson, F. P. (2007). Integrating motivational, social, and contextual work design features: A meta-analytic summary and theoretical extension of the work design literature. *Journal of Applied Psychology*, *92*, 1332–1356.
Jeong, S. S. Y., & Ryan, C. (2022). A critical review of child perfectionism as it relates to music pedagogy. *Psychology of Music*, *50*(4), 1312–1327.
Kellmann, M., Bertollo, M., Bosquet, L., Brink, M., Coutts, A. J., Duffield, R., Erlacher, D., Halson, S. L., Hecksteden, A., Heidari, J., Kallus, K. W., Meeusen, R., Mujika, I., Robazza, C., Skorski, S., Venter, R., & Beckmann, J. (2018). Recovery and performance in sport: Consensus statement. *International Journal of Sports Physiology and Performance*, *13*(2), 240–245.
Kenny, D. T., & Ackermann, B. J. (2015). Performance-related musculoskeletal pain, depression and music performance anxiety in professional orchestral musicians: A population study. *Psychology of Music*, *43*(1), 43–60.
Kenny, D. T., & Ackermann, B. J. (2016). Hitting the high notes: Healthy aging in professional orchestral musicians. In A.-S. Antoniou, R. J. Burke, & S. C. L. Cooper (Eds.), *The aging workforce handbook* (pp. 355–376). Emerald Group Publishing Limited.
Kleynhans, R., Nel, P., & Maree, K. (2024). Performing artists' career trajectory from a career construction perspective. *British Journal of Guidance & Counselling*, *52*(5), 1023–1037.

Kok, L. M., Haitjema, S., Groenewegen, K. A., & Rietveld, A. B. M. (2016). The influence of a sudden increase in playing time on playing-related musculoskeletal complaints in high-level amateur musicians in a longitudinal cohort study. *PloS ONE*, *11*(9), e0163472. https://doi.org/10.1371/journal.pone.0163472

Kozai, A., & Ambegaonkar, J. P. (2020). Health literacy for collegiate dancers: Provision and perceptions of health-related education in university dance programs. *Journal of Dance Medicine & Science*, *24*(3), 118–125.

Laumonier, T., & Menetrey, J. (2016). Muscle injuries and strategies for improving their repair. *Journal of Experimental Orthopaedics*, *3*(1), 15. https://doi.org/10.1186/s40634-016-0051-7

Leong, N. L., Kator, J. L., Clemens, T. L., James, A., Enamoto-Iwamoto, M., & Jiang, J. (2020). Tendon and ligament healing and current approaches to tendon and ligament regeneration. *Journal of Orthopaedic Research*, *38*(1), 7–12.

Leventhal, G. S. (1976). Fairness in social relationships. In J. W. Thibaut, J. T. Spence, & R. C. Carson (Eds.), *Contemporary topics in social psychology* (pp. 211–239). General Learning Press.

Manville, C., Akremi, A. E., Niezborala, M., & Mignonac, K. (2016). Injustice hurts, literally: The role of sleep and emotional exhaustion in the relationship between organizational justice and musculoskeletal disorders. *Human Relations*, *69*(6), 1315–1339.

Maugue, A., & Steiner, D. D. (2023, December 7–9). *The particular case of professional orchestra musicians: Justice perceptions, health, and instrumental performance in a context with multiple demands* [Paper presentation]. Research Meeting on Determinants of the Physical, Mental, and Social Health of Professional Musicians and Proposals for Prevention, Nice, France.

Maxwell, I., Seton, M., & Szabo, M. (2015). *The Australian actors' well-being study: A preliminary report.* In About Performance (No. 13, pp. 69–113). Sydney: Centre for Performance Studies. Retrieved March 04, 2025 from https://search.informit.org/doi/pdf/10.3316/informit.499926749273237?casa_token=zdh-NhDVB3YAAAAA%3AgKSNar5Lrzs0jGd2MDVDsVtzR-RR8YJvNyouAv5kqCMKCXeAtcbIAFmAjXIQ6M2Uyzofhjqv-WLt

McCrary, J. M., Redding, E., & Altenmüller, E. (2021). Performing arts as a health resource? An umbrella review of the health impacts of music and dance participation. *PloS ONE*, *16*(6), e0252956. https://doi.org/10.1371/journal.pone.0252956

Middlebrook, N., Heneghan, N. R., Falla, D., Silvester, L., Rushton, A. B., & Soundy, A. A. (2021). Successful recovery following musculoskeletal trauma: Protocol for a qualitative study of patients' and physiotherapists' perceptions. *BMC Musculoskeletal Disorders*, *22*, 163. https://doi.org/10.1186/s12891-021-04035-9

Morgeson, F. P., & Humphrey, S. E. (2006). The Work Design Questionnaire (WDQ): Developing and validating a comprehensive measure for assessing job design and the nature of work. *Journal of Applied Psychology*, *91*, 1321–1339.

Munro, D. (2014). Injury patterns and rates amongst students at the national institute of circus arts: An observational study. *Medical Problems of Performing Artists*, *29*(4), 235–240.

Nordin-Bates, S. M. (2020). Striving for perfection or for creativity? A dancer's dilemma. *Journal of Dance Education*, *20*(1), 23–34.

Nutbeam, D., & McGill, B. (2019). Improving health literacy in clinical and community populations. In O. Okan, U. Bauer, U. D. Levin-Zamir, P. Pinheiro, & K. Sørensen (Eds.), *International handbook of health literacy: Research, practice and policy across the lifespan* (pp. 219–232). Policy Press.

Piasecki, C., & Steiner, D. D. (2019). La justice organisationnelle comme levier pour promouvoir la qualité de vie au travail [Organizational justice as a means for promoting quality of life at work]. *Psychologie du Travail et des Organisations*, *25*, 116–126.

Prakash, A., Mahesh, K., & Akilesh, V. (2024). Umbrella review of musculoskeletal injury burden in dancers: Implication for practice and research. *The Physician and Sportsmedicine*, *52*(1), 12–25.

Prior, R., Maxwell, I., Szabo, M., & Seton, M. (2015). Responsible care in actor training: Effective support for occupational health training in drama schools. *Theatre, Dance and Performance Training*, *6*(1), 59–71.

Ranelli, S., Straker, L., & Smith, A. (2011). Playing-related musculoskeletal problems in children learning instrumental music: The association between problem location and gender, age, and music exposure factors. *Medical Problems of Performing Artists*, *26*(3), 123–139.

Ren, S. (2024). The influence mechanism of social support and health literacy on Chinese residents' physical and mental health. *American Journal of Health Behavior*, *48*(5), 1423–1437.

Robbins, J. M., Ford, M. T., & Tetrick, L. E. (2012). Perceived unfairness and employee health: A meta-analytic integration. *Journal of Applied Psychology*, *97*(2), 235–272.

Shah, S. (2019). Treating the performing artist: Special considerations. In L. E. Elson (Ed.), *Performing arts medicine* (pp. 9–14). Elsevier.

Shrier, I., Mattiello, R., Caron, M., Verhagen, E., & Steele, R. J. (2022). Observed injury rates did not follow theoretically predicted injury risk patterns in professional human circus artists. *Clinical Journal of Sport Medicine*, *32*(6), e627–e634.

Shrier, I., Meeuwisse, W. H., Matheson, G. O., Wingfield, K., Steele, R. J., Prince, F., Hanley, J., & Montanaro, M. (2009). Injury patterns and injury rates in the circus arts: An analysis of 5 years of data from Cirque du Soleil. *The American Journal of Sports Medicine*, *37*(6), 1143–1149.

Skarlicki, D. P., & Latham, G. P. (2005). How can training be used to foster organizational justice? In J. Greenberg & J. A. Colquitt (Eds.), *Handbook of organizational justice* (pp. 499–522). Lawrence Erlbaum Associates Publishers.

Smith, D. J. (2003). A framework for understanding the training process leading to elite performance. *Sports Medicine*, *33*(15), 1103–1126.

Solar, O., & Irwin, A. (2010). *A conceptual framework for action on the social determinants of health*. WHO Document Production Services. Retrieved March 04, 2025 from https://www.who.int/publications/i/item/9789241500852

Sonnentag, S., Kark, R., & Venz, L. (2024). Leader support for recovery: A multi-level approach to employee psychological detachment from work. *Journal of Occupational and Organizational Psychology*, *97*(4), 1762–1788.

Sørensen, K., Pelikan, J. M., Röthlin, F., Ganahl, K., Slonska, Z., Doyle, G., Fullam, J., Kondilis, B., Agrafiotis, D., Uiters, E., Falcon, M., & Brand, H. (2015). Health literacy in Europe: Comparative results of the European health literacy survey (HLS-EU). *The European Journal of Public Health*, *25*(6), 1053–1058.

Steiner, D. D. (2017). Organizational justice for understanding employee health and well-being. In C. Moliner, R. Cropanzano, & V. Martínez-Tur (Eds.), *Organizational justice: International perspectives and conceptual advances* (pp. 160–180). Routledge.

Steiner, D. D. (2020). *Organizational justice*. Oxford research encyclopedia of psychology. Retrieved March 04, 2025 from https://oxfordre.com/psychology/view/10.1093/acrefore/9780190236557.001.0001/acrefore-9780190236557-e-555

Sun, Y., & Liu, H. (2024). Prevalence and risk factors of musculoskeletal injuries in modern and contemporary dancers: A systematic review and meta-analysis. *Frontiers in Public Health*, *12*, 1325536. https://doi.org/10.3389/fpubh.2024.1325536

Thibaut, J., & Walker, L. (1975). *Procedural justice: A psychological analysis*. Lawrence Erlbaum.

van den Bos, K. (2005). What is responsible for the fair process effect? In J. Greenberg & J. A. Colquitt (Eds.), *Handbook of organizational justice* (pp. 273–300). Lawrence Erlbaum.

Vassallo, A. J., Pappas, E., Stamatakis, E., & Hiller, C. E. (2019). Injury fear, stigma, and reporting in professional dancers. *Safety and Health at Work*, *10*(3), 260–264.

Vastamäki, M., Heliövaara, M., Vastamäki, H., & Ristolainen, L. (2023). Orchestra musicians' work environment and health versus general workforce. *Journal of Occupational and Environmental Medicine*, *65*(4), 344–348.

Vieker, J. (2013). *The lip rip blues*. Retrieved March 04, 2025 from https://lipripblues.com/

Whitman, D. S., Caleo, S., Carpenter, N. C., Horner, M. T., & Bernerth, J. B. (2012). Fairness at the collective level: A meta-analytic examination of the consequences and boundary conditions of organizational justice climate. *Journal of Applied Psychology*, *97*, 776–791.

Wijsman, S., & Ackermann, B. J. (2019). Educating Australian musicians: Are we playing it safe? *Health Promotion International*, *34*(4), 869–876.

Willis, S., Neil, R., Mellick, M. C., & Wasley, D. (2019). The relationship between occupational demands and well-being of performing artists: A systematic review. *Frontiers in Psychology*, *10*, 393. https://doi.org/10.3389/fpsyg.2019.00393

Windt, J., & Gabbett, T. J. (2017). How do training and competition workloads relate to injury? The workload—injury aetiology model. *British Journal of Sports Medicine*, *51*(5), 428–435.

World Health Organization. (2010). *A conceptual framework for action on the social determinants of health*. Retrieved March 04, 2025 from https://iris.who.int/bitstream/handle/10665/44489/?sequence=1

3

DEVELOPING MONITORING SYSTEMS FOR THE PERFORMING ARTS

Theoretical and practical applications

Annie C. Jeffries and Aaron J. Coutts

Introduction

The performing arts encompass a variety of disciplines, including dance, orchestral music, drama, and circus. Achieving optimal performance across all disciplines requires a complex interaction of aesthetic, artistic, technical, and psychological components (Kuno et al., 1996), often involving extreme physical demands and a high level of athletic ability (Gamboa et al., 2008; Khan et al., 1995). Given the intensive physical, cognitive, and technical demands, monitoring training and recovery is critical to allow for optimal performance and reduced risk of injury and illness. However, despite these risks, monitoring systems are relatively uncommon in the performing arts, particularly in comparison to high-performance sport. While performing arts and sport both involve physical activity and skill, they differ significantly in purpose and presentation. For example, the performing arts are inherently artistic and subjective, with performers interpreting and expressing emotions, stories, and concepts (Arnold, 1995). Performances often emphasise creativity, technique, and an emotional connection with the audience. Subjectivity lies in how audiences perceive and react to the nuances of the performance, such as the interpretation of a character in a play or the expressiveness and artistry of a dance piece. While technical skills are critical, artistry and expression also play major roles across all performing arts disciplines. In contrast, sports are primarily goal-oriented

Jeffries, A. C., & Coutts, A. J. (2026). Developing monitoring systems for the performing arts: Theoretical and practical applications. In E. Altenmüller, M. Kellmann, J. Beckmann, & G. M. Moyle (Eds.), *Recovery and well-being in the performing arts* (pp. 41–59). Routledge.

DOI: 10.4324/9781003566885-4

and competitive, with clear rules and measurable outcomes. As such, the clear, objective nature of goals and performance metrics in sport enhances the ability to monitor training progress compared to the more subjective and interpretive elements in the performing arts.

Performing artists face significant challenges, particularly dancers, including extremely high training loads, nearly double that of some elite athletes, minimal recovery periods, and high rates of injury and illness (Jeffries, Wallace, Coutts, Cohen et al., 2020). For example, injury incidence rates range from 4.6 to 5.86 per 1,000 hours in professional classical ballet and contemporary dancers (Allen et al., 2012; Jeffries, Wallace, Coutts, Cohen et al., 2020). Overuse injuries, particularly affecting the lower limbs, especially the foot and ankle, are the most common among both amateur and professional dancers (Smith et al., 2016). Among these, bone stress and stress fractures are most frequently observed and are likely associated with factors such as low energy availability and low body composition (Jotwani et al., 2022). Therefore, the high training demands, together with high injury and illness incidence, increase the risk of poor health outcomes, highlighting the need for better monitoring and support systems for performing artists. The purpose of this chapter is to examine the training theory that underpins performing artist monitoring and the integral components of a monitoring system. Additionally, a discussion of case studies and practical recommendations will also be provided.

Theoretical basis of performing artist monitoring

The primary objective of training in the performing arts is to stimulate improvements in artistic performance. This requires the optimal development of physical abilities alongside technical and cognitive skills. For physical capacity improvements to occur, a careful balance between training load

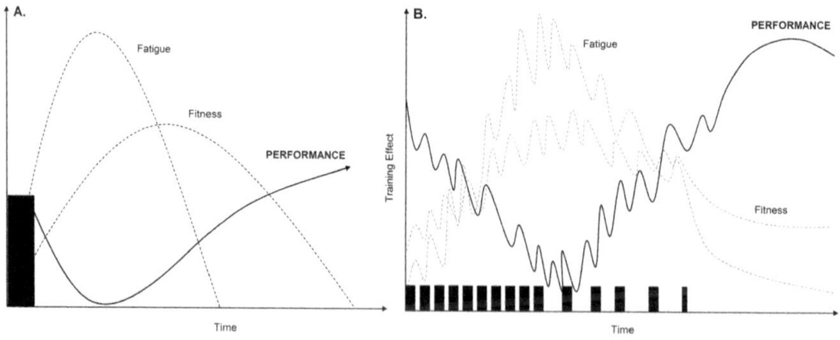

FIGURE 3.1 The modelled fitness and fatigue responses to (a) a single bout and (b) a sequence of training bouts.

and recovery is necessary (Matveyev, 1977). While it is challenging to model adaptations in artistic (technical) and cognitive performance, physical performance responses can be explained by the fitness-fatigue model (Banister et al., 1975). The fitness-fatigue model provides a straightforward method to quantify the dose-response relationship of training load to fitness, fatigue, and performance. This model has been described as fundamental for athlete monitoring systems and thus should also be relevant for monitoring systems for athletic artistic performers. Original work by Banister et al. (1975) applied a systems theory to analyse the response of physical training through a function (see Equation 3.1) that includes both a fitness response to enhance performance and a fatigue response that decreases performance.

Modelled Performance = (fitness from training model) – K (fatigue from training model)

Equation 3.1 Banister's original systems theory approach to analyse training. K = The constant that adjusts for the magnitude of the fatigue effect relative to the fitness effect.

The fitness-fatigue model illustrates the training-recovery dynamics of physical training sessions. Figure 3.1a depicts the theoretical fitness and fatigue response to a single training session, while Figure 3.1b demonstrates the modelled responses to a series of sessions (i.e., a training programme). Figure 3.1b clearly indicates that during periods of intensified physical training, where heavy training loads are undertaken without an appropriate balance of recovery, there is a resultant decline in performance.

While the training-recovery cycle may appear straightforward, individual variations in genetic and environmental characteristics, as well as the complex psychobiological adaptations resulting from training, make it challenging to predict the fitness and fatigue effects for each performer. Consequently, it has become common practice for sport scientists to regularly examine these dose-response relationships to inform decisions on training content for individual performers. Additionally, despite an increasing body of applied research in high-performance sport, there remains a relatively limited understanding of the most appropriate tools and methods to assess how individuals are coping with training. There is even less information available regarding the best tools to use with performing artists.

There are no universal criterion measures of training load, fitness, and fatigue applicable to all performers across the broad range of artistic disciplines. It is crucial that such a system be developed based on established conceptual frameworks and implemented in a manner that considers the cultural and logistical limitations present in the performance setting (i.e., selecting input measures feasible for the organisation/setting). We also advise consulting performers when selecting or developing monitoring systems and tools in recognition of the crucial importance of preserving their self-determination

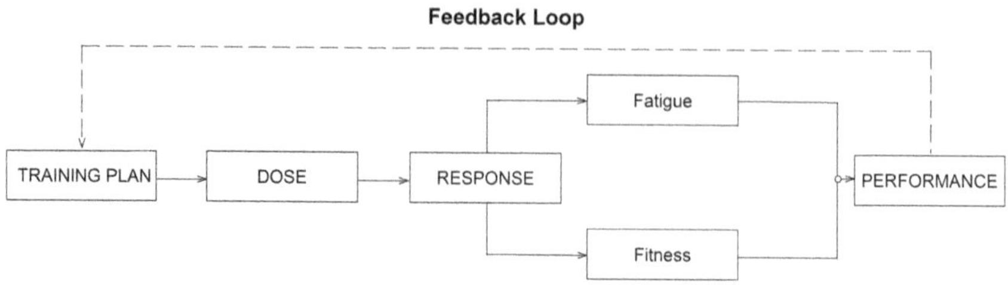

FIGURE 3.2 Conceptual model for developing athlete monitoring systems.

and autonomy throughout these processes (Ryan & Deci, 2000). Educating performers about their purpose and use will help build trust with the performers, as their buy-in will be central to the success of the system (Neupert et al., 2024). Regardless of the environment, essential components of this system should include quantifying training load measures for each performer and their fitness and fatigue responses to that training.

Figure 3.2 provides a simple model demonstrating the relationships between aspects of training load, fitness, and fatigue that combine to provide an iterative monitoring system applicable to most performers. For a more detailed discussion of the conceptual framework underpinning this simplified model, readers should refer to Jeffries et al. (2022).

Fundamental components of a performer monitoring system

The fundamental concepts utilised in the development of athlete monitoring systems for high-performance athletes (Coutts & Cormack, 2014) are relevant to monitoring performing artists. As training imposes stress on an athlete, their physical and psychological well-being move along a continuum that progresses from homeostasis through to stages of acute fatigue, overreaching, overtraining syndrome, and ultimately time-loss injury (Fry et al., 1991; Johnson & Ivarsson, 2011). Such maladaptation may arise through both poor training load management and interaction with psychological (e.g., performance pressure) and/or non-sport stressors (Fry et al., 1991; Johnson & Ivarsson, 2011). These maladaptive responses are common in professional performing artists, indicating the importance of such a system for these individuals.

Performing arts

The integration of sports science into performing arts training systems emphasises precise monitoring of key constructs such as training load, fitness, and fatigue to enhance performance outcomes. External training load, encompassing physical demands, is quantified using technologies like inertial measurement units (IMUs), while internal training load is assessed through validated methods such as session rating of perceived exertion (sRPE). Fitness monitoring, though underutilised, requires scientifically validated, cost-effective tools tailored to the specific needs of performers. The multifaceted nature of fatigue necessitates robust, validated instruments to measure training effects and recovery, ensuring accurate insights into physiological and psychological responses.

Training load

Training load is the most frequently manipulated input variable within a training system that is used to elicit the desired training response. Accordingly, the quantification and monitoring of training load form the basis of any monitoring system. The application of sports science principles is still a growing area in the preparation of performing artists, including the control of the stress applied or the measurement of the adaptive response. The following sections provide an overview of various constructs of training load and how they may be integrated into performing artist monitoring.

External training load

Dance in particular places significant demands on both the cardiovascular and musculoskeletal systems, reflecting its dual nature as an art form and a physically intensive activity. Dance often involves intermittent bursts of high-intensity activity, requiring a well-developed cardiovascular system to sustain performance. The cardiovascular load varies depending on the dance style, intensity, and duration. For example, high-energy styles like jazz or contemporary dance can elevate heart rates (HRs) significantly, while slower forms like ballet may involve more controlled exertion (Twitchett et al., 2009). Additionally, the musculoskeletal system is heavily engaged in dance, with repetitive movements, jumps, and turns placing stress on joints, muscles, and tendons. As such, dancers are prone to overuse injuries, particularly in the lower limbs (Bronner et al., 2003), due to the high physical demands and repetitive nature of their training (Jeffries, Wallace, Coutts, Cohen et al., 2020).

External training load can be defined constitutively as 'what the performing artist does' (e.g., work, speed, or distance covered) and operationally accommodates quantification in a variety of manners. Within the disciplines of dance and circus, wearable micro technologies, such as IMUs and accelerometers, have been used to measure external training loads during training and performance environments (Barker et al., 2020; Jeffries et al., 2017). These devices provide detailed information on aspects of external load, such as the number of accelerations/decelerations, body loads experienced in three dimensions, and count discrete activities such as changes of direction and twisting activities. Other devices frequently used in other sports include Global Positioning System (GPS), Local Position Systems (LPS), or computer vision systems, which provide detailed information on the external load such as position changes and derived metrics, such as distance travelled and the number of accelerations/decelerations. However, these systems are not suitable for dance activities due to limitations of training in an indoor environment (i.e., GPS connectivity limitations), their high financial cost and that metrics obtained from position changes per se do not properly reflect the physical demands of dance. As such, LPS with integrated IMUs are likely the ideal technology for quantifying the external training load demands of dance. However, a challenge in the application of IMUs for the measurement of external training load in performing artists is the practicality of a suitable placement of the device that does not interfere with motion. Additionally, if multiple sensors are utilised, this may increase costs, impact participant adherence, together with the requirement of expert knowledge for data analysis and interpretation (Coutts, 2014). Collectively, while these devices can provide detailed information on the external loads completed by performing artists, however, these issues may limit their effective use in practice.

Internal training load

Internal training load refers to the physiological and psychological responses experienced during a training session or performance. It can be quantified through validated measures, such as perceptual indicators (e.g., rating of perceived exertion) or physiological markers (e.g., HR). In the realm of dance, internal training load has been validated in pre-professional contemporary and professional classical ballet dancers using the sRPE method (Jeffries et al., 2017; Shaw et al., 2020). These studies have demonstrated that sRPE is a reliable indicator of internal training load across various populations of dancers and may serve as a practical tool for developing periodisation strategies. However, the most commonly used measure in dance for assessing training load is 'training time', which acts as a surrogate for training exposure (Volkova et al., 2023). Anecdotally, dance instructors often rely on training hours combined with their experience, intuition, and perception to gauge the intensity and training load experienced by dancers. It is important to note that subjective assessments made by dance teachers without validated assessment tools, along with the use of time as a measure of work volume, are not evidence-based or controllable.

Alternative methods for measuring internal training load include HR monitoring, oxygen consumption, and blood lactate assessment (Schantz & Astrand, 1984). However, practical limitations such as cost and technical expertise render these methods impractical for regular use. In summary, the sRPE method is a validated measure of internal training load that can be effectively employed in the performing arts to quantify performers' training. This simple yet valid tool allows coaches to combine training loads from different modalities into consistent units, providing an accurate reflection of the total training load.

Fitness

While measuring changes in fitness is an essential component of an athlete monitoring system, it remains an area largely overlooked across the performing arts disciplines. As such, without regular fitness measures, it is challenging to accurately determine a positive (or negative) response to training or assess if the performers' fitness status has been adequately developed. Gold standard fitness assessment procedures such as maximal oxygen uptake ($\dot{V}O_{2max}$) typically require expensive laboratory equipment and maximal effort, which can be challenging to implement within an artist's performance schedule. A fitness test utilised in a performing arts monitoring system should meet several criteria including being valid and reliable, accurately reflecting training status, cost-effective, and having minimal interruption to training and performing routines. Various studies have aimed to develop dance and non-dance-specific fitness tests, with dance-specific fitness tests targeted to more closely mimic the demands of dance and improve the specificity of the test (Redding et al., 2009; Twitchett et al., 2011). For example, Redding et al. (2009) developed a high-intensity, dance-specific fitness test to measure cardiovascular fitness in professional contemporary dancers by observing changes in HR, oxygen uptake, and blood lactate levels. Additionally, a multistage, ballet-specific aerobic fitness test using classical ballet movements has been found to be reliable and valid for assessing aerobic fitness in a dance studio setting (Twitchett et al., 2011).

Despite the availability of various protocols to assess fitness within a dance context, research on the measurement properties of these protocols remains limited (Tiemens et al., 2023). Additionally, many of these fitness tests involve maximal or submaximal effort. Within sport, resting HR, HR response to exercise (HRex), and HR recovery following an exercise bout are simple measures that can be collected in a training setting and have been suggested to have some utility for assessing athlete fitness (Shushan et al., 2023). For instance, since HR is closely linked to oxygen uptake during sustained exercise, a lower exercise HRex serves as a reliable indicator of an athlete's aerobic fitness level, which can be assessed through a short, standardised submaximal exercise bout (Coutts et al., 2022). As such, monitoring of HR may provide a relatively simple solution to assessing fitness that is non-invasive, time-efficient, and fairly low-cost. Therefore, simple HR measures may provide useful insight into the fitness-related changes to training in performing artists. Future research is required to assess the feasibility of this approach to monitoring the fitness status of performing artists.

Fatigue

Fatigue is a complex and multifaceted symptom. Fatigue lacks a single, universally accepted definition, with the definition being context-dependent such as, such as clinical, physiological, or psychological (Pattyn et al., 2018). However, in the context of athlete or performer monitoring fatigue is operationally defined as a "psychobiological state associated with an inability to complete a physical task that was once achievable within a recent time frame and is usually associated with altered perceptions of effort, along with feelings of tiredness and/or exhaustion" (Coutts et al., 2022, p. 22). Although the physiological and psychological mechanisms underpinning fatigue are not fully understood, there is agreement that measuring subjective fatigue is a crucial component of athlete monitoring.

Table 3.1 summarises the most common instruments. To assess fatigue, there are many psychometric tools available commonly termed Athlete-Reported Outcome Measures (AROMs). Within research and practice, AROMs are frequently used to measure the training response and include both multiple and single-item scales. Although traditional multiple-item scales may have superior psychometric properties, there are several reasons for the use of single items including reducing respondent burden and criterion contamination and increasing face validity (Jeffries, Wallace, Coutts, McLaren

TABLE 3.1 Common athlete-reported outcome measures.

Instrument	*Instrument properties*
Fatigue and recovery (Jeffries et al., 2023)	Single-item fatigue and recovery validated in dancers.
Multi-Component Training Distress Scale (Main and Grove, 2009)	22-item questionnaire assessing six factors: depression, vigour, physical symptoms, sleep disturbances, stress, and fatigue.
Recovery-Stress Questionnaire for Athletes (Kellmann and Kallus, 2001, 2025)	76-item questionnaire assessing physical and mental impact of training stress and frequency of recovery-associated activities.
Acute Recovery and Stress Scale (Kellmann and Kölling, 2019)	32-item questionnaire assesses the physical, mental, emotional, and overall recovery and stress states of athletes.
Short Recovery and Stress Scale (Kellmann and Kölling, 2019)	Derived from the Acute Recovery and Stress Scale, consists of eight items which are grouped into the Short Recovery Scale and the Short Stress Scale.

et al., 2020). Additionally, symptoms such as fatigue can be used to measure the training effect construct to assess how a performing artist is responding to the demands imposed by training. Furthermore, single-item AROMs have greater sensitivity to acute and chronic training loads than commonly used objective measures (Saw et al., 2016). Within the performing arts disciplines, it is common to rely on instruments used in sport for the measurement of fatigue; however, this should require independent validation specific to each population. Currently, there are few valid and practical methods for monitoring training effects across the performing arts disciplines. Within dance, there is preliminary evidence of construct validity, reliability, and agreement for the single item of fatigue and recovery (Jeffries et al., 2023). Additionally, comprehension and interpretation of fatigue within a dance population has been explored using a concept identification approach. This approach aims to understand the respondent's perspective when evaluating the fatigue construct. Notably, the main concepts that present for fatigue are 'tiredness', 'muscle soreness', and 'energy'. Therefore, given the complex nature of fatigue, it is suggested that individuals are provided with a definition of the term, or there is a risk that they may not be responding to the intended concept. Given that performing artists, dancers in particular, undertake very high training loads, together with potentially inadequate recovery (Jeffries, Wallace, Coutts, Cohen et al., 2020), a purposefully validated instrument to assess the fatigue construct may be useful to monitor training effects.

Other components

Effective monitoring of performing artists requires a multifaceted approach, including day-to-day qualitative assessments of health, injury, and well-being to address the high physical demands and intense schedules. Incorporating established frameworks and reliable measures, monitoring systems must guide training adjustments while considering the unique challenges of the performing arts. Contextualising training load through models such as the fitness-fatigue model aids in balancing performance readiness with injury prevention. A personalised approach that integrates training history, acute and chronic effects, and contextual data ensures informed decision-making to optimise health and performance.

Qualitative assessments, individual day-to-day health/injury

An important component of performing artist monitoring is individual day-to-day clinical and health care assessments. Specifically, monitoring musculoskeletal injury, illness and well-being is crucial, due to the high training volumes, physical demands, together with touring schedules that may not allow for adequate rest and recovery periods. Additionally, performing artists will often persist with training and performance while injured and ill, potentially reflecting their high level of commitment. As such, an individual person-centred approach to monitoring and assessment by a skilled clinician is warranted and may provide a qualitative method to understand how a performing artist is coping with training and performance demands and help guide an individual's musculoskeletal health and well-being.

Analysing data

It is critical for athlete/performer monitoring systems to be underpinned by established conceptual or reference frameworks and incorporate valid and reliable measures (Jeffries et al., 2022). However, their effectiveness is contingent upon the extent to which the data can be effectively applied to inform coaching and training decisions (Coutts & Cormack, 2014). Across the performing arts disciplines, there may be challenges regarding the implementation of monitoring systems and decisions around manipulating training due to the unique demands and environment. Ultimately, 'the show must go on', as the pursuit of excellence and commitment to performance often requires overcoming obstacles, adapting in real-time, and ensuring that the audience experiences the art as intended, no matter the difficulties faced behind the scenes.

Contextualising training load

Understanding the relationship between training load and performance is essential. There are several methods used to analyse how training impacts performance, fitness, and fatigue, which can indicate the likelihood of injury or illness risk, readiness to perform, and performance outcomes (Crowcroft et al., 2015; Foster et al., 1996; Gabbett, 2016; Jeffries, Wallace, Coutts, Cohen et al., 2020). The following section briefly describes some commonly used methods to contextualise training load data in sports and apply them to the performing arts.

The fitness-fatigue model quantifies the relationship between training load and performance. Although this model has been used to predict performance, fitness, and fatigue, its application in practical settings may be limited due to the oversimplification of the complex, non-linear dose-response relationship. Despite these drawbacks, the model provides a useful foundation for planning training and reducing errors.

Another method used to contextualise training load data is the acute-to-chronic workload ratio (ACWR). This method is based on the fitness-fatigue model, where fatigue equals an acute workload (e.g., seven-day rolling average workload) and fitness equals a chronic workload (e.g., 28-day rolling average workload). The ACWR was initially developed to plan and predict performance and later suggested as a method to predict injury (Gabbett, 2016; Hulin et al., 2017). However, it has been shown that associations to predict injury are actually statistical artefacts related to the use of the ratio score (Impellizzeri et al., 2021). Rather than relying on metrics like the ACWR to inform training load decisions, it is important for practitioners to carefully manage the training loads of performing artists and ensure adequate recovery and rest periods, especially during periods of heavy workloads or training.

We suggest paying careful attention to performers during prolonged periods of high cumulative loading or when there are sudden increases in training load. Ultimately, managing a performing artist's training load is key to preparing for performance. Instead of using generic metrics to make decisions about current and future training, practitioners should consider an artist's training history, responses to both acute and chronic training effects (objective and subjective), along with contextual information. We also suggest interpreting athlete response measures in the context of both the acute and cumulative training load for individual performers. These elements together can inform best practices when making decisions about a performer's training.

Cultural challenges

There are several cultural challenges within the performing arts disciplines when it comes to managing training load, including the control of the stress applied and the measurement of the adaptive response. These challenges are unique to the performing arts and often stem from hierarchical structures, integrating training load data with artistic interpretation, resources, perfectionism, and traditional training approaches.

Hierarchical organisational structures in the performing arts may hinder open communication regarding training load management. For example, where decisions are made by artistic directors, choreographers, and company managers, this top-down approach can create barriers in transparent communication. Additionally, performers may fear negative consequences, such as job security risks, leading to underreporting of workload, injury, or fatigue, further increasing the risk of detrimental health outcomes. To address this, we recommend fostering a culture of open communication and trust between leadership and performers where performers feel comfortable sharing concerns (Beckmann & Kellmann, 2003). As there may be no specific sport science-trained staff to monitor training data, initial check-ins with health and medical teams can help discuss training and fatigue status. These teams should receive targeted training to enhance their support capabilities. Overall, we advocate for a collaborative decision-making process involving performers, coaches, choreographers, and medical professionals.

Performing artists engage in a diverse range of activities, each placing different physical and mental demands on the body. As such, a one-size-fits-all monitoring system may not be effective, and it can be difficult to design a system that accurately captures the specific needs of different disciplines. Additionally, the subjective nature of performance, where creativity, emotion, and expression are central, can make it difficult to quantify performance-related data. Monitoring systems that rely on objective measures may not capture the full scope of an artist's abilities or exertion, particularly when it comes to psychological or emotional health. Therefore, a potential solution is the development of discipline-specific measures that reflect the unique demands of each art form. The selection of measures to be included in a monitoring system should be guided by a conceptual model (Jeffries et al., 2022) and informed by the preferences of performers, as well as input from expert clinicians and sport scientists. Utilising internal training load measures such as sRPE combined with individual training effect measures may help better capture performing artists' training and performance-related data. A performer-centred approach with strong trust and open dialogue is also central to successfully implementing a monitoring system within this context.

Another challenge in developing and maintaining a comprehensive monitoring system is the cost, particularly for smaller companies or independent performers who may lack financial resources. This includes the need for specialised test equipment and personnel to interpret monitoring data and provide actionable feedback. Additionally, successful implementation requires collaboration between performing arts professionals (such as choreographers, musicians, and actors), healthcare providers, and data scientists. Coordinating this interdisciplinary approach can be difficult due to differing or competing priorities. Furthermore, even with comprehensive monitoring data, translating information into actionable insights for improving performance or preventing injury is complex. Without clear guidelines on applying the data practically and beneficially, the system's effectiveness may be compromised. Securing funding for specialists in this role presents an additional barrier to implementing best practice performer monitoring.

Within the performing arts, there is a culture of perfectionism, stoicism, and an underlying expectation to 'push through' pain and fatigue (Soundy & Lim, 2023). There may be external and internal pressure for performers to ignore their bodies' signals and continue training even when experiencing pain, fatigue, or discomfort (Soundy & Lim, 2023). Unfortunately, this can result in chronic injuries, poor health, and ultimately burnout. We suggest that more work is required on educating performers, coaches, and artistic management about the benefits and importance of recovery for optimising performance. For example, the promotion of healthy training environments that prioritise long-term artist development over short-term gains is encouraged. Performers should also be encouraged to 'listen to their bodies' and actively seek medical attention when necessary.

Finally, underpinning all these issues is cultural resistance. Many performing arts disciplines rely on established training methods passed down through generations (e.g., classical ballet). Often performing arts value tradition, individual expression, and intuition over quantitative measures. These long-standing traditions may create resistance and limit the adoption of new technologies and data-driven approaches to training load management. As such, performing artists may prioritise intuition and subjectivity over objective data, leading to scepticism about the benefit of measuring monitoring systems. Performers may resist the idea of systematic health monitoring, feeling that it undermines the artistic process or compromises personal autonomy. Potential solutions are the introduction of simple metrics like sRPE and single-item psychometric measures (e.g., pain, soreness, recovery, etc.) before the integration of more complex physiological measures. Addressing all these cultural challenges requires tailored monitoring systems that integrate both physical, psychological, and artistic aspects of performing arts.

Case study of contemporary dance

In this section, we present a case study focused on monitoring the performing artist in the discipline of dance. The case study will specifically examine professional contemporary dance, providing background and context and identifying key issues affecting dancers' health and well-being. Additionally, we propose practical solutions that can be integrated into artist monitoring systems to enhance health outcomes for dancers. Furthermore, the insights gained from this case study can be applied to other disciplines within the performing arts, offering a comprehensive roadmap for effective implementation across various artistic fields.

Achieving peak performance in contemporary dance requires the integration of aesthetic, artistic, and technical elements and involves a high level of athletic ability. To achieve peak performance, professional contemporary dancers routinely undertake very high volumes of training. For example, in comparison to many other high-level athletes, the mean accumulated weekly training loads for professional contemporary dancers are almost double those reported in professional Australian football players (Jeffries et al., 2017). Moreover, there are very few recovery periods within and between training cycles (Jeffries, Wallace, Coutts, Cohen et al., 2020). This stands in contrast to athlete monitoring in sports, where recovery is seen as an integral component in optimising performance, preventing injury, and promoting overall well-being (Kellmann et al., 2018). In addition, dancers also experience high injury rates, both in terms of medical attention and time-loss injuries. This is likely due to repetitive movements, high-impact landings, high training volumes, and the physical strain of training and performances (Jeffries, Wallace, Coutts, Cohen et al., 2020).

Professional contemporary dance is also associated with high illness rates and lengthy durations of upper respiratory tract illness symptoms (Jeffries, Wallace, Coutts, Cohen et al., 2020). Additionally, while dancers experience upper respiratory tract illness symptoms, there are typically few modifications to training or time loss (e.g., sick leave; Jeffries, Wallace, Coutts, Cohen et al., 2020). Given that dancers persist with training and performance despite injury and illness, this may reflect their high level of commitment and stoic nature. However, persistent illness can have a negative effect on health and performance, which is concerning, particularly when dancers are undertaking high levels of strenuous exercise. Collectively, this is the (im)perfect combination for increased injury and illness risk and poor health outcomes in this population and should be addressed. Understanding these challenges is crucial for developing solutions and designing effective monitoring systems that can enhance dancers' overall health outcomes. To address these issues effectively, we propose several solutions.

First, from a practical perspective, one potential intervention involves sensible training load distribution. This can be achieved by applying well-established training principles such as progressive overload, balancing load with recovery activities, and individualising each performer's training programme based on their response to training. For instance, incorporating recovery periods within and between training cycles can be beneficial. Given that professional dancers may need to undertake high training loads to achieve optimal performance, adapting the training load distribution and including recovery days and short periods of reduced load are immediate potential interventions. Other physical and psychological recovery activities may also be beneficial.

Second, there are population-specific validated tools to monitor training load (e.g., sRPE) and acute training effects (e.g., single items of fatigue and recovery; Jeffries et al., 2023). These tools are simple, low-cost, and easy to implement into a monitoring system. For example, weekly or biweekly measures of the acute effects of fatigue and recovery using single-item instruments may provide a foundation for adapting training distribution and incorporating recovery periods. This approach offers an effective method to guide coaching and medical decision-making.

Finally, given dancers' typically stoic nature and strong work ethic (e.g., the desire to continue working despite illness and injury), practitioners need to carefully monitor the incidence of injury and illness and actively adjust training loads accordingly. Implementing an injury and illness surveillance system, along with trained personnel to administer it, may assist in identifying patterns, managing risks, and improving preventive measures. Therefore, considering the high training loads, frequent injuries, and illnesses, along with dancers' propensity to continue training despite pain or health setbacks, these solutions may be employed to monitor individual responses to training and inform future training decisions (Box 3.1).

BOX 3.1 RECOMMENDATIONS FOR IMPROVING MONITORING IN ARTISTIC PERFORMERS.

1 **Incorporate more evidence-based practices:** Emphasise the importance of evidence-based monitoring based on established conceptual models and validated measurement tools. Rely on training programmes based on established scientific theory rather than on traditional methods. Highlight how integrating scientific research into monitoring the training loads and training responses can lead to better health outcomes and performance improvements for dancers.
2 **Focus on performer-centred approaches:** Ensure that the monitoring systems and interventions are tailored to the specific needs and experiences of the performers, their coaches and medical staff. This includes involving performers in the development process and considering their feedback when designing training programmes.
3 **Build trust and buy-in from performers:** Address the importance of building trust and gaining buy-in from performers. This can be achieved by clearly communicating the benefits of monitoring systems, providing education on their importance, and involving performers in decision-making processes.
4 **Promote a culture of open communication:** Encourage open communication between performers, coaches, and medical professionals. Create an environment where performers feel comfortable sharing concerns about training loads, injuries, and fatigue without fear of negative consequences.
5 **Implement cost-effective monitoring tools:** Use simple, low-cost monitoring tools such as the sRPE and single-item psychometric measures. These tools are easy to implement and can provide valuable insights into training loads and acute training effects.
6 **Address cultural challenges:** Acknowledge the cultural challenges within the performing arts, such as perfectionism and resistance to change. Provide strategies to overcome these challenges, such as promoting the benefits of rest and recovery and gradually introducing new monitoring technologies.
7 **Enhance injury and illness surveillance:** Implement an injury and illness surveillance system to identify patterns, manage risks, and improve preventive measures. This can help practitioners make informed decisions about training loads and reduce the risk of injury and illness.
8 **Provide clear guidelines for data interpretation:** Ensure that there are clear guidelines for interpreting monitoring data and applying it to training decisions. This includes contextualising training load, fitness, and fatigue measures in relation to one another to understand how dancers are responding to training.

Developing multidimensional monitoring systems

Developing effective monitoring systems requires interpreting the relevant variables within the context of the performing artist's training phase and load. This is especially crucial during periods of intensified training, such as leading up to performances, where it is important to contextualise perceptual measures alongside training load. For instance, during such intensified phases like preseason rehearsals, a significant negative change in subjective measures (e.g., very high fatigue) may occur due to the increased training load (Saw et al., 2017). Conversely, if the same change happens without negative subjective measures, it could indicate positive training adaptations and a potential improvement in performance. Therefore, it is essential to consider changes in training load, fitness, and fatigue measures in relation to one another to understand how a performing artist is responding to training.

Conclusion and recommendations for practice

Performing arts monitoring systems are still relatively uncommon, especially in comparison to high-performance sports. Effective monitoring should be grounded in evidence derived from studies conducted in dance, rather than tradition-based monitoring, ensuring that training programmes are informed by the latest research and best practices. The goal of a monitoring system is to understand how individual performing artists are responding to training and help inform decisions about future training (Box 3.1).

A well-designed monitoring system should be performer-focussed and prioritise the performer's needs and experiences, ensuring that it is tailored to their specific requirements. Building trust and buy-in from performers is critical for the success of any monitoring system. This can be achieved by involving performers in the development process, clearly communicating the benefits, and providing education on the importance of monitoring for their health and performance.

Finally implementing a monitoring system often requires a culture change and education within the organisation. Educating both artists and coaches about the value of evidence-based monitoring and the positive impact it can have on performance and well-being can facilitate this transition. The essential measures that should be incorporated into a monitoring system include quantifying training load and proxy measures of artist 'fitness' and 'fatigue'. Although 'fitness' remains an area largely overlooked across the performing arts disciplines, it is essential for overall performance and injury prevention.

References

Allen, N., Nevill, A., Brooks, J., Koutedakis, Y., & Wyon, M. (2012). Ballet injuries: Injury incidence and severity over 1 year. *Journal of Orthopaedic & Sports Physical Therapy*, 42(9), 781–790.

Arnold, P. J. (1995). Objectivity, expression, and communication in dance as a performing art. *Journal of Aesthetic Education*, *29*(1), 61–68.
Banister, E. W., Calvert, T. W., Savage, M. V., & Bach, T. (1975). A systems model of training for athletic performance. *IEEE Transactions on Systems, Man, and Cybernetics*, *7*(3), 57–61.
Barker, L., Burnstein, B., & Mercer, J. (2020). Acceleration profile of an acrobatic act during training and shows using wearable technology. *Sports Biomechanics*, *19*(2), 201–211.
Beckmann, J., & Kellmann, M. (2003). Procedures and principles of sport psychological assessment. *The Sport Psychologist*, *17*(3), 338–350.
Bronner, S., Ojofeitimi, S., & Rose, D. (2003). Injuries in a modern dance company: Effect of comprehensive management on injury incidence and time loss. *American Journal of Sports Medicine*, *31*(3), 365–373.
Coutts, A. J. (2014). In the age of technology, Occam's razor still applies. *International Journal of Sports Physiology and Performance*, *9*(5), 741.
Coutts, A. J., & Cormack, S. (2014). Monitoring the training response. In D. Joyce & D. Lewindon (Eds.), *High-performance training for sports* (pp. 71–84). Human Kinetics.
Coutts, A. J., Crowcroft, S., & Kempton, T. (2022). Developing athlete monitoring systems: Theoretical basis and practical applications. In M. Kellmann & J. Beckmann (Eds.), *Recovery and well-being in sport and exercise* (pp. 17–31). Routledge.
Crowcroft, S., Duffield, R., McCleave, E., Slattery, K., Wallace, L. K., & Coutts, A. J. (2015). Monitoring training to assess changes in fitness and fatigue: The effects of training in heat and hypoxia. *Scandinavian Journal of Medicine & Science in Sports*, *25*(Suppl. 1), 287–295.
Foster, C., Daines, E., Hector, L., Snyder, A. C., & Welsh, R. (1996). Athletic performance in relation to training load. *Wisconsin Medical Journal*, *95*(6), 370–374.
Fry, R. W., Morton, A. R., & Keast, D. (1991). Overtraining in athletes. An update. *Sports Medicine*, *12*(1), 32–65.
Gabbett, T. J. (2016). The training-injury prevention paradox: Should athletes be training smarter and harder? *British Journal of Sports Medicine*, *50*(5), 273–280.
Gamboa, J. M., Roberts, L. A., Maring, J., & Fergus, A. (2008). Injury patterns in elite preprofessional ballet dancers and the utility of screening programs to identify risk characteristics. *The Journal of Orthopaedic and Sports Physical Therapy*, *38*(3), 126–136.
Hulin, B. T., Gabbett, T. J., Johnston, R. D., & Jenkins, D. G. (2017). Wearable microtechnology can accurately identify collision events during professional rugby league match-play. *Journal of Science & Medicine in Sport*, *20*(7), 638–642.
Impellizzeri, F. M., Woodcock, S., Coutts, A. J., Fanchini, M., McCall, A., & Vigotsky, A. D. (2021). What role do chronic workloads play in the acute to chronic workload ratio? Time to dismiss acwr and its underlying theory. *Sports Medicine*, *51*(3), 581–592.
Jeffries, A. C., Marcora, S. M., Coutts, A. J., Wallace, L., McCall, A., & Impellizzeri, F. M. (2022). Development of a revised conceptual framework of physical training for use in research and practice. *Sports Medicine*, *52*(4), 709–724.
Jeffries, A. C., Novak, A. R., Coutts, A. J., McCall, A., McLaren, S. J., & Impellizzeri, F. M. (2023). Development and validation of single items for fatigue and recovery in dancers. *International Journal of Sports Physiology & Performance*, *18*(5), 474–487.

Jeffries, A. C., Wallace, L., & Coutts, A. J. (2017). Quantifying training loads in contemporary dance. *International Journal of Sports Physiology & Performance*, *12*(6), 796–802.

Jeffries, A. C., Wallace, L., Coutts, A. J., Cohen, A. M., McCall, A., & Impellizzeri, F. M. (2020). Injury, illness, and training load in a professional contemporary dance company: A prospective study. *Journal of Athletic Training*, *55*(9), 967–976.

Jeffries, A. C., Wallace, L., Coutts, A. J., McLaren, S. J., McCall, A., & Impellizzeri, F. M. (2020). Athlete-reported outcome measures for monitoring training responses: A systematic review of risk of bias and measurement property quality according to the COSMIN guidelines. *International Journal of Sports Physiology & Performance*, *15*(9), 1203–1215.

Johnson, U., & Ivarsson, A. (2011). Psychological predictors of sport injuries among junior soccer players. *Scandinavian Journal of Medicine & Science in Sports*, *21*(1), 129–136.

Jotwani, V., Aflatooni, J., Barter, L., & Harris, J. (2022). Management of stress fractures in ballet. *Journal of the American Academy of Orthopaedic Surgeons*, *30*(12), 543–553.

Kellmann, M., Bertollo, M., Bosquet, L., Brink, M., Coutts, A. J., Duffield, R., Erlacher, D., Halson, S. L., Hecksteden, A., Heidari, J., Kallus, K. W., Meeusen, R., Mujika, I., Robazza, C., Skorski, S., Venter, R., & Beckmann, J. (2018). Recovery and performance in sport: Consensus statement. *International Journal of Sports Physiology and Performance*, *13*, 240–245.

Kellmann, M., & Kallus, K. W. (2001). *The Recovery-Stress Questionnaire for Athletes; manual*. Human Kinetics.

Kellmann, M., & Kallus, K. W. (Eds.). (2025). *The Recovery-Stress Questionnaires: A user manual*. Routledge.

Kellmann, M., & Kölling, S. (2019). *Recovery and stress in sport: A manual for testing and assessment*. Routledge.

Khan, K., Brown, J., Way, S., Vass, N., Crichton, K., Alexander, R., Baxter, A., Butler, M., & Wark, J. (1995). Overuse injuries in classical ballet. *Sports Medicine*, *19*(5), 341–357.

Kuno, M., Fukunaga, T., Hirano, Y., & Miyashita, M. (1996). Anthropometric variables and muscle properties of Japanese female ballet dancers. *International Journal of Sports Medicine*, *17*(2), 100–105.

Main, L. C., & Grove, J. (2009). A multi-component assessment model for monitoring training distress among athletes. *European Journal of Sport Science*, *9*(4), 195–202.

Matveyev, L. (1977). *Fundamentals of sports training*. Fizkultura i Sport Publisher.

Neupert, E., Tim, H., Luke, G., & Jobson, S. A. (2024). More than metrics: The role of socio-environmental factors in determining the success of athlete monitoring. *Journal of Sports Sciences*, *42*(4), 323–332.

Pattyn, N., van Cutsem, J., Dessy, E., & Mairesse, O. (2018). Bridging exercise science, cognitive psychology, and medical practice: Is "cognitive fatigue" a remake of "the emperor's new clothes"? *Frontiers in Psychology*, *9*, 1246. https://doi.org/10.3389/fpsyg.2018.01246

Redding, E., Weller, P., Ehrenberg, S., Irvine, S., Quin, E., Rafferty, S., Wyon, M., & Cox, C. (2009). The development of a high intensity dance performance fitness test. *Journal of Dance Medicine and Science*, *13*(1), 3–9.

Ryan, R. M., & Deci, E. L. (2000). Self-determination theory and the facilitation of intrinsic motivation, social development, and well-being. *American Psychologist*, *55*(1), 68–78.

Saw, A. E., Kellmann, M., Main, L. C., & Gastin, P. B. (2017). Athlete self-report measures in research and practice: Considerations for the discerning reader and fastidious practitioner. *International Journal of Sports Physiology and Performance*, *12*(Suppl. 2), S2127–S2135.

Saw, A. E., Main, L. C., & Gastin, P. B. (2016). Monitoring the athlete training response: Subjective self-reported measures trump commonly used objective measures: A systematic review. *British Journal of Sports Medicine*, *50*(5), 281–291.

Schantz, P. G., & Astrand, P. O. (1984). Physiological characteristics of classical ballet. *Medicine and Science in Sports and Exercise*, *16*(5), 472–476.

Shaw, J. W., Springham, M., Brown, D. D., Mattiussi, A. M., Pedlar, C. R., & Tallent, J. (2020). The validity of the session rating of perceived exertion method for measuring internal training load in professional classical ballet dancers. *Frontiers in Physiology*, *11*, 480. https://doi.org/10.3389/fphys.2020.00480

Shushan, T., Lovell, R., Buchheit, M., Scott, T. J., Barrett, S., Norris, D., & McLaren, S. J. (2023). Submaximal fitness test in team sports: A systematic review and meta-analysis of exercise heart rate measurement properties. *Sports Medicine - Open*, *9*(1), 21. https://doi.org/10.1186/s40798-023-00564-w

Smith, T. O., Davies, L., de Medici, A., Hakim, A., Haddad, F., & Macgregor, A. (2016). Prevalence and profile of musculoskeletal injuries in ballet dancers: A systematic review and meta-analysis. *Physical Therapy in Sport*, *19*, 50–56.

Soundy, A., & Lim, J. Y. (2023). Pain perceptions, suffering and pain behaviours of professional and pre-professional dancers towards pain and injury: A qualitative review. *Behavioral Sciences*, *13*(3), 268. https://doi.org/10.3390/bs13030268

Tiemens, A., van Rijn, R. M., Koes, B. W., & Stubbe, J. H. (2023). A systematic review of cardiorespiratory fitness tests used in dance. *Journal of Dance Medicine and Science*, *27*(1), 27–40.

Twitchett, E., Koutedakis, Y., & Wyon, M. (2009). Physiological fitness and professional classical ballet performance: A brief review. *Journal of Strength and Conditioning Research*, *23*, 2732–2740.

Twitchett, E., Nevill, A., Angioi, M., Koutedakis, Y., & Wyon, M. (2011). Development, validity, and reliability of a ballet-specific aerobic fitness test. *Journal of Dance Medicine and Science*, *15*(3), 123–127.

Volkova, V. G., Räisänen, A., Benson, L. C., Ferber, R., & Kenny, S. (2023). Systematic review of methods used to measure training load in dance. *BMJ Open Sport & Exercise Medicine*, *9*(3), e001484. https://doi.org/10.1136/bmjsem-2022-001484

PART II

Recovery and well-being of performing artists

4

MANAGING THE PRACTICE LOAD

Recovery-stress balance and injury risk in performing arts

Derrick Brown-Appenzeller, Jamie Tallent, and Matthew Wyon

Introduction

In two systematic reviews the relationship between training load, stress, and recovery in pre-professional and professional dancers was highlighted as reciprocal and interdependent (Kenny et al., 2016; Shaw et al., 2021). Effective management of training load is crucial for optimising performance and reducing the risk of injuries, while inadequate recovery can lead to increased physiological stress and overuse injuries (Mattiussi et al., 2021). Evidence suggests that dance training rarely stresses their physiological engine resulting in a relatively under-developed cardiorespiratory system compared with equivalent athletes (Wyon et al., 2016) and that it is only during performance periods that positive adaptation occurs (Wyon & Redding, 2005; Wyon et al., 2004). Research has revealed a decrement in dance performance over time when repetitive injury, overuse, overtraining, prolonged or high-volume dancing seasons, and a functional work-life balance are not maintained (Liederbach & Compagno, 2023). The ability to quantify training stress and understand the relationship between training stress, stressors, and the subsequent adaptive or maladaptive responses is equally important in pre- and professional dancers. The relationship between training load, stress, and recovery is complex and multifaceted particularly in dance where the association between physical, aesthetic and artistic demands varies across

Brown-Appenzeller, D., Tallent, J., & Wyon, M. (2026). Managing the practice load: Recovery-stress balance and injury risk in performing arts. In E. Altenmüller, M. Kellmann, J. Beckmann, & G. M. Moyle (Eds.), *Recovery and well-being in the performing arts* (pp. 63–77). Routledge.

DOI: 10.4324/9781003566885-6

genres (DiPasquale et al., 2021; Koutedakis & Jamurtas, 2004). Kellmann (2010) emphasised the importance of preventing overtraining in high-intensity sports by monitoring stress and recovery. Overtraining can lead to decreased performance, increased risk of injury, and psychological distress across all artistic and or athletic physical activities (Kellmann et al., 2018).

Training load

There are many ways to contextualise the concept of training load (Impellizzeri et al., 2023; Jeffries & Coutts, this volume, Chapter 3). Rather than one definition it is perhaps more helpful to consider the concept from a categorical perspective. Thus, in a dancing context, internal training loads can be defined as the relative biological (both physiological and psychological) stressors imposed on the (performing, e.g., artistic) athlete during training or competition or performance. External loads in contrast encompass objective measures of the work performed by the athletic training, competition or performance and can be assessed independently of internal workloads (Impellizzeri et al., 2019).

A key factor in understanding training load is the concept of adaptation (Jeffries & Coutts, this volume, Chapter 3). In pre- and professional dancers in particular dancing sessions (e.g., daily class, rehearsals, and performance) impose body-mind stresses, disrupting the body's homeostasis, causing a temporary response. Initially this leads to a decrement in neuromuscular performance after a bout of training (Lambert, 2012). However, after a recovery period, a supercompensation effect occurs, such that a subsequent training session of the same intensity would ideally not disrupt homeostasis. However, repeated physiological stress over time stimulates a chronic adaptive response, resulting in semi-permanent physiological changes (Soligard et al., 2016). If rest and recovery are insufficient following a training session, the dance artist's capacity for load may decrease as additional training stress is applied. Importantly, it should be acknowledged that training (e.g., dance class and performance) or physiological and mechanical responses are not a consequence of training alone, rather a myriad of psycho-social-physiological factors (締 Herta & Hassmén, 2002); lifestyle, nutrition, sleep, work-life balance, all of which must be integrated into a complex puzzle of training load management, injury prevention and reduction as well as recovery (Figure 4.1).

Given the high training loads in dance, it has been suggested that priority should be given to workload management through structured timetabling, reducing total training hours where possible and minimising large week-to-week fluctuations (Jeffries et al., 2020; Shaw et al., 2023; Wyon & Allard, 2022). However, implementing such changes in the performing arts remains challenging. Therefore, a multifaceted approach to recovery is essential, incorporating targeted interventions to mitigate overreaching and

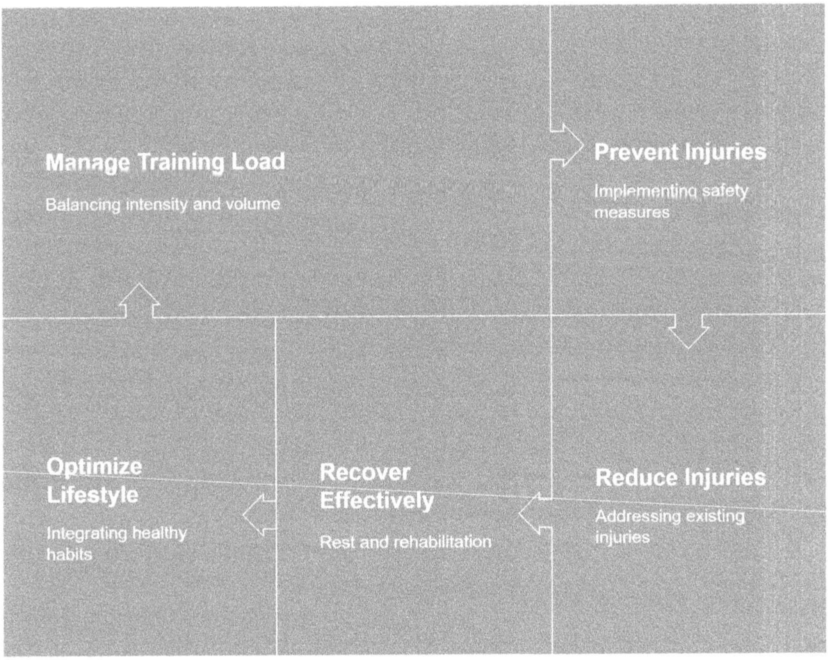

FIGURE 4.1 Psycho-social-physiological factors of dance training.

support overall well-being and performance. Additionally, improving aerobic fitness should not be overlooked, as it has been shown to reduce the fatigue response to strenuous exercise in athletes (Bogdanis, 2012), though these recommendations remain challenging for a variety of reasons outlined below.

Current injury risks linked to practice load

The link between injury and workload in dance has been reported since the 1960s (Robertson, 1967). Although initial research was focused on classical ballet (Howse, 1972), further survey-based studies were more encompassing of other dance genres (Brinson & Dick, 1996; Dang et al., 2020; Laws, 2004; Riding-McCabe et al., 2014; Tsiouti & Wyon, 2021). These studies reported fatigue and workload to be the two main perceived causes of injury reported by surveyed dancers. In the 1980s more objective data on the physical demands of dance were reported initially using heart rate monitors (Cohen, Segal, & McArdle, 1982; Cohen et al., 1982) and gas analysis of limited dance sequences using Douglas bags (Schantz & Åstrand, 1984). The cardiorespiratory fitness levels of ballet and contemporary dancers indicated comparatively low maximal aerobic values compared to equivalent sports (Laws, 2005; Wyon et al., 2016), though DanceSport, street dance, and musical theatre dancers reported similar values (Liiv et al., 2013; Stephens & Wyon, 2020; Wyon et al., 2018). This is probably due to the high skill level and fine motor control required for ballet that preclude exercising at the intensities required to cause adaptation of the cardiorespiratory system. The development of wearable breath-by-breath gas analysis technology has allowed longer and more in-depth analysis of dance classes, rehearsals and performances (dress rehearsals) (Rodrigues-Krause et al., 2014; Wyon et al., 2004). These studies have reported that contemporary dance class and rehearsal have mainly low aerobic demands with short periods of high-intensity activity lasting between 15 and 120 seconds. This contrasts with data from dance performances where longer periods (two- to five-minute bouts) were spent at high intensities (above 60% of VO_{2max}). Unlike the relative homogeneity observed with a specific sport's performances (Teixeira et al., 2024), the physical demands of performances in a single dance company can vary hugely as they are dependent on the choreographers engaged with the company within any given performance season.

Although data on isolated training sessions are useful and provide detailed information, how they integrate into a training day or season has not had been adequately examined. The monitoring of training and performance workloads in sport has become an integral part of professional sports' coaching culture, with players being constantly monitored via 'wearables' (McGuigan et al., 2020). A few studies have tried to utilise wearables by the participants wearing accelerometers, using metabolic equivalents (METs) as a measure of training load (Kozai et al., 2020; Twitchett et al., 2010). This apparatus can be worn during training (class and rehearsals) but not during performance. The data indicated large daily and weekly variations in workload for individual dancers and between ballet ranks and sex (Kozai et al., 2020). The use of session rate of perceived exertion (sRPE; Foster et al., 1996) has had some traction and evidence of efficacy with heart rate during dance being good (Fuller et al., 2024; Stubbe et al., 2022; Surgenor & Wyon, 2019); the underlying premise is that the correlation between heart rate and oxygen consumption is strong as the link was developed during steady state exercise. Dance is not steady state and therefore the link with oxygen consumption is not as strong due to the heart rate remaining high during rest periods (Redding et al., 2004). An alternative is the use of school timetables and company schedules to calculate injury incidence (injuries/1,000 hrs). The limitation with this method is that presumptions are made on the length of each session as well as the amount and intensity of activity for each dancer during that session. This is particularly true for ballet companies where second or third casts may be just observing or marking the choreography and thus spending less time physically moving during that session.

Accelerometer data reinforced the reported indirect gas analysis data, with the majority of the dancers' workdays spent between 3 and 6 METs and only minutes spent at intensities between 6 and 9 METs and rarely intensities above 9 METs were observed (Twitchett et al., 2010). The study also highlighted the fact that dancers rarely used their contracted one-hour lunch break. Anecdotal evidence from this study and the authors' experiences working in numerous companies suggest this was due to rehearsals over running. A further accelerometer study (Kozai et al., 2020) noted that dancers were carrying out as much activity outside of their working day as they were in it. Sleep data indicated large variations among the participants with the average being 6 hrs 40 min; 10% of sleep periods were below five hrs, and only 16% achieved eight hrs. These two studies highlight two key factors with regard to physiological recovery; firstly, dancers' planned (contracted) breaks are often encroached on by artistic staff with no leeway given to subsequent rehearsals if a preceding one overran. Secondly, the dancers themselves have not learned to optimise their 'down' periods by not resting or taking in optimal nutrition and liquids. Previous research on dancers' perception of the causes of injury indicated overwork and fatigue (Laws, 2005) but the accelerometer data (Kozai et al., 2020) suggests that the dancers themselves were in control of half their workload and could implement strategies (reducing activity intensity, prioritising eating, and increasing sleep hours) to avoid the reported physical fatigue. A lack of education, a culture of long training hours and the perception that they are artists rather than athletes compound this problem. Contrary to work practices during the season, holidays are used as recovery periods where the dancers are often very inactive with no or very little dance or other physical activity. Koutedakis et al. (1999) noted that dancers were probably 'burnt out' at the end of the season but they recovered from these physical deficits after their six-week summer break.

Another area of concern has been timetabling, the organisation of class, rehearsal, and performance schedules. Although performance schedules are planned years in advance, due to the need to book theatres, class and rehearsal schedules are planned on a weekly basis and published the preceding Friday. The accelerometer study (Kozai et al., 2020) noted large daily and weekly variations in dance hours and workload and this was reinforced by Shaw et al. (2021)'s study on a single company that reported week-to-week change in workload was positively associated with over-use injuries. Allen et al. (2013) indirectly reinforced this when they observed that an increase in acute injuries was due to an intervention that decreased chronic injuries; they surmised that the chronic injuries provided reduced workloads in the dancers' schedules, and when this was 'lost', dancers were becoming more fatigued leading to the observed acute injuries. At a pre-professional level, Fuller et al. (2024), using sRPE, noted that spikes in injury coincided with workload spikes and changes in training schedule over an academic year; these data were mimicked in a study on a small professional contemporary dance company (Jeffries et al., 2020).

An area of growing concern within dance is the prevalence of dancers with relative energy deficiency syndrome (REDs) or female athlete triad (Allen et al., 2024). At its most basis definition this is an intentional or unintentional mismatch between energy expenditure (workload) and energy input (food). As mentioned above, the work schedule with few planned or achieved breaks means that fuelling during the day is very difficult for dancers. This is accompanied by an environment that often promotes the aesthetic looks of a dancer's body over their athletic ability from an early age (Pickard, 2013) leading to high incidence of disordered eating and eating disorders and eating habits that avoid 'looking full' when wearing tight body-hugging clothing (Silverii et al., 2022). Within the context of this chapter the work schedule accompanied by poor fuelling leads to an increased risk of injury (Biernacki et al., 2021) and as Twitchett et al. (2008) noted dancers with low body fat were more prone to injury and took longer to recover.

The generalisability of the data reported above needs to be viewed with an amount of caution as there has been little if any replication. Recent systematic reviews have all highlighted the lack of strong evidence and the need for more prospective longitudinal studies (Biernacki et al., 2021; Kenny et al., 2016). The dance environment is also undergoing change, with supplemental physical fitness training becoming more normal within dance schools and companies, though not necessarily part of a dancer's contracted hours (Rosenthal et al., 2021).

Recovery interventions

Elite ballet dancers have physical profiles comparable to those of elite athletes, often exceeding the training hours of endurance athletes (Haugen et al., 2022; Shaw et al., 2023). Consequently, recovery interventions are crucial for restoring both physical and psychological capacity and maintaining performance. In sport, and as mentioned above athletes are often unaware of the impact of recovery interventions on physical performance restoration (Crowther et al., 2017) with the implementation of the latest exercise science research findings often not translating to practical changes in sport (Fullagar et al., 2019). There is a clear opportunity to improve artistic directors, dance teachers/coaches and dancers' understanding of recovery through structured education, which could enhance both their perceived recovery and performance outcome.

Funding

Although this chapter does not compare sport and dance contexts it is important to acknowledge the funding disparity between elite arts and sport. These disparities in resource are likely to be a key contributor for the differences in practises between dancers and athletes. With only about 4% of total US sponsorship spending allocated to the arts, sports sponsorship dominates the market due to its stronger commercial appeal, whereas arts sponsorship is often positioned more philanthropically (Toscani & Prendergast, 2019). Potential reasons for underfunding may include lack of advocacy, misconceptions about dance, and the perception of dance as a luxury rather than a necessity. The lack of funding limits investment in dedicated healthcare teams to manage timetables, track workload, and support recovery. A few leading ballet companies have developed healthcare provisions comparable to those in elite sport, these remain in the minority, arguably due to funding.

Sports clubs have invested considerable time and money in optimising players' timetables and recovery strategies, including providing onsite food, the latest recovery tools, and dedicated staff to manage workloads. Given the limited funding in the arts, it makes it challenging to create a similar environment for dancers. Instead, the focus should be on implementing basic, cost-effective measures such as tracking studio time, providing food where possible, and educating dancers, teachers, and healthcare professionals on key recovery strategies, such as appropriate nutrition. Appropriate nutrition support would be essential to aid recovery and a key building block for dance. For example, Rigoli et al. (2024) demonstrated that pre-professional dancers often struggle with low energy availability and inadequate nutrient intake, which are crucial for health and recovery. Simple education programmes such as ensuring that dancers have the appropriate nutritional intake may have a positive influence on recovery in dancers and can be cost-effective.

Theatre and choreographer availability

Theatre availability often restricts when dancers can perform, unlike in elite ballet companies where studio access is not an issue. For example, a studio and its dancers may only be available in the evenings and on weekends. As a result, workloads can become condensed into short periods, such as Friday evenings leading into the weekend. While dance companies do not face these specific availability issues, they must still navigate scheduling challenges, particularly around choreographer availability. This can be further complicated when multiple choreographers work within the same company, as a lack of communication between them may lead to spikes in workload and insufficient recovery. Wanke and colleagues (2015) have conducted research on the physical and mental workloads of professional dance teachers and work-related musculoskeletal disorders among dance teachers in Germany (Schmidt et al., 2023); their findings highlight the challenges and potential health risks faced by dance professionals due to factors such as condensed workloads, scheduling constraints, and physical demands.

Travel

Work schedules have a significant impact on dancers' health and recovery. Professional dancers typically follow rigid timetables, rehearsing for six to eight hours per day, which can increase to up to ten hours during performance periods, often extending late into the evening (Wyon, 2010). After finishing a performance past 22:00, dancers are expected to return to the company the following morning, leaving limited time for recovery. Commute times further influence recovery, as some dancers may travel over an hour each way, particularly if commuting from a city centre (Kozai et al., 2020). Research supports this concern, showing that dancers experience reduced sleep efficiency and shorter sleep duration over a 67-day rehearsal period leading up to a premiere performance (Fietze et al., 2009). Additionally, injury rates are 1.7 times higher among athletes who sleep less than eight hours per night compared to those who sleep more (Milewski et al., 2014). Given these challenges, optimising travel schedules in professional ballet companies to support better sleep hygiene could be a key strategy for enhancing dancers' health and performance.

Touring companies face unique challenges. Unlike some dance companies with dedicated recovery facilities and pre-planned schedules, touring companies move from city to city with limited access to recovery support. The added stress of travel, frequent hotel changes, and late-night performances often followed by early-morning rehearsals, which further increase demands on dancers and reduce their ability to recover effectively (Duffield & Fowler, 2022).

Another important group to consider is independent dancers (Sjölin, 2023). They often experience periods of intense performing with minimal recovery. While they have control over their schedules and can theoretically manage their workload, the need to secure consistent work means they frequently take on any available opportunities, often at the expense of adequate rest and recovery (Hopper et al., 2020).

Schools: Periodisation

The physical and skill requirements of a graduating pre-professional dancer have diversified enormously over the past 15 years with dance companies rarely now solely performing in one dance genre, sex divisions in choreographed movement being removed (Alterowitz, 2014; Oliveira Souza et al., 2022) and ranges of movement of the lower limbs increasing (Storm et al., 2018). This has led to pressure on pre-professional dance institutions to increase and expand their training provision resulting in more hours dancing for the students and subsequently increased incidence of injury and drop out (Ekegren et al., 2014). The implementation of periodisation into pre-professional training is possible, though as Wyon (2004) noted artistic directors of schools are worried that changing how dancers are trained could affect the employment rates of graduates and the schools' reputations. In a ten-year intervention Wyon and Allard (2022) demonstrated how periodisation could have a beneficial effect on employment opportunities for dancers and more importantly positively affect injury incidence and drop out.

Companies: Performance scheduling

Few studies have investigated timetable management within dance. Shaw et al. (2023) provide a valuable framework for the periodisation of rehearsal and performance schedules in professional ballet. Shaw et al. (2023) recommend scheduling time-efficient productions between more demanding or newly created works to facilitate volume offload and avoid rehearsal and performance congestion. These findings also underscore the importance of forecasting rehearsal hours to allow gradual progressions in dance volume, particularly at the start of rehearsals or during rehabilitation. Mixed bills and newly created shorter ballets, which often require disproportionately high rehearsal hours, should be paired with established, time-efficient productions to manage overall workload. These insights not only provide practical guidance for managing professional company timetables but also highlight the potential for further research into scheduling and training loads across other dance companies and schools, including those with unique demands like touring or year-to-year variability in dancers' workloads (Figure 4.2).

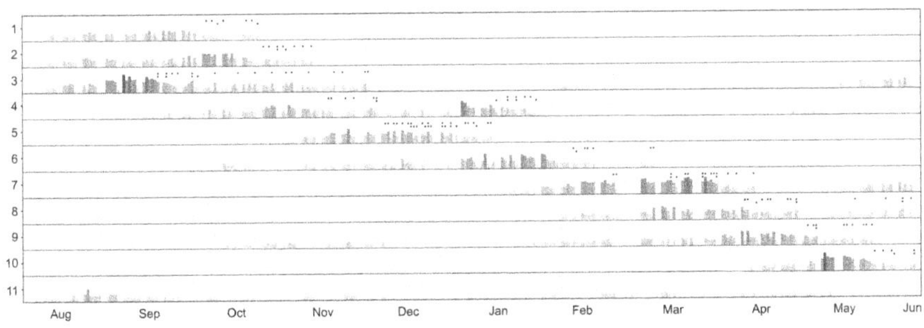

FIGURE 4.2 A representative season timeline (2015–2016) showing each production on the y-axis and the time course of the season on the x-axis. Column height and darkness represent the daily rehearsal time for the production, while lower and upper dots indicate matinees and evening performances, respectively.

Note: The end of the season was immediately followed by a four-week touring period. Productions: 1–Raven Girl/Connectome; 2–Quadruple Bill; 3–Romeo and Juliet; 4–Triple Bill; 5–The Nutcracker; 6–Triple Bill; 7–Giselle; 8–The Winter's Tale; 9–Frankenstein; 10–Triple Bill; and 11–Non-main rep Shaw et al. (2023).

Historically, dancers have been perceived as expendable commodities, with little regard for their long-term health and well-being (Lewis et al., 1997; Rönkkö et al., 2007; Smith et al., 2017). This perception is in part due to the belief that injuries were considered an inevitable part of the profession (Robertson, 1967). However, over the past few decades, there has been a gradual shift in attitudes, with a growing recognition of the importance of dancer health and injury prevention.

Howse (1972) challenged the notion of dancers as expendable highlighting the need for orthopaedic support and medical care for ballet dancers. As mentioned previously in this chapter, subsequent research delved deeper into the physical demands and injury risks associated with dance across different genres. The work environment of Western stage dance, with its long training hours and large number of performances, places dancers at a high risk of injuries, particularly to the lower extremities (Biernacki et al., 2021; Jeffries et al., 2020; Kenny et al., 2016). Furthermore, the aesthetic demands of the profession often lead to unhealthy weight management practices (Nascimento et al., 2012), increasing the risk of REDs (Allen et al., 2024).

Furthermore, more emphasis is now placed on the long-term health and well-being of dancers, particularly those in established dance companies and institutions. This includes providing access to medical professionals, implementing injury prevention programmes, and fostering a supportive environment that encourages open communication about physical and mental health concerns (Rosenthal et al., 2021).

Conclusion and recommendations for practice

In conclusion, the attitudes towards dancers have undergone a significant transformation, with a growing recognition of the physical demands and injury risks associated with the profession. While challenges persist in adhering to societal norms and maintaining long-term health, the dance community has made strides in addressing these issues through research, injury prevention strategies, and a greater emphasis on dancer well-being. Dance companies play a crucial role in supporting their performers and ensuring a sustainable and healthy environment for artistic expression.

Shaw et al. (2021) demonstrated how scheduling can increase injury risk in dance companies. Dance companies know their performance schedules years in advance as theatres and choreographers need to be booked. This should allow greater schedule planning, rather than the normal current practice of publishing rehearsal schedules a week in advance. Pre-professional dance schools can also pre-plan training loads and performance periods across the training years and also make sure that dancers are taught about health, nutrition, self-care and supplemental training (Wyon & Allard, 2022).

References

Allen, N., Kelley, S., Lanfear, M., Mountjoy, M., Reynolds, A., Clarke, R., Wyon, M., & Wolman, R. (2024). Relative Energy Deficiency in Dance (RED-D): A consensus method approach to REDs in dance. *BMJ Open Sport & Exercise Medicine*, *10*, e001858. https://doi.org/10.1136/bmjsem-2023-001858

Allen, N., Nevill, A., Brooks, J., Koutedakis, Y., & Wyon, M. (2013). The effect of a comprehensive injury audit program on injury incidence in ballet: A 3-year prospective study. *Clinical Journal of Sport Medicine*, *25*(3), 373–378.

Alterowitz, G. (2014). Embodying a queer worldview: The contemporary ballets of Katy Pyle and Deborah Lohse. *Dance Chronicle*, *37*(3), 335–366.

Biernacki, J. L., Stracciolini, A., Fraser, J., Micheli, L. J., & Sugimoto, D. (2021). Risk factors for lower-extremity injuries in female ballet dancers: A systematic review. *Clinical Journal of Sport Medicine*, *31*(2), e64–e79.

Bogdanis, G. C. (2012). Effects of physical activity and inactivity on muscle fatigue. *Frontiers in Physiology*, *3*, 142. https://doi.org/10.3389/fphys.2012.00142

Brinson, P., & Dick, F. (1996). *Fit to dance?* Calouste Gulbenkian Foundation.

Cohen, J. L., Segal, K. R., & McArdle, W. D. (1982). Heart rate response to ballet stage performance. *The Physician and Sportsmedicine*, *10*(11), 120–133.

Cohen, J. L., Segal, K. R., Witriol, I., & McArdle, W. D. (1982). Cardiorespiratory responses to ballet exercise and VO_{2max} of elite ballet dancers. *Medicine and Science in Sports and Exercise*, *14*(3), 212–217.

Crowther, F., Sealey, R., Crowe, M., Edwards, A., & Halson, S. (2017). Team sport athletes' perceptions and use of recovery strategies: A mixed-methods survey study. *BMC Sports Science, Medicine and Rehabilitation*, *9*, 6. https://doi.org/10.1186/s13102-017-0071-3

Dang, Y., Koutedakis, Y., & Wyon, M. (2020). Fit to dance survey: Elements of lifestyle and injury incidence in Chinese dancers. *Medical Problems in Performing Artists*, *35*(1), 10–18.

DiPasquale, S., Wood, M. C., & Edmonds, R. (2021). Heart rate variability in a collegiate dance environment: Insights on overtraining for dance educators. *Research in Dance Education*, *22*(1), 108–125.

Duffield, R., & Fowler, P. M. (2022). Domestic and international travel: Implications for performance and recovery in team-sport athletes. In M. Kellmann & J. Beckmann (Eds.), *Recovery and well-being in sport and exercise* (pp. 169–184). Routledge.

Ekegren, C. L., Quested, R., & Brodrick, A. (2014). Injuries in pre-professional ballet dancers: Incidence, characteristics and consequences. *Journal of Science and Medicine in Sport*, *17*(3), 271–275.

Fietze, I., Strauch, J., Holzhausen, M., Glos, M., Theobald, C., Lehnkering, H., & Penzel, T. (2009). Sleep quality in professional ballet dancers. *Chronobiology International*, *26*(6), 1249–1262.

Foster, C., Daines, E., Hector, L., Snyder, A. C., & Welsh, R. (1996). Athletic performance in relation to training load. *Wisconsin Medical Journal*, *95*(6), 370–374.

Fullagar, H. H., McCall, A., Impellizzeri, F. M., Favero, T., & Coutts, A. J. (2019). The translation of sport science research to the field: A current opinion and overview on the perceptions of practitioners, researchers and coaches. *Sports Medicine*, *49*, 1817–1824.

Fuller, M., Moyle, G. M., & Minett, G. (2024). Weekly injury rates within semesters of a three-year tertiary dance program, and prospective training monitoring across one semester of training: A longitudinal study. *Research in Dance Education*, *25*(2), 158–175.

Haugen, T., Sandbakk, Ø., Seiler, S., & Tønnessen, E. (2022). The training characteristics of world-class distance runners: An integration of scientific literature and results-proven practice. *Sports Medicine - Open*, *8*(1), 46. https://doi.org/10.1186/s40798-022-00438-7

Hopper, L. S., Blevins, P., Erskine, S., Hendry, D., Hill, R., & Longbottom, R. (2020). Sustaining dancer wellbeing through independent professional dance careers. *Theatre, Dance and Performance Training*, *11*(4), 470–486.

Howse, A. (1972). Orthopaedists aid ballet. *Clinical Orthopaedics and Related Research*, *89*, 52–63.

Impellizzeri, F. M., Marcora, S. M., & Coutts, A. J. (2019). Internal and external training load: 15 years on. *International Journal of Sports Physiology and Performance*, *14*(2), 270–273.

Impellizzeri, F., Shrier, I., McLaren, S., Coutts, A., McCall, A., Slattery, K., Jeffries, A., & Kalkhoven, J. (2023). Understanding training load as exposure and dose. *Sports Medicine*, *53*(9), 1667–1679.

Jeffries, A., Wallace, L., Coutts, A., Cohen, A., McCall, A., & Impellizzeri, F. (2020). Injury, illness, and training load in a professional contemporary dance company: A prospective study. *Journal of Athletic Training*, *55*(9), 967–976.

Kellmann, M. (2010). Preventing overtraining in athletes in high-intensity sports and stress/recovery monitoring. *Scandinavian Journal of Medicine and Science in Sports*, *20*, 95–102.

Kellmann, M., Bertollo, M., Bosquet, L., Brink, M., Coutts, A., Duffield, R., Erlacher, D., Halson, S. L., Hecksteden, A., Heidari, J., Kallus, K. W., Meeusen, R., Mujika, I., Robazza, C., Skorski, S., Venter, R., & Beckmann, J. (2018). Recovery and performance in sport: Consensus statement. *International Journal of Sports Physiology and Performance*, *13*, 240–245.

Kenny, S., Whittaker, J., & Emery, C. (2016). Risk factors for musculoskeletal injury in preprofessional dancers: A systematic review. *British Journal of Sports Medicine*, *50*(16), 997–1003.

Kenttä, G., & Hassmén, P. (2002). Underrecovery and overtraining: A conceptual model. In M. Kellmann (Ed.), *Enhancing recovery: Preventing underperformance in athletes* (pp. 57–79). Human Kinetics.

Koutedakis, Y., & Jamurtas, A. (2004). The dancer as a performing athlete: Physiological considerations. *Sports Medicine*, *34*(10), 651–661.

Koutedakis, Y., Myszkewycz, L., Soulas, D., Papapostolou, V., Sullivan, I., & Sharp, N. C. (1999). The effects of rest and subsequent training on selected physiological parameters in professional female classical dancers. *International Journal of Sports Medicine*, *20*(6), 379–383.

Kozai, A., Twitchett, E., Morgan, S., & Wyon, M. (2020). Workload intensity and rest periods in professional ballet: Connotations for injury. *International Journal of Sports Medicine*, *41*(6), 373–379.

Lambert, M. I. (2012). Quantification of endurance training and competition loads. In I. Mujika (Ed.), *Endurance training: Science and practice* (pp. 211–228). Vitoria-Gasteiz.

Laws, H. (2004). *Healthier Dance Survey II: Initial findings*. 14th Annual Meeting: October 150–17, 2004 San Francisco, California, USA. International Association for Dance Medicine & Science.
Laws, H. (2005). *Fit to dance 2- Report of the second national inquiry into dancers' health and injury in the UK*. Newgate Press.
Lewis, R., Dickerson, J., & Davies, G. (1997). Lifestyle and injuries of professional ballet dancers: Reflections in retirement. *Journal of the Royal Society of Health*, *117*(1), 23–31.
Liederbach, M., & Compagno, J. (2023). Psychological aspects of fatigue-related injuries in dancers. *Journal of Dance Medicine & Science*, *5*(4), 116–120.
Liiv, H., Wyon, M. A., Jürimäe, T., Saar, M., Mäestu, J., & Jürimäe, J. (2013). Anthropometry, somatotypes, and aerobic power in ballet, contemporary dance, and dancesport. *Medical Problems of Performing Artists*, *28*(4), 207–211.
Mattiussi, A. M., Shaw, J. W., Williams, S., Price, P. D., Brown, D. D., Cohen, D. D., Clark, R., Kelly, S., Retter, G., & Pedlar, C. (2021). Injury epidemiology in professional ballet: A five-season prospective study of 1596 medical attention injuries and 543 time-loss injuries. *British Journal of Sports Medicine*, *55*(15), 843–850.
McGuigan, H., Hassmén, P., Rosic, N., & Stevens, C. J. (2020). Training monitoring methods used in the field by coaches and practitioners: A systematic review. *International Journal of Sports Science & Coaching*, *15*(3), 439–451.
Milewski, M. D., Skaggs, D. L., Bishop, G. A., Pace, J. L., Ibrahim, D. A., Wren, T. A., & Barzdukas, A. (2014). Chronic lack of sleep is associated with increased sports injuries in adolescent athletes. *Journal of Pediatric Orthopaedics*, *34*(2), 129–133.
Nascimento, A. L., Luna, J. V., & Fontenelle, L. F. (2012). Body dysmorphic disorder and eating disorders in elite professional female ballet dancers. *Annals of Clinical Psychiatry*, *24*(3), 191–194.
Oliveira Souza, M., Pedroso, B., Della Giustina Dos Reis, F., & Mendes Capraro, A. (2022). Ballet, gender and sexuality: A systematic review in the scopus and web of science databases. *Research in Dance Education*, *25*(4), 425–442.
Pickard, A. (2013). Ballet body belief: Perceptions of an ideal ballet body from young ballet dancers. *Research in Dance Education*, *14*(1), 3–19.
Redding, E., Wyon, M., Shearman, J., & Doggart, L. (2004). Validity of using heart rate as a predictor of oxygen consumption in dance. *Journal of Dance Medicine and Science*, *8*(3), 69–72.
Riding-McCabe, T., Ambegaonkar, J., Redding, E., & Wyon, M. (2014). Fit to dance survey: A comparison with DanceSport injuries. *Medical Problems in Performing Artists*, *29*(2), 102–110.
Rigoli, A., Dang, E., Michael, V., Gifford, J., & Davies, A. (2024). What do we know about the energy status and diets of pre-professional and professional dancers: A scoping review. *Nutrients*, *16*(24), 4293. https://doi.org/10.3390/nu16244293
Robertson, I. (1967). Injuries of the lower limb in football: Ballet injuries. *Proceedings of the Royal Society of Medicine*, *60*(6), 530–532.
Rodrigues-Krause, J., dos Santos Cunha, G., Alberton, C., Follmer, B., Krause, M., & Reischak-Oliveira, A. (2014). Oxygen consumption and heart rate responses to isolated ballet exercise sets. *Journal of Dance Medicine and Science*, *18*(3), 99–105.
Rönkkö, R., Markku, H., Malmivaara, A., Roine, R., Seitsalo, S., Sainio, P., & Kettunen, J. (2007). Musculoskeletal pain, disability and quality of life among retired dancers. *Journal of Dance Medicine & Science*, *11*(4), 105–109.

Rosenthal, M., McPherson, A. M., Docherty, C. L., & Klossner, J. (2021). Perceptions and utilization of strength training and conditioning in collegiate contemporary and ballet dancers: A qualitative approach. *Medical Problems of Performing Artists*, *36*(2), 78–87.

Schantz, P., & Åstrand, P.-O. (1984). Physiological characteristics of classical ballet. *Medicine and Science in Sports and Exercise*, *16*(5), 472–476.

Schmidt, M., Reer, R., Groneberg, D. A., Holzgreve, F., & Wanke, E. M. (2023). Work-related musculoskeletal disorders of dance teachers in Germany: A retrospective cross-sectional study. *Applied Sciences*, *13*(3), 1454. https://doi.org/10.3390/app13031454

Shaw, J. W., Mattiussi, A. M., Brown, D. D., Williams, S., Kelly, S., Springham, M., Pedlar, C. R., & Tallent, J. (2021). Dance exposure, individual characteristics, and injury risk over five seasons in a professional ballet company. *Medicine and Science in Sports and Exercise*, *53*(11), 2290–2297.

Shaw, J. W., Mattiussi, A. M., Brown, D. D., Williams, S., Springham, M., Pedlar, C. R., & Tallent, J. (2023). Rehearsal and performance volume in professional ballet: A five-season cohort study. *Journal of Dance Medicine & Science*, *27*(1), 3–12.

Silverii, G. A., Cosentino, C., Santagiuliana, F., Rotella, F., Benvenuti, F., Mannucci, E., & Cresci, B. (2022). Effectiveness of low-carbohydrate diets for long-term weight loss in obese individuals: A meta-analysis of randomized controlled trials. *Diabetes, Obesity & Metabolism*, *24*(8), 1458–1468.

Sjölin, C. (2023). Embracing a precarious life. *Nordic Journal of Dance*, *14*(2), 16–21.

Smith, T., de Medici, A., Oduoza, U., Hakim, A., Paton, B., Retter, G., Haddad, F. S., & Macgregor, A. (2017). National survey to evaluate musculoskeletal health in retired professional ballet dancers in the United Kingdom. *Physical Therapy in Sport*, *23*, 82–85.

Soligard, T., Schwellnus, M., Alonso, J. M., Bahr, R., Clarsen, B., Dijkstra, H. P., Gabbett, T., Gleeson, M., Hägglund, M., Hutchinson, M. R., Janse van Rensburg, C., Khan, K. M., Meeusen, R., Orchard, J. W., Pluim, B. M., Raftery, M., Budgett, R., & Engebretsen, L. (2016). How much is too much? (Part 1) International Olympic Committee consensus statement on load in sport and risk of injury. *British Journal of Sports Medicine*, *50*(17), 1030–1041.

Stephens, N., & Wyon, M. (2020). Physiological characteristics of musical theatre performers and the effect on cardiorespiratory demand whilst singing and dancing. *Medical Problems of Performing Artists*, *35*(1), 54–58.

Storm, J., Wolman, R., Bakker, E., & Wyon, M. (2018). The relationship between range of motion and injuries in adolescent dancers and sportspersons: A systematic review. *Frontiers in Psychology*, *9*, 287. https://doi.org/10.3389/fpsyg.2018.00287

Stubbe, J. H., Soerel, B., Oudejans, R., Kegelaers, J., & van Rijn, R. M. (2022). Quantifying internal load in pre-professional contemporary dancers: The association between objective heart-rate derived outcome measures and subjective dancers' and teachers' perceptions. *Journal of Dance Medicine & Science*, *26*(1), 59–65.

Surgenor, B., & Wyon, M. (2019). Measuring training load in dance: The construct validity of session-RPE. *Medical Problems in Performing Artists*, *34*(1), 1–5.

Teixeira, J. E., Branquinho, L., Leal, M., Morgans, R., Sortwell, A., Barbosa, T. M., Monteiro, A. M., Afonso, P., Machado, G., & Encarnação, S. (2024). Match-to-match variation on high-intensity demands in a Portuguese professional football team. *Journal of Functional Morphology and Kinesiology*, *9*(3), 120. https://doi.org/10.3390/jfmk9030120

Toscani, G., & Prendergast, G. (2019). Arts sponsorship versus sports sponsorship: Which is better for marketing strategy? *Journal of Nonprofit & Public Sector Marketing*, *31*(4), 428–450.

Tsiouti, N., & Wyon, M. (2021). Injury occurrence in hip hop dance: An online cross-sectional cohort study of breakers. *Journal of Dance Medicine & Science*, *25*, 2–8.

Twitchett, E., Angioi, M., Koutedakis, Y., & Wyon, M. (2010). The demands of a working day among female professional ballet dancers. *Journal of Dance Medicine & Science*, *14*(4), 127–132.

Twitchett, E., Angioi, M., Metsios, G., Koutedakis, Y., & Wyon, M. (2008). Body composition and ballet injuries: A preliminary study. *Medical Problems in Performing Artists*, *23*(3), 93–98.

Wanke, E. M., Schmidt, M., Leslie-Spinks, J., Fischer, A., & Groneberg, D. A. (2015). Physical and mental workloads in professional dance teachers. *Medical Problems of Performing Artists*, *30*(1), 54–60.

Wyon, M. (2004). Challenging habit: Planning and preparation, the art of periodisation and optimising performance. In M. van der Linden (Ed.), *Not just anybody and soul* (pp. 66–71). Uitgeveij International Theatre and Film Books.

Wyon, M. (2010). Preparing to perform periodization and dance. *Journal of Dance Medicine & Science*, *14*(2), 67–72.

Wyon, M., Abt, G., Redding, E., Head, A., & Sharp, N. (2004). Oxygen uptake during of modern dance class, rehearsal and performance. *Journal of Strength and Conditioning Research*, *18*(3), 646–649.

Wyon, M., & Allard, G. (2022). *Periodization: A framework for dance training*. Bloomsbury.

Wyon, M., Allen, N., Cloak, R., Beck, S., Davies, P., & Clarke, F. (2016). Assessment of maximum aerobic capacity and anaerobic threshold of elite ballet dancers. *Medical Problems in Performing Artists*, *31*(3), 145–149.

Wyon, M., Harris, J., Adams, F., Cloak, R., Clarke, F., & Bryant, J. (2018). Cardiorespiratory profile and performance demands of elite hip-hop dancers: Breaking and new style. *Medical Problems in Performing Artists*, *33*(3), 198–204.

Wyon, M., & Redding, E. (2005). The physiological monitoring of cardiorespiratory adaptations during rehearsal and performance of contemporary dance. *Journal of Strength and Conditioning Research*, *19*(3), 611–614.

5

MINDFULNESS AS A TOOL FOR ENHANCING RECOVERY IN THE PERFORMING ARTS

Peta Blevins, Shona Erskine, and Luke Hopper

Introduction

Performing artists, including dancers, musicians, actors, and circus artists, operate under intense physical, emotional, and cognitive demands shaped not only by their personal practices but also by the training environments, institutions, and cultural norms they inhabit. Recovery, a cornerstone of sustainable performance, requires both individual strategies like mindfulness and systemic support to thrive, yet its conceptualisation in the performing arts is less developed than in sports science (Saw et al., 2015). While physical recovery often takes precedence, psychological recovery is equally critical to mitigate mental fatigue and enhance well-being. Though recovery is frequently framed as an individual concern, dancers train and perform within interconnected systemic frameworks – schools, companies, and sociocultural contexts – that influence their capacity to recover (Meadows, 2008). This chapter explores mindfulness as an individual recovery strategy, focusing on its application in dance, while emphasising how broader systems must align to enhance dancer health and well-being, fostering change across training, organisations, and cultural norms.

Recovery in the performing arts

In a performance context, recovery can be defined as a dynamic and multifaceted process involving intentional activities aimed at restoring depleted resources across physical, psychological, and social domains, culminating in a

Blevins, P., Erskine, S., & Hopper, L. (2026). Mindfulness as a tool for enhancing recovery in the performing arts. In E. Altenmüller, M. Kellmann, J. Beckmann, & G. M. Moyle (Eds.), *Recovery and well-being in the performing arts* (pp. 78–96). Routledge

DOI: 10.4324/9781003566885-7

state of renewed functioning and well-being (Kellmann et al., 2018). This definition underscores the dual nature of recovery, highlighting the importance of both the processes undertaken and the outcomes achieved. Recovery processes in the performing arts are ideally tailored to the specific challenges of each discipline, such as the high-impact physicality of dance, the cognitive precision of music, or the emotional intensity of acting, emphasising psychological flexibility, mental focus, and physical resilience. This variability underscores the need for nuanced strategies to achieve recovery (i.e., facilitate restoration and adaptation) that address these multifaceted demands and lead to optimal functioning across physical, psychological, and social domains.

Diverse training and recovery demands

Training and recovery needs vary significantly across performing arts disciplines, shaped by both individual efforts and systemic influences. Dancers often face high physical demands, with repetitive high-impact movements and long rehearsal hours leading to musculoskeletal strain and physical and psychological fatigue (Blevins et al., 2019; Wyon, 2010). Specific examples include pointe work in ballet, stressing feet and lower legs, and contemporary dance movements requiring repeated jumps and floor work. These demands are compounded by systemic factors, such as rigid rehearsal schedules or cultural pressures to perform through fatigue, which can limit dancers' ability to prioritise recovery (Lakes, 2005). In contrast, musicians face cognitive and motor demands from intricate fingerwork and prolonged practice, often resulting in upper limb pain and injuries (Sheibani-Rad et al., 2013). Ackermann and Altenmüller (2021) note these injuries stem not just from individual practice but also from institutional expectations of extended static posture, highlighting how recovery depends on both personal habits and the systems structuring their work.

Mindfulness, defined as intentional, nonjudgemental awareness of the present moment (Kabat-Zinn, 1990), helps artists manage recovery-stress imbalance by fostering cognitive rest, emotional regulation, and physiological restoration. For dancers, it can mitigate overtraining risks by enhancing mental clarity amid repetitive strain. For musicians, it supports focus and relaxation despite prolonged practice, and for actors, it builds resilience against emotional fatigue. With its emphasis on individual focus, adaptability to flexible schedules, minimal cost and easy access (requiring little more than intentional practice) mindfulness offers a practical, discipline-specific approach to replenishing resources and optimising performance across the arts.

Recovery-stress balance framework

Kellmann and Kallus' (2001) *Scissors-model of the interrelation of stress states and recovery demands* offers a comprehensive framework, emphasising the interplay between stressors and recovery strategies within a dynamic system. Recovery is not merely the absence of stress but a process of replenishing resources to build resilience and optimise performance, as well as a resultant state achieved following effective recovery processes, influenced by both individual actions and environmental contexts (Kellmann, 2002a). The *Scissors-model* of recovery (see Altenmüller et al., this volume, Chapter 1) provides an effective visual representation of the widening gap between rising stress and inadequate recovery. The top blade of the scissors symbolises increasing stress (e.g., training demands, performance pressure), while the bottom blade represents recovery. When recovery efforts do not match the level of stress, the blades diverge – indicating a growing imbalance and an elevated risk of underrecovery, fatigue, or burnout (Kellmann et al., 2018).

In dance, achieving recovery-stress balance means navigating personal stressors like overtraining alongside systemic pressures, such as expectations to rehearse or perform without rest, forming feedback loops where inadequate recovery amplifies stress (Meadows, 2008). Practices like yoga and mindfulness can mitigate these risks by supporting recovery processes and reducing the scissor gap. For musicians, the model applies to managing mental stress and repetitive strain, exacerbated by rehearsal structures lacking restorative breaks. Mindfulness exercises, in particular, can foster present-moment awareness, emotional regulation, focus, and relaxation within these systemic constraints, thereby enhancing psychological recovery.

An imbalance between stress and recovery can lead to conditions such as burnout, underrecovery, and injury. For instance, Meeusen and colleagues (2013) highlight how inadequate recovery in athletes can exacerbate motor coordination issues, a finding that parallels overtraining syndrome in dancers. Similarly, dance students who failed to engage in adequate recovery face increased risk of injury, fatigue, and mental exhaustion (Blevins et al., 2019). Introducing formal frameworks for scheduling recovery phases into artist training and performance schedules has the potential to substantially improve artist well-being (Hopper et al., 2020).

Recovery phases within a training cycle are critical for fostering adaptation and improving performance (Norris & Smith, 2002). Athletes often employ various recovery strategies, such as hydrotherapy, massage, compression garments, and mental skills, to mitigate the stress and fatigue associated with training demands (Venter, 2014). Specific recovery needs will be unique to the individual, dependent on the activity undertaken. For example, an end-of-year dance performance may provoke considerable physical and psychological stress for dance students; however, effective recovery from this event will depend upon the specific needs of the student. According to Kellmann (2002a) recovery strategies can be active (e.g., physical activities aimed to relieve physical fatigue, such as cool-down after dance class), passive (e.g., activities requiring minimal individual effort such as massage or cold baths), or pro-active (e.g., self-initiated, purposeful actions putting the individual in control). Engaging in recovery strategies mindfully, whether active, passive, or pro-active in approach, will assist the individual in selecting the most appropriate recovery strategy to address their needs and monitor outcomes. For example, a mindfully attuned dancer who notices a change in their emotional state may pro-actively select to take time to catch up with friends, compared to their peer who has noticed they are experiencing increased physical soreness and increases their cool-down activities at the end of class.

Environmental factors must also be considered in the recovery process as they can impact recovery outcomes. In the performing arts specifically, an example where environmental factors may influence recovery can be when performing artists are expected to attend opening night celebrations immediately post-performance and do not have the capacity to engage in post-performance cool-down activities. In situations such as these, performers would benefit from having built up a stress buffer in anticipation of reduced capacity for recovery strategies post-performance.

As illustrated in the *Scissor-model* (Kallus & Kellmann, 2000), when demands lead to heightened stress, and recovery is insufficient, individuals may experience a recovery-stress imbalance. Prolonged exposure to stressors without adequate recovery can result in a gradual deterioration of the recovery-stress state, creating an imbalance between stress and recovery (Heidari et al., 2022). Restoring this balance requires addressing a range of contributing factors, including lifestyle elements (e.g., sleep, nutrition, recreational activities), training parameters (e.g., duration, intensity, periodisation), health considerations (e.g., injury, illness), environmental influences (e.g., school or university), and psychosocial dynamics (e.g., support from family, teammates, or coaches/teachers; Kellmann, 2002a). Research suggests that underrecovery is a precursor to adverse training outcomes, such as overtraining syndrome and burnout, and that early identification of underrecovery in the training cycle, as well as during a performance season, could help prevent more severe maladaptation (Gustafsson et al., 2008; Kellmann, 2002b; Meeusen et al., 2013).

Shifting attention from stress overload to recovery facilitates a deeper exploration of psychological and psychosocial variables influencing recovery. While overtraining research predominantly focuses on physical responses to training, recovery is often addressed through interventions targeting physical fatigue (e.g., compression garments, massage, cold-water therapies). However, examining the psychological dimensions of recovery may help explain aspects that physiological data cannot (Lemyre & Fournier, 2013). Psychological monitoring may also offer a simpler and more efficient method for detecting early-warning signs of recovery-stress imbalance compared to physiological testing (Knettä & Hassmén, 1998). Adopting a holistic, biopsychosocial approach to recovery is therefore recommended to address the complex and multifaceted recovery needs of individuals (Heidari et al., 2022; Lemyre & Fournier, 2013).

Dance research has started identifying methods to improve the psychological recovery of dance students from the stressors they encounter during vocational training. Research in sports science has shown that mindfulness can effectively reduce the impact of stress on collegiate and elite athletes (Petterson & Olson, 2017). Additionally, mindfulness has been found to stabilise emotions in athletes (Baltzell & Akhtar, 2014) and is associated with increased positive affect and decreased negative affect (Weinstein et al., 2009). Affective (emotional) states serve as indicators of training adaptation, with low mood linked to poor training adaptation (Lemyre et al., 2006; Terry et al., 2007) and intense negative emotions correlated with inadequate recovery (Lemyre & Fournier, 2013). Empirical support has been demonstrated for the integration of mindfulness training in vocational dance education, linking mindfulness with improved psychological recovery and affective states (Blevins, 2019). In the context of Kellmann and Kallus's (2001) recovery-stress framework and *Scissors-model*, mindfulness can be viewed as both a recovery strategy and a modulating factor, enhancing psychological flexibility, emotional regulation, and awareness of personal limits.

Mindfulness as a recovery strategy

In the context of the recovery-stress framework, mindfulness offers a foundational approach to managing the complex and fluctuating demands placed on performing artists. Central to effective recovery is the ability to notice and interpret one's own internal state – physically, mentally, and emotionally – and to recognise when recovery is needed (Kellmann & Kallus, 2001; Kellmann et al., 2018). Since psychological recovery often relies on subjective self-report rather than objective physiological data (Lemyre & Fournier, 2013), mindfulness becomes an essential skill that supports accurate, moment-to-moment assessment of one's experiences. For dancers, this includes tuning into physical fatigue and emotional strain, while for actors it may mean noticing the residual effects of performance, such as the need to 'de-role' or recover from vocal or expressive exertion. The multifaceted nature of artistic work, shaped by individual differences, creative processes, and systemic pressures, necessitates recovery strategies that are not only diverse but also contextually relevant and personally meaningful. Mindfulness has emerged as a flexible and evidence-informed method that enables individuals to implement recovery strategies with greater intentionality and adaptability (Baltzell & Akhtar, 2014; Petterson & Olson, 2017). While mindfulness is one of several recovery strategies available to performers, we propose it should be considered a foundational skill – an underlying capacity from which other recovery practices can be mindfully selected, applied, and refined to suit the unique needs of the artist and the environments in which they work.

Defining mindfulness

Mindfulness involves intentional, nonjudgemental focus on the present moment, fostering awareness of thoughts, emotions, and bodily sensations (Kabat-Zinn, 1990). Originating from Eastern philosophical and spiritual roots, mindfulness has become an area of growing interest in research within clinical and normative populations over the past 30 years. While dancers can cultivate mindfulness individually, its effectiveness may hinge on training environments that allow time for such practices, facilitated by systemic support often absent in high-pressure dance cultures (Roche & Huddy, 2015).

Attention to and awareness of the present moment are central to any definition of mindfulness (Brown & Ryan, 2003). While stress reduction is not the primary objective of mindfulness practice, research has shown it to be a beneficial side effect (Palmer & Rodger, 2009; Petterson & Olson, 2017). Moreover, increased mindfulness has been associated with enhanced focus on tasks, reduced performance anxiety, diminished stress related to task demands, and improved overall well-being among elite performers (Bühlmayer et al., 2017; Sappington & Longshore, 2015). Mindfulness skills provide athletes with strategies to manage the challenges of elite performance, facilitating the acquisition and execution of critical skills (Röthlin et al., 2016). Given these benefits, it is reasonable to suggest that mindfulness skills could similarly support performing artists in navigating the demands of their training and performance.

Evidence across disciplines

The benefits of mindfulness have been demonstrated in a number of domains (e.g., clinical, educational, and sport), and across various outcomes including improvements in stress, pain, emotion regulation, and well-being (Baer, 2003; Brown & Ryan, 2003; Noetel et al., 2017). A recent review of empirical studies examining the impact of mindfulness on psychological health found a positive relationship between mindfulness and various psychological health outcomes. These include increased positive affect, improved emotion regulation, and reduced levels of perceived stress and burnout across correlational, clinical intervention, and experimental research (Keng et al., 2011). Furthermore, mindfulness has been linked to heightened positive affect and diminished negative affect among university students (Brown & Ryan, 2003). Evidence also suggests that mindfulness training can effectively reduce stress and anxiety (Kaufman et al., 2018; Khoury et al., 2015), making it a valuable tool for stress management and recovery enhancement.

In sports research, mindfulness enhances athletic performance and psychological well-being, thriving where coaching systems encourage its use (Gardner & Moore, 2017). In dance, similar institutional backing could amplify its impact, suggesting a need for systemic integration beyond individual adoption

(Roche & Huddy, 2015). Mindfulness and acceptance-based approaches to performance differ from traditional psychological skills training by emphasising the acceptance of one's current thoughts and feelings, rather than attempting to control them (Gardner & Moore, 2012). Studies involving elite junior and collegiate athletes have found that higher levels of dispositional mindfulness act as a buffer against stress (Gustafsson et al., 2015). Additionally, mindfulness has been demonstrated to be an important factor in improved recovery-stress states and sleep regulation, not only through long-term training but also via daily fluctuations in mindfulness that predict sleep quality and recovery dynamics (Birnkraut et al., 2025). Mindfulness interventions have also been shown to positively influence performance outcomes and reduce stress levels (Petterson & Olson, 2017).

In the performing arts, mindfulness can serve as both a preventative measure and a recovery tool, enhancing emotional regulation, cognitive clarity, and resilience. By training individuals to engage fully with the present, mindfulness reduces the cognitive load associated with performance anxiety and enhances their ability to recover from high-stress situations. For instance, Acceptance and Commitment Therapy (ACT; Hayes et al., 2016), a mindfulness-based approach, has been effective in reducing performance anxiety among musicians (Juncos et al., 2017) and qualitative feedback from participants in an ACT-based mindfulness programme within tertiary dance training curriculum indicated mindfulness meditation has a positive impact on performance and general well-being (Moyle, 2016).

Further, mindfulness interventions have shown efficacy in reducing stress and enhancing performance in both dance and music contexts. For instance, mindfulness techniques for musicians have reduced anxiety and enhanced mental clarity during performance (Czajkowski et al., 2022). Mindfulness and acceptance approaches have also been linked to improvements in emotion regulation and acceptance, and the ability to manage performance anxiety in dancers, musicians, and actors (Lubert et al., 2023). Additionally, mindfulness has been linked to improved sleep quality, reduced somatic complaints, and greater resilience to stress in musicians and dancers alike. For example, a randomised control trial on university music students found that a six-week mindfulness programme significantly reduced performance-related stress (Juncos et al., 2017).

Mechanisms of action

Mindfulness enhances psychological recovery in the performing arts by addressing the interplay of cognitive, emotional, and physical demands, offering dancers and other artists a tool to restore balance amid intense training and performance schedules. It reduces mental fatigue by quieting rumination and performance anxiety, allowing artists like dancers to regain clarity through practices such as focused breathing (Blevins, 2019). This cognitive rest is vital in high-pressure environments where systemic expectations, such as relentless rehearsal demands, often amplify stress. Emotionally, mindfulness fosters regulation by encouraging nonjudgemental awareness, helping performers manage stage nerves and emotional reactivity with fewer fluctuations (Czajkowski & Greasley, 2015; Czajkowski et al., 2021). Physiologically, it activates the parasympathetic nervous system via techniques like body scans, reducing tension and enhancing sleep quality; key for dancers combating overuse injuries within rigid training structures (Batson, 2009). Additionally, mindfulness sharpens focus, enabling a flow state that enhances choreography execution in dance or task absorption across disciplines, a benefit echoed in sport research (Petterson & Olson, 2017). These mechanisms collectively support individual recovery, though their efficacy often depends on systemic support, such as time for practice within institutional frameworks.

Application of mindfulness in dance

Within the high-demand environment of dance training, mindfulness offers a powerful means of bridging awareness and recovery. While dancers are conditioned to develop acute bodily awareness (attuning to posture, movement, and rhythm), they are equally socialised to ignore the warning signs of overtraining, including pain, fatigue, and emotional exhaustion (Blevins et al., 2019). This paradoxical training culture can undermine dancers' ability to effectively respond to recovery needs. Positioned within the broader recovery-stress framework (Kellmann & Kallus, 2001, 2025), mindfulness extends beyond passive awareness to become a practical, adaptive recovery tool – one that must be implemented intentionally and in ways that account for individual, contextual, and systemic factors. Mindfulness may enable dancers to better perceive internal cues, self-assess their recovery states, and mindfully engage with appropriate strategies (Blevins et al., 2022). This foundation supports more accurate self-monitoring and recovery implementation, especially critical in dance environments where recovery-stress imbalances are often overlooked or normalised (Blevins et al., 2019). As such, mindfulness serves as a foundational layer upon which other recovery strategies can be built and tailored, supporting the longer-term goals of resilience, emotional regulation, and sustainable performance.

Mindfulness in vocational dance: Insights from empirical research

The authors of this chapter conducted two studies to investigate mindfulness as a tool for psychological recovery among pre-professional vocational dance students. The research included an investigation of the relationships between mindfulness, recovery-stress balance, and well-being among pre-professional vocational dance students studying at universities in Australia (Blevins et al.,

2022) as well as an evaluation of the effectiveness of a mindfulness and acceptance training programme (MATP) for first-year students (Blevins, 2019).

In the initial study (Blevins et al., 2022), 72 dance students at two Australian universities completed online self-report measures of mindfulness, recovery-stress states, and affect, with findings indicating mindfulness can reduce stress and have a positive effect on recovery, as well as enhancing emotional well-being. Students with higher mindfulness levels experienced significantly lower levels of both general and dance-specific stress, highlighting mindfulness as a protective factor against the high demands of vocational training. Further, mindfulness positively correlated with dance-specific recovery, suggesting that students with a greater capacity for mindful awareness are better equipped to manage training-related stressors. Mindfulness was also significantly associated with increased positive affect and reduced negative affect, emphasising its role in fostering emotional balance. Group comparisons were conducted, indicating that students with high mindfulness reported better recovery-stress outcomes and fewer negative emotions compared to their low-mindfulness counterparts. These findings underscore mindfulness' potential as a powerful tool for improving both psychological recovery and overall well-being in dance training contexts.

Based on these findings, a second study (Blevins, 2019) was conducted to evaluate the effects of a five-week MATP for first-year university dance students. The aim of the MATP was to introduce the general concepts of mindfulness to the dance students and to provide them with the opportunity to practice mindfulness skills that could benefit their dance practice. The MATP utilised an acceptance-based approach drawing primarily from ACT and mindful acceptance commitment (MAC; Gardner & Moore, 2007) protocols. A summary of the weekly sessions is presented in Table 5.1.

Key outcomes from this study included reduced stress levels, stabilised emotional states, and enhanced recovery and resilience. Participants reported significantly lower dance-specific stress levels following the programme, indicating mindfulness can mitigate the psychological strain of intensive training. However, qualitative feedback revealed challenges applying MATP skills in group-based dance settings, where rigid schedules and cultural norms prioritise output over recovery limit integration (Blevins et al., 2020). This suggests mindfulness's full potential requires systemic adjustments, such as embedding it into class structures. The group-based nature of dance training, unlike sports' tailored programmes, underscores a systemic tension: individual recovery tools thrive only when supported by the broader training ecosystem (Heidari et al., 2022).

Together, these studies provide evidence supporting the integration of mindfulness practices in dance training and highlight mindfulness's efficacy in reducing stress, promoting recovery, and improving emotional and psychological

TABLE 5.1 Details of sessions in the mindfulness training programme.

Session theme	*Session goals & psychoeducational component*	*Experiential exercises*	*Between sessions exercises*
Week 1: Introduction to mindfulness	Questionnaire completion. Introduce key concepts of mindfulness; rational for mindfulness skills in dance; develop rapport with students	Brief centring exercise	Take ten breaths; Notice five things; Mindful eating; Mindful morning routine (Harris, 2009)
Week 2: Mindfulness of thoughts	Introduce cognitive defusion	Cognitive defusion techniques; Leaves on a stream (Harris, 2009)	Continued practice of preferred defusion techniques; 'Getting Hooked' worksheet (Harris, 2009)
Week 3: Mindfulness of emotions	Define emotions and their function in human experience	Accepting emotions; body scan	Continued practice of body scan; 'Struggling vs Opening Up' worksheet (Harris, 2009)
Week 4: Contact with the present moment	Introduction to concept of thinking self vs observing self, enhancing present moment awareness	Anchoring – 'The Mindful S.T.O.P.' (Harris, 2018); mindful walking exercise	Continued mindful movement practice, encouraged to apply it to dance practice in classes or rehearsals
Week 5: Values and Goals	Definitions of values and goals, explanation of how to use values to guide goal setting and end-of-study questionnaires	Performance Obituary; Setting Values-Based Goals (Harris, 2009); Willingness & Action Plan (Harris, 2009)	

well-being among students navigating the challenges of intensive training programmes. A valuable avenue for both further empirical research and practical applications of mindfulness in performing arts environments is to explore the embedding and systematic integration of mindfulness practices within training to harness their full potential within supportive systems.

Implications and recommendations in dance

Considering the research investigating recovery-stress balance and the role of mindfulness in enhancing psychological recovery in dance, three overarching themes can be extrapolated.

Empowering the individual

Recognising individual differences in stress responses is vital. Dancers' unique stress responses highlight the need for self-monitoring tools, but these are most effective when training systems – unlike their traditional rigidity – adapt to individual needs, mirroring sports' athlete-centred approaches (Heidari et al., 2022). Dancers perceive stressors uniquely, influenced by personal attitudes and mindfulness levels, yet coping strategies vary, with adaptive behaviours (e.g., prioritising rest) linked to positive outcomes and maladaptive ones (e.g., ignoring fatigue) contributing to injuries and burnout.

Athlete monitoring is common in elite-level sport (Coutts et al., 2022); however, dance has yet to embrace this element of high-performance training (Jeffries & Coutts, this volume, Chapter 3). Monitoring systems assist individuals to appraise changes in mood, mental, and physical states for the early detection of recovery-stress imbalances (Heidari et al., 2022). There is an inherent tension, however, in how to balance the individual needs of the dancer within dance training environments, which are usually group-based and follow a more rigid structure (and therefore less easily adapt to individual needs) than team training environments in sport.

It has been recommended that athlete monitoring in team sports develop position- and person-specific training programmes (Heidari et al., 2022). This approach may not be easily applied to dance training environments because dancers do not train for specific positions within the group in the same way that an athlete may. Dance training tends to follow a traditional group-based teaching format, where teachers deliver a single task to the group pitched at a general level of ability, rather than targeted to individual needs and skill level (Buckroyd, 2000). Considering the group-based nature of dance training, it may therefore be beneficial to educate dance students about self-monitoring practices to manage their individual responses to training.

Likewise, implementing mindfulness training programmes in dance training environments may be challenging due to the individual differences of the dancers within the group. Research is yet to identify the ideal total length of a mindfulness training programme, the ideal duration of individual sessions within the programme, timing and mode of delivery of content (Baltzell & Akhtar, 2014; Kaufman et al., 2018). Further, on the integration of somatic practices to dance training (Roche & Huddy, 2015), standalone classes in mindfulness may not allow dancers to easily adapt mindfulness principles to dance-specific situations. Movement-based mindfulness skills and activities may produce greater changes in levels of mindfulness in dancers as they more readily mimic the learning and training environments that dancers are accustomed to. Research into different modes of delivery for mindfulness skills would be a valuable area of pursuit.

The role of dance organisations

Building on mindfulness's individual benefits, organisations must evolve from output-driven models to ones embedding recovery into curricula, such as mindful movement classes, to sustain dancer health. Institutions play a crucial role in balancing performance development with recovery, integrating support systems throughout training to foster sustainable careers. The inclusion of recovery monitoring alongside training curriculum and performance seasons can play an essential role in providing performers with information about their individual recovery needs, and can assist companies in managing performers' well-being during rehearsal and performance seasons (Hopper et al., 2020).

Evidence suggests movement-based mindfulness activities can seamlessly integrate into traditional training formats, enhancing applicability (Roche & Huddy, 2015). Mindful stretching, yoga, or pilates help dancers integrate mindfulness into their physical routines. These practices promote body awareness, reduce tension, and enhance flexibility, key attributes for dancers.

Sociocultural considerations

Dance's cultural bias towards perseverance over well-being, reinforced by organisational norms, requires systemic reform – starting with early education – to align with recovery science (Lakes, 2005). Systems theory underscores this: recovery is co-constructed by dancers and their ecosystems, with feedback loops (e.g., overwork expectations) perpetuating stress unless subsystems like studio policies or peer networks shift to prioritise rest (Meadows, 2008). Dance culture often reinforces behaviours linked to overtraining and underrecovery, such as valuing aesthetic ideals over functionality and promoting sustained perseverance through pain, with limited attention paid to recovery (Blevins et al., 2019). Early intervention is needed to address ingrained beliefs and support healthier attitudes towards recovery, starting at community dance school levels.

Research indicates that by the time a dancer reaches pre-professional dance training environments, they have likely already developed strongly held beliefs about approaches to dance training and expected behaviours regarding training loads; early warning signs of injury or pain; and responding to illness, injury, and fatigue (Blevins et al., 2022). Further research would be beneficial to explore how sociocultural norms shape dancers' health-related behaviours and identify strategies to shift these norms towards promoting well-being.

Another potential area for future research is the improved understanding of the role of organisations in developing dance culture and ideologies, particularly in relation to health and well-being in vocational dance training and professional dance environments. Blevins and colleagues (2020) found that some dance training organisations were perceived to endorse behaviours related to overtraining, such as the need to be constantly training or being pressured to return early from injury for significant performances. When considered alongside research indicating that dance training may promote harmful norms such as pushing through pain, injury, and fatigue (McEwan & Young, 2011), as well as authoritarian teaching approaches (Lakes, 2005), these findings suggest that cultural transformation within dance organisations may be necessary to reduce risks to dancers' health and well-being.

Overcoming barriers to recovery

Common barriers to integrating recovery are based on misconceptions about its relevance and lack of time. Barriers like time scarcity reflect systemic issues; rehearsal-heavy schedules leave little room for recovery strategies. These issues stem from training environments that prioritise performance over recovery, creating stress-reinforcing feedback loops (Meadows, 2008). While there are many recovery strategies available to performing artists, mindfulness has shown promise as a tool to benefit performance and wellbeing in both dance and music (Bartos et al., 2021; Blevins, 2019). Strategies to overcome barriers include improving education through workshops, using mobile apps providing mindfulness programmes and resources (e.g., Headspace, a federally funded app in Australia) for consistent practice, and embedding mindfulness in curricula as a subsystem intervention to normalise recovery and disrupt these loops (Roche & Huddy, 2015). Creating peer-support groups can also encourage sustained engagement with mindfulness practices.

Conclusion and recommendations for practice

Mindfulness empowers dancers to manage mental fatigue and enhance recovery, as shown in individual practices and MATP outcomes (Blevins, 2019). Yet, as systems theory reveals, its efficacy depends on supportive subsystems – training environments, organisational policies, and cultural norms (Meadows, 2008). Future efforts must integrate mindfulness into these systems, ensuring dancer health and artistic excellence are mutually reinforced through a transformed dance ecosystem that prioritises recovery as essential to elite performance. Drawing from the recovery-stress framework and research presented in this chapter, the following recommendations support the integration of mindfulness as a foundational tool to enhance psychological recovery across diverse performing arts disciplines.

Position mindfulness as a foundational recovery skill

Mindfulness should be integrated not as an isolated well-being initiative, but as a core capability that underpins all recovery strategies – physical, psychological, and social. Performing artists must be supported to cultivate the capacity to notice internal cues (e.g., fatigue, stress, emotional strain) and use this awareness to make intentional, adaptive decisions about recovery (Blevins et al., 2022; Kellmann et al., 2018). This foundational role makes mindfulness not only a recovery strategy in itself, but also a mechanism for optimising the selection and effectiveness of other strategies.

Train artists to build a recovery buffer through mindfulness

Mindfulness can serve as a pro-active tool to build a 'recovery buffer' – a psychological reserve that helps artists better absorb acute stressors, such as performance pressure or disrupted recovery opportunities (e.g., post-show obligations). Training should emphasise regular mindfulness practices (e.g., brief daily grounding exercises, breathwork, mindful movement) to support the accumulation of recovery capacity, rather than relying solely on reactive recovery following high-stress events (Blevins, 2019).

Encourage mindful self-monitoring and recovery planning

Support performers in developing mindful self-monitoring routines that help them track fluctuations in stress and recovery states. This may include reflective journaling, guided body scans, or the use of standardised monitoring tools (e.g., Recovery-Stress Questionnaire; Kellmann & Kallus, 2001, 2025) to facilitate recognition of recovery needs. These practices help artists engage in intentional, context-specific recovery planning, whether through active strategies (e.g., movement-based cool-downs), passive approaches (e.g., rest, massage), or pro-active psychosocial recovery (e.g., connecting with peers).

Embed mindfulness-based recovery practices into artistic training

Where possible, embed brief, discipline-relevant mindfulness practices into the regular structure of classes, rehearsals, or warm-up/cool-down routings. For example, mindful breathing or sensory awareness exercises can be integrated into acting rehearsals, instrumental warm-ups, or dance technique classes. This approach enhances ecological validity and promotes habit formation while minimising additional time demands (Roche & Huddy, 2015).

Tailor mindfulness training to artistic and individual contexts

Mindfulness interventions must reflect the diverse demands of performance domains and the specific needs of the individual artist. For example, a circus artist working with dynamic physical risk may benefit from present-moment anchoring, while a vocalist experiencing performance anxiety may benefit from emotion-focused acceptance strategies. One-size-fits-all programmes are unlikely to be effective. Instead, offer flexible delivery formats (e.g., brief audio exercises, guided movement meditations) that align with existing training modalities (Blevins et al., 2020).

Support institutional integration of recovery and mindfulness practices

Organisations should adopt a systems approach by embedding mindfulness and recovery education into training curricula, staff development, and scheduling practices. This includes allocating time for recovery, normalising conversations about fatigue and emotional strain, and encouraging reflective recovery planning. Without structural support, individual efforts to implement mindfulness-based recovery strategies risk being undermined by performance-oriented cultural norms (Heidari et al., 2022; Meadows, 2008).

Educate teachers and coaches in mindfulness-informed recovery support

Teachers, choreographers, music directors, and coaches play a key role in shaping the recovery culture of training environments. Professional development should include training in mindfulness-informed recovery support, helping staff recognise signs of underrecovery, model mindful behaviours, and facilitate recovery conversations without judgement. This cultural shift can help disrupt performance-at-all-costs narratives and foster sustainable practices across disciplines (Blevins, 2019).

Use mindfulness to bridge psychological and physical recovery

Encourage artists to use mindfulness to link psychological and physical recovery processes. For instance, a dancer recovering from physical soreness might incorporate mindful stretching and body scans to promote parasympathetic activation, while also using mindfulness to acknowledge emotional frustration or performance concerns related to injury. This integrated approach acknowledges the biopsychosocial complexity of recovery in high-performance artistic contexts (Batson, 2009).

References

Ackermann, B. J., & Altenmüller, E. (2021). The development and use of an anatomy-based retraining program (MusAARP) to assess and treat focal hand dystonia in musicians – A pilot study. *Journal of Hand Therapy*, *34*(2), 309–314.

Baer, R. A. (2003). Mindfulness training as a clinical intervention: A conceptual and empirical review. *Clinical Psychology: Science and Practice*, *10*(2), 125–143.

Baltzell, A., & Akhtar, V. L. (2014). Mindfulness meditation training for sport (MMTS) intervention: Impact of MMTS with division I female athletes. *The Journal of Happiness & Well-Being*, *2*(2), 160–173.

Bartos, L. J., Funes, M. J., Ouellet, M., Pilar Posadas, M., & Krageloh, C. (2021). Developing resilience during the COVID-19 pandemic: Yoga and mindfulness for the well-being of student musicians in Spain. *Frontiers in Psychology*, *12*, 642992. https://doi.org/10.3389/fpsyg.2021.642992

Batson, G. (2009). Somatic studies and dance. *International Journal of Dance Medicine & Science*, *11*(2), 35–42.

Birnkraut, T., Kellmann, M., & Jakowski, S. (2025). Effect of daily mindfulness fluctuations on sleep and recovery-stress states in elite level judoka: An observational study. *Frontiers in Sports and Active Living*, *7*, 1583058. https://doi.org/10.3389/fspor.2025.1583058

Blevins, P. (2019). *Dancing through it: Enhancing psychological recovery in dance* [Doctoral dissertation, Edith Cowan University]. Research Online. https://ro.ecu.edu.au/theses/2207

Blevins, P., Erskine, S., Hopper, L., & Moyle, G. M. (2019). Finding your balance: An investigation of recovery-stress balance in vocational dance training. *Journal of Dance Education*, *20*(1), 12–22.

Blevins, P., Erskine, S., Moyle, G. M., & Hopper, L. (2020). Student and teacher attitudes towards overtraining and recovery in vocational dance training. *Theatre, Dance and Performance Training*, *11*(1), 5–24.

Blevins, P., Moyle, G. M., Erskine, S., & Hopper, L. (2022). Mindfulness, recovery-stress balance, and well-being among university dance students. *Research in Dance Education*, *23*(1), 142–155.

Brown, K. W., & Ryan, R. M. (2003). The benefits of being present: Mindfulness and its role in psychological well-being. *Journal of Personality and Social Psychology*, *84*(4), 822–848.

Buckroyd, J. (2000). *The student dancer*. Dance Books Ltd.

Bühlmayer, L., Birrer, D., Röthlin, P., Faude, O., & Donath, L. (2017). Effects of mindfulness practice on performance-relevant parameters and performance outcomes in sports: A meta-analytical review. *Sports Medicine*, *47*(11), 2309–2321.

Coutts, A. J., Crowcroft, S., & Kempton, T. (2022). Developing athlete monitoring systems: Theoretical basis and practical applications. In M. Kellmann & J. Beckmann (Eds.), *Recovery and well-being in sport and exercise* (pp. 17–31). Routledge.

Czajkowski, A.-M., & Greasley, A. E. (2015). Mindfulness for musicians: A mixed methods study. *International Journal of Music Education*, *33*(4), 439–453.

Czajkowski, A.-M., Greasley, A. E., & Allis, M. (2021). Mindfulness for singers: A mixed methods replication study. *Music & Science*, *4*, 1–16.

Czajkowski, A.-M., Greasley, A. E., & Allis, M. (2022). Mindfulness for musicians: A mixed methods study investigating the effects of 8-week mindfulness courses on music students at a leading conservatoire. *Musicae Scientiae*, *26*(2), 259–270.

Gardner, F. L., & Moore, Z. E. (2007). *The psychology of enhancing human performance: The mindfulness-acceptance-commitment (MAC) approach*. Springer.

Gardner, F. L., & Moore, Z. E. (2012). Mindfulness and acceptance models in sport psychology: A decade of basic and applied scientific advancements. *Canadian Psychology/Psychologie Canadienne*, *53*(4), 309–318.

Gardner, F. L., & Moore, Z. E. (2017). Mindfulness-based and acceptance-based interventions in sport and performance contexts. *Current Opinion in Psychology, 16*, 180–184.

Gustafsson, H., Hassmén, P., Kenttä, G., & Johansson, M. (2008). A qualitative analysis of burnout in elite Swedish athletes. *Psychology of Sport and Exercise, 9*(6), 800–816.

Gustafsson, H., Skoog, T., Davis, P., Kenttä, G., & Haberl, P. (2015). Mindfulness and its relationship with perceived stress, affect, and burnout in elite junior athletes. *Journal of Clinical Sport Psychology, 9*, 263–281.

Harris, R. (2009). *ACT made simple: An easy-to-read primer on acceptance and commitment therapy*. New Harbinger Publications.

Harris, R. (2018). *The complete set of client handouts and worksheets* [Unpublished manuscript, provided during ACT practitioner training].

Hayes, S. C., Strosahl, K. D., & Wilson K. G. (2016). *Acceptance and commitment therapy: The process and practice of mindful change* (2nd ed.). Guilford Press.

Heidari, J., Jakowski, S., & Kellmann, M. (2022). The value of recovery-stress monitoring for athletes' well-being. In M. Kellmann & J. Beckmann (Eds.), *Recovery and well-being in sport and exercise* (pp. 3–16). Routledge.

Hopper, L. S., Blevins, P., Erskine, S., Hendry, D., Hill, R., & Longbottom, R. (2020). Sustaining dancer wellbeing through independent professional dance careers. *Theatre, Dance and Performance Training, 11*(4), 470–486.

Juncos, D. G., Heinrichs, G. A., Towle, P., Duffy, K., Grand, S. M., Morgan, M. C., & Kalkus, E. (2017). Acceptance and commitment therapy for the treatment of music performance anxiety: A pilot study with student vocalists. *Frontiers in Psychology, 8*, 986. https://doi.org/10.3389/fpsyg.2017.00986

Kabat-Zinn, J. (1990). *Full catastrophe living: Using the wisdom of your body and mind to face stress, pain, and illness*. Delacorte.

Kallus, K. W., & Kellmann, M. (2000). Burnout in athletes and coaches. In Y. Hanin (Ed.), *Emotions in sport* (pp. 209–230). Human Kinetics.

Kaufman, K. A., Glass, C. R., & Pineau, T. R. (2018). *Mindful sport performance enhancement: Mental training for athletes and coaches*. American Psychological Association.

Kellmann, M. (2002a). Underrecovery and overtraining: Different concepts – Similar impact? In M. Kellmann (Ed.), *Enhancing recovery: Preventing underperformance in athletes* (pp. 3–24). Human Kinetics.

Kellmann, M. (2002b). Psychological assessment of underrecovery. In M. Kellmann (Ed.), *Enhancing recovery: Preventing underperformance in athletes* (pp. 37–55). Human Kinetics.

Kellmann, M., Bertollo, M., Bosquet, L., Brink, M., Coutts, A. J., Duffield, R., Erlacher, D., Halson, S. L., Hecksteden, A., Heidari, J., Kallus, K. W., Meeusen, R., Mujika, I., Robazza, C., Skorski, S., Venter, R., & Beckmann, J. (2018). Recovery and performance in sport: Consensus statement. *International Journal of Sports Physiology and Performance, 13*(2), 240–245.

Kellmann, M., & Kallus, K. W. (2001). *Recovery-Stress Questionnaire for Athletes: User manual*. Human Kinetics.

Kellmann, M., & Kallus, K. W. (Eds.). (2025). *The Recovery-Stress Questionnaires: A user manual*. Routledge.

Keng, S.-L., Smoski, M. J., & Robins, C. J. (2011). Effects of mindfulness on psychological health: A review of empirical studies. *Clinical Psychology Review, 31*, 1041–1056.

Kenttä, G., & Hassmén, P. (1998). Overtraining and recovery. *Sports Medicine*, *26*(1), 1–16.

Khoury, B., Sharma, M., Rush, S. E., & Fournier, C. (2015). Mindfulness-based stress reduction for healthy individuals: A meta-analysis. *Journal of Psychosomatic Research*, *78*, 519–528.

Lakes, R. (2005). The messages behind the methods: The authoritarian pedagogical legacy in western concert dance technique training and rehearsals. *Arts Education Policy Review*, *106*(5), 3–20.

Lemyre, P.-N., & Fournier, C. (2013). Psychological aspects of recovery. In C. Hausswirth & I. Mujika (Eds.), *Recovery for performance in sport* (pp. 43–52). Human Kinetics.

Lemyre, P.-N., Treasure, D. C., & Roberts, G. C. (2006). Influence of variability in motivation and affect on elite athlete burnout susceptibility. *Journal of Sport & Exercise Psychology*, *28*(1), 32–48.

Lubert, V. J., Nording-Bates, S. M., & Gröpel, P. (2023). Effects of tailored interventions for anxiety management in choking-susceptible performing artists: A mixed-methods collective case study. *Frontiers in Psychology*, *14*, 1164273. https://doi.org/10.3389/fpsyg.2023.1164273

McEwen, K., K., & Young, K. (2011). Ballet and pain: Reflections on a risk-dance culture. *Qualitative Research in Sport, Exercise and Health*, *3*(2), 152–173.

Meadows, D. H. (2008). *Thinking in systems: A primer.* Chelsea Green Publishing.

Meeusen, R., Duclos, M., Foster, C., Fry, A., Gleeson, M., Nieman, D., Raglin, J., Rietjens, G., Steinacker, J., Urhausen, A., European College of Sport Science, & American College of Sports Medicine (2013). Prevention, diagnosis, and treatment of the overtraining syndrome: Joint consensus statement of the European College of Sport Science and the American College of Sports Medicine. *Medicine and Science in Sports and Exercise*, *45*(1), 186–205.

Moyle, G. M. (2016). Mindfulness and dancers. In A. Baltzell (Ed.), *Mindfulness and performance* (pp. 367–388). Cambridge University Press.

Noetel, M., Ciarrochi, J., Van Zanden, B., & Lonsdale, C. (2017). Mindfulness and acceptance approaches to sporting performance enhancement: A systematic review. *International Review of Sport and Exercise Psychology*, *12*, 139–175.

Norris, S. R., & Smith, D. J. (2002). Planning, periodization, and sequencing of training and competition: The rationale for a competently planned, optimally executed training and competition program, supported by a multidisciplinary team. In M. Kellmann (Ed.), *Enhancing recovery: Preventing underperformance in athletes* (pp. 121–141). Human Kinetics.

Palmer, A., & Rodger, S. (2009). Mindfulness, stress, and coping among university students. *Canadian Journal of Counselling*, *43*(3), 198–212.

Petterson, H., & Olson, B. L. (2017). Effects of mindfulness-based interventions in high school and college athletes for reducing stress and injury, and improving quality of life. *Journal of Sport Rehabilitation*, *26*, 578–587.

Roche, J., & Huddy, A. (2015). Creative adaptations: Integrating Feldenkrais principles in contemporary dance technique to facilitate the transition into tertiary dance education. *Theatre, Dance and Performance Training*, *6*(2), 145–158.

Röthlin, P., Horvath, S., Birrer, D., & Holtforth, M. G. (2016). Mindfulness promotes the ability to deliver performance in highly demanding situations. *Mindfulness*, *7*, 727–733.

Sappington, R., & Longshore, K. (2015). Systematically reviewing the efficacy of mindfulness-based interventions for enhanced athletic performance. *Journal of Clinical Sport Psychology*, *9*, 232–262.

Saw, A. E., Main, L. C., & Gastin, P. B. (2015). Monitoring the athlete training response: Subjective self-reported measures trump commonly used objective measures: A systematic review. *British Journal of Sports Medicine*, *49*(4), 231–238.

Sheibani-Rad, S., Wolfe, S., & Jupiter, J. (2013). Hand disorders in musicians. *The Bone & Joint Journal*, *95–B*(2), 146–150.

Terry, P. C., Galambos, S. A., West, J., & Iizuka, C. A. (2007). Psychological correlates of training load among athletes. *Australian Journal of Psychology*, *59* (Suppl. 1), 347.

Venter, R. E. (2014). Perceptions of team athletes on the importance of recovery modalities. *European Journal of Sport Science*, *14*(S1), 569–576.

Weinstein, N., Brown, K. W., & Ryan, R. M. (2009). A multi-method examination of the effects of mindfulness on stress attribution, coping, and emotional well-being. *Journal of Research in Personality*, *43*, 374–385.

Wyon, M. (2010). Preparing to perform: Periodization and dance. *Journal of Dance Medicine & Science*, *14*(2), 67–72.

6

RECOVERY IN PROFESSIONAL MUSICIANS

Maria Schuppert and Eckart Altenmüller

Introduction

From the audience's perspective, professional instrumental and vocal performance appears to be accomplished with physical ease, flexibility, and dynamic flow. However, a 'close-up' on speed and precision of finger and hand movements, fine control of orofacial muscles, or breath control of singers and wind instrumentalists unveils an analogy between the art of music making and elite athletes' performance: indeed, regarding the sensorimotor and musculoskeletal system as well as mental strength, musicians are virtually 'peak-performance athletes'. In this chapter, we aim to elucidate parallels as well as differences between professional music making and high-performance sports and illustrate the distinctive (neuro-) physiological aspects of lifelong practising and performance in music. This will allow for a targeted approach to address the unique needs of musicians regarding health promotion and recovery. With respect to recovery, we take a perspective that goes beyond regeneration or 'being cured' or 'being normal again' (Beckmann et al., 2023). This broader perspective addresses recovery as a resource that enables individuals not only to recover from stress but also to develop resilience to health-threatening stress. Kallus (2016, p. 42) defined recovery as "an inter- and intraindividual multilevel (e.g., psychological, physiological, social) process in time for the re-establishment of personal resources and their full functional capacity". Recovery thus is understood as an expanded concept

Schuppert, M., & Altenmüller, E. (2026). Recovery in professional musicians. In E. Altenmüller, M. Kellmann, J. Beckmann, & G. M. Moyle (Eds.), *Recovery and well-being in the performing arts* (pp. 97–114). Routledge.

DOI: 10.4324/9781003566885-8

of building resilience. In this chapter we focus on strategies musicians may adopt to improve recovery and prevent stressful activities. Furthermore, we will exemplify how resilience is put into practice.

Neural mechanisms underlying musical skills

Making music is highly complex. The sensorimotor, auditory, visual, and emotional skills for musical instrument playing and singing are acquired through persistent practice. This includes developing motor control programmes for the required movements, along with the intuitive acquisition of structural knowledge to understand musical compositions. Additionally, it involves the practice of emotionally expressive playing and singing, whether individually or in an ensemble. To attain the artistic and technical level necessary for admission to a university of music, sustained and long-term practice during childhood and adolescence is required, amounting to about 10,000 hours (Ericsson et al., 1993; Hambrick et al., 2020). Further prerequisites of success include the quality of practice: a combination of goal-oriented, structured and effortful practising with motivation, resources and focused attention from an early age on lays the ground for successful musicianship. This long-term attitude has been labelled 'deliberate practice' by Ericsson and Lehmann (1996). Extraordinarily skilled musicians therefore exert a great deal more effort and concentration during their practice than less skilled musicians, and are more likely to plan, imagine, monitor and control their playing by focusing their attention on what they are practising and how it can be improved. Furthermore, they can be eager to build up a network of supportive peers, frequently involving family and friends.

Skills musicians must develop include not only the ability to reliably recall movement sequences, exhibiting both temporal and spatial precision, but also performative qualities and expressing emotional authenticity (Akkermans et al., 2019). Life-long continuous practice is necessary not only to acquire these expert musical skills, but also to maintain them. In the professional domain, making music consistently demands peak performance under intense social scrutiny and therefore needs well-planned recovery processes.

Some physiological and psychological aspects of professional musicianship

Musicians do not generally face elevated health risks and should not be stigmatised or perceived as particularly prone to illness; however, as in athletes, the quality of performance relies on physical and mental health and on general well-being. Therefore, the unique demands of their musical development and professional activities necessitate customised prevention programmes and specialised medical care:

- Although musicians are not affected by fundamentally different diseases than non-musicians (Zalpour et al., 2021), the localisation and manifestation of their health issues often follow patterns specific to their musical activity (i.e., nerve compression syndromes due to wrist position when playing the instrument) or the associated working environment (i.e., narrow seating, loudness).
- Concerning instrument design, playing techniques, and work environments, ergonomic conditions often fail to align with the natural physical capabilities of the human body. Instrumental performance can therefore be associated with considerable musculoskeletal strain, depending on the individual's constitution, posture, playing style, repertoire, and actual workplace. For singers, factors such as poor stage conditions, stage directions and non-physiological vocal demands of a role can result in excessive vocal strain (Norris, 1993).
- Musical instrument playing and singing push physical and mental limits. It involves intricate, rapid sequences of movement, precisely predetermined in timing and spatial precision, and relies on the unique interplay of motor function, sensory processing, the auditory system, timing, memory, and emotions (Furuya & Altenmüller, 2015). Furthermore, practising and performing are associated with an overall strain in terms of physical endurance, a factor that is often underestimated. Long hours of daily practice are required, and usually both practising and performing must be sustained over decades. This is a key distinction from athletes who frequently retire early (Dick et al., 2013).
- This balance of perfection in sensorimotor extremes is highly susceptible to disruption and can be impaired by even minor changes in muscle tone, fatigue, emotional states, metabolic fluctuations, or the effects of medication (Zão et al., 2025). Even minimal functional impairments of physiological systems often first become evident during music-making, directly affecting the quality of professional performance. However, performance quality is subject to continuous monitoring. Consequently, health-related performance declines not only have the potential to compromise professional status but are also the source of anxieties (Kenny et al., 2018).
- Due to a socialisation that has usually focused on music since childhood, professional musicians define themselves strongly through their artistic abilities. Consequently, issues that affect their performance result in significant distress and anxiety (Sickert et al., 2022).

In summary, probably no other profession demands such complex skills over a span of six to seven decades, while maintaining consistent peak performance that is evaluated by external observers.

Musicians' health issues and strategies for recovery

Lifetime prevalence of playing-related medical problems can amount up to 80% of professional instrumental musicians (Elam et al., 2022). The most common complaints are playing-related musculoskeletal disorders (PRMDs) and pain syndromes, psychological disorders – in particular performance anxiety (Spahn et al., 2002) – and neurological conditions, namely nerve compression syndromes and focal dystonia. Diseases of the vocal tract are more prevalent in singers; however, hoarseness and laryngeal pain may also occur in wind instrumentalists. Noise-related hearing deterioration, chronic tinnitus, internal diseases, dental, ophthalmological, or dermatological diseases also play a role. Like occupational medicine, musician's medicine extends across the entire spectrum of medical specialities. For an exhaustive overview of medical problems in musicians we refer to the textbook *Performing Arts Medicine* by Sataloff et al. (2010).

Playing-related musculoskeletal disorders

PRMDs are very common in musicians. PRMD is commonly used as an umbrella term that comprises musculoskeletal disorders and musculoskeletal pain. Fishbein et al. (1988) included 2,212 of a total of 4,025 musicians surveyed from 48 US professional orchestras in a questionnaire focusing on playing-related pain complaints. Of these, 49% reported musculoskeletal pain, which was localised differently depending on the instrument and the postural workload. In a more recent study of 408 musicians from ten German orchestras, approximately 40% complained of frequent or constant pain associated with playing their instruments, and up to 43% reported more than five affected pain regions over more than three months, indicating a high rate of chronification (Steinmetz et al., 2015). Women were found to be at a higher risk of experiencing playing-related pain than men. This is consistent with data from general pain research (Dao & LeResche, 2000). Interestingly, these numbers and gender distribution do not only hold for classical musicians, but also for jazz, rock and pop musicians (Stanhope & Weinstein, 2020).

Recovery from PRMDs needs a multimodal approach, especially in chronic conditions, defined as lasting more than three months. A key requirement is to take and to make time for it. The first step is to interrupt or stop the stressful activity to terminate or at least reduce the stress which provoked PRMDs. Important is reflection about the PRMDs provoking stressful events. These are frequently 'overuse-injuries', namely practising a too demanding repertoire too long without pauses. Information must be given about general mechanisms provoking pain and strategies to overcome pain, especially with respect to 'overwriting' pain-memory. Additionally, supportive psychotherapy should be offered to reduce frustration, anxieties, anger, and shame linked to the inability to perform, and to rebuild self-confidence and optimism (Ioannou et al., 2018). Furthermore, return to playing should start early. As soon as the pain subsides, the instrument should be played again as an active recovery approach. Here, starting with several five-to-ten-minute practice sessions spread throughout the day is beneficial. Technically simpler pieces that are demanding in terms of sound quality and involve a wide range of movements are suitable for this. Each practice session should end before more severe pain occurs, but at the same time an attempt is made to gradually extend the practice time. Mental practice is highly effective and helps to quickly rebuild the repertoire (Bernardi et al., 2013). In addition, methods such as *Feldenkrais* or the *Alexander Technique* are used to improve body awareness and normalise the restricted movement patterns when making music. Physiotherapy with expertise in musicians, especially manual therapy, is often recommended to restore mobility in muscles and joints and to create the necessary fluidity of movement sequences when making music. In addition, the recovery process can be supported by antidepressant medication heightening pain thresholds in the central nervous system and promoting learning processes (Zamorano et al., 2015). In summary, active recovery strategies and increasing resilience by overcoming negative emotions, building up confidence, self-efficacy and a self-concept of enabling to return to work is the general path, how resilience is put into practice in PRMDs.

Performance anxiety

A common psychosocial reaction among professional musicians is performance anxiety (Kenny, 2023). Symptoms of performance anxiety occur at the cognitive, emotional, physical, and behavioural levels (Kenny, 2011). Summarising, the causes of performance anxiety are diverse and individual. In addition to preparation for the performance, practice, performance experience, audience characteristics, and physical and emotional-biographical factors play a role. According to the learning theory model, performance anxiety can also arise after bad reviews or unsuccessful performances through the rules of classical and instrumental conditioning. Music educators should therefore try to avoid negative performance experiences (Fernholz et al., 2019). In our experience, one of the most destructive causes of performance anxiety, especially in highly successful musicians is dysfunctional perfectionism, characterised by excessively high standards, unrealistic expectations for oneself or others, and the belief that anything less than perfect is unacceptable. These beliefs are frequently linked to the fear of failure and mistakes, which are seen as a sign of personal worthlessness (Alpheis et al., 2022). Overgeneralised self-criticism is frequently learned in training institutions, since criticising a performance is frequently part of traditional teaching strategies (Arbinaga, 2023).

Recent studies on the treatment of severe performance anxiety have shown some success of such programmes, with a significant decrease in anxiety parameters, especially if it is client-tailored and problem-oriented (Spahn et al., 2016). Coaching strategies adapted from sports (Lubert et al., 2023) and an awareness of 'self-compassion', i.e., treating oneself well (Frost et al., 2024), are nowadays part of the toolbox for dealing with performance anxiety.

Recovery strategies and building of resilience for performance anxiety include basic information about stress reactions and performance, a positive communication style, constructive handling of mistakes, stage presence training using video feedback and performance evaluation, and teaching meaningful preparation methods. In addition, there is a broad spectrum of cognitive, mental, behavioural, and physical measures, accompanied by relaxation techniques, which should be implemented from the beginning of professional training at the music schools. Multimodal intervention programmes and simulation settings of performance situations are widely used, including the use of virtual reality (Bellinger et al., 2023; Gómez-López & Sánchez-Cabrero, 2023). With respect to the ability to support the stresses of performing in public under scrutiny of the audiences, the development of a positive self-concept is important. This includes the implementation of self-care, rest, social networks, hobbies and a strong sense of meaningfulness and connectedness (Bengel & Lyssenko, 2012).

Musicians' dystonia

Musicians' dystonia ('musicians' cramp') is characterised by the degradation or loss of fine motor control of movements that require a high degree of temporal and spatial precision. Its lifetime prevalence among German musicians is between 2% and 5% (Dressler et al., 2022). This movement disorder occurs task-specifically during music-making, affects usually hand or embouchure, and is mostly not linked to pain, although perception of strain while playing is not unusual. Symptoms of hand dystonia often manifest in involuntary curling or spreading of individual fingers during instrumental playing. For brass players, unreliable control of intonation in a particular pitch register can be the first sign of embouchure dystonia. When fully developed, the diagnosis is easy to make by examining the musician while playing the instrument. The remaining neurological and neuroradiological findings are unremarkable (Altenmüller & Jabusch, 2009).

The cause of the disease is multifactorial and lies in a disruption of the central nervous system's sensorimotor control programmes. It is presently considered a neural network disease, involving the sensorimotor and the limbic pathways in the brain (Alpheis et al., 2023). Consequently, a task-specific lack of balance between inhibition and excitation of neural networks leads to task-related overshooting motor activation of critical muscle groups involved in high-resolution temporo-spatial control during playing. Younger men, classical musicians, guitarists and pianists are most often affected. Among other things, starting to play an instrument late and a tendency towards anxiety and perfectionism are considered risk factors (Altenmüller et al., 2015).

For recovery, a long-term perspective and time must be taken. Since the disorder develops because of a period of maladaptive learning, prompted and aggravated by a complex set of risk factors, some of these, such as genetic predisposition, are impliable. Others, such as practice organisation and strategies, general performance-related health, and psychosocial factors within the learning environment, are malleable and can be positively influenced in educational settings (Detari & Altenmüller, in press). In other words, resilience to protect against musician's dystonia can be taught. Reduction of perfectionist attitudes, general well-being, and strategies to cope with stressors are the bases of the recovery according to our understanding.

For convalescence, retraining, and sensory-motor unlearning of the dysfunctional movement patterns stored firmly in procedural memory needs months to years (Ackermann & Altenmüller, 2021). At the beginning of the retraining process, creative artistic research into new functional movement patterns at the instrument under heightened self-awareness is useful. This is accompanied by slow-down exercises, followed by stepwise increasing tempo of movements under scrutiny of proprioception and audition, avoiding subjective feelings of tension and degraded sound quality (Altenmüller et al., 2015; Enke & Poskey, 2018). Thus, 70% of musicians who have suffered dystonia stay in their profession (Lee et al., 2015).

Prevention

The distinctive background and unique characteristics of music learning and professional music-making, along with the associated health issues faced by musicians, clearly underscore the necessity for health services tailored to the particular needs and working conditions of musicians. To address the challenges of recovery and well-being throughout an artist's career, salutogenetic approaches must be prioritised. The key questions in this context are:

- Which factors contribute to musicians' health and resilience?
- What health-related elements positively influence the development of artistic potential?
- What fosters sustained motivation for practice and performance?
- Which mechanisms support full and lasting recovery from physical and mental strain or illness in musicians?

Adopting our salutogenetic understanding of recovery, which is not only a process of replenishing resources but also a resource that generates resilience, sustained well-being in musicians requires multidisciplinary and systemic approaches. It touches the areas of prevention, expert diagnostics and treatment, as well as research. Prevention clearly stands out as the most effective long-term strategy and must remain the top priority in performing arts healthcare (Araújo & Spahn, 2022).

The key preventive strategies for musicians can be outlined as follows:

- *Adapting posture, ergonomics, playing technique, and repertoire* to individual physical conditions. It is imperative to identify and respect potentially unfavourable individual factors, such as biomechanical restrictions or unique physical characteristics.

  A collection of ergonomic equipment for musicians is available from Bertsch (2021).
- *Preventing myofascial overload and muscular imbalances* through regular physical training, which should include
  - Exercises for mobilisation, coordination, gentle stretching, and gentle strengthening (Türk-Espitalier, 2016),
  - Routine full-body as well as instrumental/vocal warm-ups before, and cool-down exercises after playing or singing (BAPAM, n.d.; Türk-Espitalier, 2016).
- *Avoiding playing through pain,* as a 'no pain, no gain' mentality poses significant physical and mental risks and is ultimately counterproductive (Stanhope et al., 2022).
- *Gradual increase of practice time* for new techniques, repertoire, or instruments.
- *Eliminating ineffective or harmful practice methods* but ensuring that practice routines are efficient, healthy, and conducive to progress (Araújo et al., 2017; Breaden Madden et al., 2023; Passarotto et al., 2023; Williams, 2017).
- *Using mental training and coaching strategies* to enhance focus and support stability.
- *Improving body awareness* by techniques such as the Alexander Technique, Feldenkrais®, or Dispokinesis to develop more efficient and economical movements.
- *Practising relaxation techniques* such as Progressive Muscle Relaxation, Autogenic Training, or Mindfulness-Based Techniques, to reduce stress and support physical and mental recovery.
- *Performing regular workouts* to improve general fitness and body coordination, which in turn will positively impact instrumental and vocal

coordination. Regular physical exercise also offers strong benefits for mental well-being and recovery.

Health prevention for musicians is only effective when based on several key pillars. This approach may be conceptualised as the *Musicians' Triad of Well-being* (Figure 6.1) and obviously is of particular significance during advanced musical education and professional practice. The following three levels are integrated within this triad, reflecting the need for systemic approaches to recovery and well-being in the performing arts:

1 Workplace/university characteristics (Table 6.1)
2 Organisational, structural, team-related factors (Table 6.2)
3 The individual's health-related behaviours and self-care (Table 6.3)

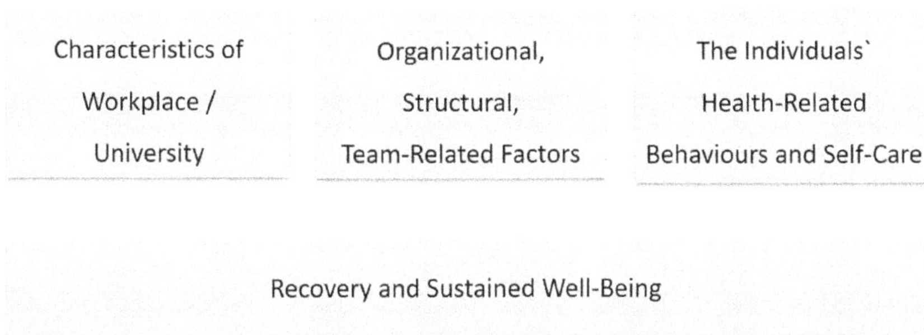

FIGURE 6.1 The Musicians' triad of well-being.

TABLE 6.1 Workplace and university characteristics.

• Adequate workload management and organisation of rehearsal schedules, teaching duties, and school projects
• Increased decision-making latitude and participation within the orchestra/school/university
• Support for individual growth and musical development, and integration of personal or group projects
• Optimisation of health-related factors in the workplace, including ergonomic conditions of the orchestra setting
• Step-by-step occupational reintegration following illness or rehabilitation
• Partial retirement options
• Fostering a culture of tolerance and respect
• Providing information on musicians' health and access to healthcare resources
• Implementing music physiology and psychological care in music university curricula

TABLE 6.2 Organisational, structural, and team-related factors.

- Job security, financial stability, and transparency
- Managerial behaviour that is communicative, appreciative, and aligned with team values
- Institutional/orchestra communication culture
- Conflict management strategies
- Supervision and coaching can be beneficial, but must be specifically tailored to the institution's/orchestra's needs
- Freelance financial and retirement protection
- Financial resources for prevention and psychological services at music universities
- Flexibility in study procedures and examination modalities for students with special health conditions/problems

TABLE 6.3 The individual's health-related behaviour and self-care.

To support recovery and resilience, self-care needs to be taken seriously and put into practice:

- Implementing active, pro-active, and passive recovery strategies, tailored to one's individual needs. These include balancing one's body through exercise and proper nutrition, as well as engaging in mental well-being practices
- Cultivating and sustaining social relationships
- Responding to new situations and opportunities with openness, flexibility, and creativity
- Finding musical/pedagogical activities outside one's job on stage, in the orchestra or in school
- Maintaining and fostering one's love of music and of performance
- Finding genuine areas of interest and individual success to enhance self-esteem and self-motivation
- Analysing, recognising, and respecting individual strengths, weaknesses, and sensitivities
- Analysing success as well as failure constructively

How should prevention be applied and integrated into the different stages of a musician's career?

Long-term effectiveness demands early prevention. Therefore, early music education for children must already incorporate and adhere to the principles of musician-specific prevention. This implies that music pedagogues should have a fundamental understanding of music physiology (Gembris et al., 2020).

With the onset of professional training, psychological attention for students and music physiology – in terms of early information, sensitisation, prevention, and intervention – needs to be intensified: implementing well-structured musicians' health programmes at music universities plays a crucial role in our efforts to promote specialised care for the lasting recovery and sustained well-being of musicians. The objective of these programmes is twofold: firstly, they focus on the personal, physical, and mental health of our students. Awareness of the underlying physiological processes in playing and singing, along with an understanding of the psychological contexts involved, are prerequisites for lifelong healthy practising and performing and for developing personal health-promoting strategies. Secondly, they seek to expand the students' pedagogical concepts as prospective music teachers. Equipping our music students with a basic understanding of music physiology will ensure they are well prepared for health-oriented music education from the outset of a child's musical training. They can then integrate the knowledge they have acquired into their own teaching of children, adolescents, or adults. This gradual process helps to close the circle, ensuring that music physiology is consistently applied in music schools and will become an integral part of music education.

We also need a range of continuing education opportunities for both employed and freelance music teachers. Pedagogues, who did not receive training in music physiology during their own studies, should have access to these fundamental concepts. In general, comprehensive and state-of-the-art courses on musicians' physical and mental health should be made available to all music teachers. In addition, there should be ample opportunity for specific training in methods such as body awareness, mental training, and relaxation techniques to ensure a broad perspective on health and well-being in music education and performance. Meanwhile, there are several valuable training opportunities in music physiology/musicians' health for professional musicians. Most of these are one-off events, but there are also certificate courses in Germany and Austria as well as two new master's programmes in Zürich (Switzerland) and Freiburg (Germany).

The orchestra comes with even more and very specific challenges – therefore we also need an array of health-focused workshops and support for orchestra musicians and conductors.

The role of musicians' health programmes at music universities

Music physiology is defined by its multiple interfaces and multidisciplinary approaches from the fields of medicine, psychology, music pedagogy, neuroscience, and sports science. So, music universities are clearly the place where music physiology and psychological attention are most important and can have the most formative impact on musicians' current and future well-being and resilience: university years represent a period when the still very young performers face significant artistic, physical, and mental challenges while also being highly receptive and willing to learn!

In designing musicians' health concepts for music universities, we must always consider the key question: how can we best support our students in their artistic and personal development? This goal cannot be achieved solely through diagnosing and treating playing-/singing-related conditions, nor does a purely preventive approach fully address the issue. Long-lasting, resilience-building support for music students goes beyond these measures – it means taking a distinctly holistic approach to their well-being and recovery.

The role of music physiology and musicians' health at our universities should be to:

- Raise students' awareness of the physical, emotional, and mental aspects of music-making,
- teach prevention strategies and foster self-responsibility for physical and mental well-being,
- educate on the intersections of music pedagogy, music physiology, musicians' health, and psychology,
- ensure medical and therapeutic help if necessary,
- provide individual guidance and support, emphasising learning facilitation, resource-oriented approaches, personal growth, and resilience.

This requires well-balanced programmes with a comprehensive concept tailored to the respective institution and infrastructure. Programmes must aim at all students, regardless of their chosen major – whether it is music pedagogy, orchestra, or soloist. They must include a compulsory, comprehensive introductory course on music physiology and musicians' health, spanning one to two semesters, and should be further complemented by elective in-depth seminars, classes on various body-oriented techniques, psychologically focused courses, and individual counselling opportunities.

The introductory course should be taught by physicians or psychologists with extensive expertise in the physical and psychological demands of playing musical instruments and singing. They should also have a deep understanding of the unique aspects of music studies and the music professions. The course follows a clinical-scientific approach, yet with a strong emphasis on functional correlations, relevance for musicians, and practical application. It provides basic knowledge of music physiology and efficient learning, along with the principles of healthy practising and performing. Lessons cover a wide range of topics, such as the characteristics of muscle activity and sensorimotor functions in music-making, the physiological capabilities and limits of posture and movement, responses to fatigue, overall principles of prevention, musicians' hearing and hearing protection, music performance anxiety, coordination skills, effective practice strategies, and specific considerations for teaching both seniors and the very young beginners. The 'Music Physiology Curriculum' suggested by the German Association for Music Physiology and Musicians' Medicine (DGfMM) is a valuable resource.

Over the past three decades, most music universities in Germany, Austria, and Switzerland have gradually introduced a range of compulsory and elective courses covering both fundamental and advanced topics in music physiology, often complemented by individual musicians' medicine counselling. While some universities also provide psychological support, there remains a notable gap in this area.

Having physicians and therapists based directly at universities of music has proven immensely beneficial, as it enables direct and immediate interaction with students, faculty, and staff. It is very helpful for students to know that they can easily access support within a protected setting on campus and under medical confidentiality. This low threshold also encourages students to seek help for physical and mental issues at a much earlier stage. In this context, it is worth noting that a considerable number of consultations for music students are not specifically related to musicians' health, but rather general student health. But all problems and stressors tend to have an early negative effect on the sensitive system involved in practising and performing in these young artists, may it be financial hardship, homesickness, a sense of uprootedness among international students, relationship strain, the additional burden of being a family caregiver, etc.

Networking both within and beyond the university is a crucial aspect for physicians and psychologists responsible for musicians' health at the respective institution: for individualised student support, exchange with university lecturers, Deans of Studies, and administrators is often beneficial or necessary. Some challenges faced by individual students are best addressed by joint efforts of the physician or psychologist and the respective pedagogue. Also, consultation with university administration may be necessary for matters such as disadvantage compensation, study exemptions, study extensions, and (partial) exam postponements. Given the wide range of medical complaints including psychological issues, referring students to external specialists and therapists is an elementary task of the attending physician.

Research: The foundation for advancements in musicians' health and well-being

A strong scientific basis is crucial for the advancement of effective prevention strategies and the development of state-of-the-art applied medicine for musicians. Over the past three decades, research in music physiology, musicians' medicine and psychology, and health-oriented music pedagogy has expanded significantly, leading to noticeable improvements in musicians' healthcare. However, there are still gaps in both clinical and basic research that need to be addressed. These include practice efficiency, music performance anxiety, neurological conditions such as chronic pain syndromes and focal dystonia, and hearing protection in the orchestra and on stage. Furthermore, there is a critical need for research on resilience and effective recovery strategies for musicians. Instrumentalists and singers face an increasingly competitive and perfection-driven professional environment, which fosters the development of anxiety, self-doubt, self-devaluation, and dissatisfaction. Long-term, multicentre research projects would be beneficial for advancing progress on these complex issues.

Conclusions and recommendations for practice

To prevent health issues and to support recovery to performance in professional musicians, we need to establish an alliance of scientists, physicians, psychologists, therapists, pedagogues, and experienced musicians. Prevention begins with the very first music lesson in childhood. It starts with the fundamentals, such as choosing the right instrument, ensuring it is the right size, teaching the proper posture and, above all, instilling a culture of practising. Music teachers and parents are the primary sources of support for healthy, joyful learning and music-making.

On the path to professionalisation in young adulthood, it is important to advise highly motivated young musicians appropriately and, in particular, to protect them from overuse due to pieces or performances that are too difficult or excessive practice times. Music teachers also have a role to play here.

Music physiology lessons are important at music colleges and music universities, and the topics should include not only physical prevention, stretching exercises, warming up and cooling down, but also stress management, dealing with failure, efficient practice techniques and mental preparation. Information about preventing or reducing performance anxiety is an absolute must during studies, as it is still the most frequently cited problem affecting the quality of life of young musicians.

For recovery, it is important to create suitable schedules and working structures during studies and in professional life. This includes guaranteeing free time during studies or professional activities to ensure adequate recovery periods. It is particularly important to provide emotional support to musicians after injuries, as such events are often accompanied by feelings of guilt, shame, anxiety and loss of self-esteem. Here, it is important to provide psychological support for musicians if needed and wanted.

In summary, interdisciplinary, research-based, and holistic healthcare concepts must be an integral part of academic training at music universities, as these institutions aim to prepare students for their future careers. By closely mentoring music students and raising their awareness of musicians' health principles, we can help build a solid foundation for managing both professional and personal stress, ultimately promoting long-term well-being and resilience.

References

Ackermann, B. J., & Altenmüller, E. (2021). The development and use of an anatomy-based retraining program (MusAARP) to assess and treat focal hand dystonia in musicians – A pilot study. *Journal of Hand Therapy*, *34*(2), 309–314.

Akkermans, J., Schapiro, R., Müllensiefen, D., Jakubowski, K., Shanahan, D., Baker, D., Busch, V., Lothwesen, K., Elvers, P., Fischinger, T., Schlemmer, K., & Frieler, K. (2019). Decoding emotions in expressive music performances: A multi-lab replication and extension study. *Cognition & Emotion*, *33*(6), 1099–1118.

Alpheis, S., Altenmüller, E., & Scholz, D. S. (2022). Influence of adverse childhood experiences and perfectionism on musician's dystonia: A case control study. *Tremor and other Hyperkinetic Movements*, *12*, 8. https://doi.org/10.5334/tohm.687

Alpheis, S., Altenmüller, E., & Scholz, D. S. (2023). Focal dystonia and the stress network: The role of stress vulnerability and adverse childhood experiences in the development of musician's dystonia. *Advances in Neurobiology*, *31*, 23–44.

Altenmüller, E., Ioannou, C. I., & Lee, A. (2015). Apollo's curse: Neurological causes of motor impairments in musicians. *Progress in Brain Research*, *217*, 89–106.

Altenmüller, E., & Jabusch, H. C. (2009). Focal hand dystonia in musicians: Phenomenology, etiology, and psychological trigger factors. *Journal of Hand Therapy*, *22*, 144–154.

Araújo, L. S., & Spahn, C. (2022). Promoting health-related lifestyle. In G. McPherson (Ed.), *The Oxford handbook of music performance* (Vol. 2, pp. 279–308). Oxford University Press.

Araújo, L. S., Wasley, D., Perkins, R., Atkins, L., Redding, E., Ginsborg, J., & Williamon, A. (2017). Fit to perform: An investigation of higher education music students' perceptions, attitudes, and behaviors toward health. *Frontiers in Psychology*, *8*, 1558. https://doi.org/10.3389/fpsyg.2017.01558

Arbinaga, F. (2023). Resilient behaviors in music students: Relationship with perfectionism and self-efficacy. *Behavioral Sciences*, *13*, 722. https://doi.org/10.3390/bs13090722

BAPAM Performing Arts Medicine. (n.d.). *Don't cramp your style*. Retrieved March 04, 2025 from https://www.bapam.org.uk/dont-cramp-your-style/

Beckmann, J., Kellmann, M., & Jakowski, S. (2023). Recovery is more than just healing: Advocating a broader perspective on recovery in physical and mental health. In M. Kellmann, S. Jakowski, & J. Beckmann (Eds.), *The importance of recovery for physical and mental health: Negotiating the effects of underrecovery* (pp. 266–270). Routledge.

Bellinger, D., Wehrmann, K., Rohde, A., Schuppert, M., Störk, S., Flohr-Jost, M., Gall, D., Pauli, P., Deckert, J., Herrmann, M. J., & Erhardt-Lehmann, A. (2023). The application of virtual reality exposure versus relaxation training in music performance anxiety: A randomized controlled study. *BMC Psychiatry*, *23*(1), 555. https://doi.org/10.1186/s12888-023-05040-z

Bengel, J., & Lyssenko, L. (2012). *Resilienz und psychologische Schutzfaktoren im Erwachsenenalter. Stand der Forschung zu psychologischen Schutzfaktoren von Gesundheit im Erwachsenenalter* [Resilience and psychological protective factors in adulthood. State of research on psychological protective factors of health in adulthood]. Forschung und Praxis der Gesundheitsförderung (Bd. 43). Bundeszentrale für gesundheitliche Aufklärung.

Bernardi, N. F., De Buglio, M., Trimarchi, P. D., Chielli, A., & Bricolo, E. (2013). Mental practice promotes motor anticipation: Evidence from skilled music performance. *Frontiers in Human Neuroscience*, *7*, 451. https://doi.org/10.3389/fnhum.2013.00451

Bertsch, M. (2021). *ERGO collection for musicians*. Retrieved March 04, 2025 from https://matthias-bertsch.at/Downloads/MB-PDF/2021e_Bertsch_ERGO-Collection-for-Musicians.pdf

Breaden Madden, G., Herff, S. A., Beveridge, S., & Jabusch, H.-C. (2023). Emotional cherry-picking: The role of personality and goal orientation in selective emotion regulation for musical practice. *Frontiers in Psychology*, *14*, 1201442. https://doi.org/10.3389/fpsyg.2023.1201442

Dao, T. T., & LeResche, L. (2000). Gender differences in pain. *Journal of Orofacial Pain*, *14*(3), 169–184.

Detari, A., & Altenmüller, E.(in press) Preventing musician's focal dystonia: A guide for music educators. *Internation Journal of Music Education*. https://doi.org/10.1177/02557614251339548

Dick, R. W., Berning, J. R., Dawson, W., Ginsburg, R. D., Miller, C., & Shybut, G. T. (2013). Athletes and the arts – The role of sports medicine in the performing arts. *Current Sports Medicine Reports*, *12*(6), 397–403.

Dressler, D., Altenmüller, E., Giess, R., Krauss, J. K., & Adib Saberi, F. (2022). The epidemiology of dystonia: The Hannover epidemiology study. *Journal of Neurology*, *269*, 6483–6493.

Elam, T., Mowen, S., & Jonas, C. (2022). Occupational injuries in musicians: A literature review. *Military Medicine*, *187*, e619–e623.

Enke, A. M., & Poskey, G. A. (2018). Neuromuscular re-education programs for musicians with focal hand dystonia: A systematic review. *Medical Problems of Performing Artists*, *33*(2), 137–145.

Ericsson, K. A., Krampe, R. T., & Tesch-Römer, C. (1993). The role of deliberate practice in the acquisition of expert performance. *Psychological Review*, *100*(3), 363–406.

Ericsson, K. A., & Lehmann, A. C. (1996). Expert and exceptional performance: Evidence of maximal adaptation to task constraints. *Annual Review of Psychology*, *47*, 273–305.

Fernholz, I., Mumm, J. L. M., Plag, J., Noeres, K., Rotter, G., Willich, S. N., Ströhle, A., Berghöfer, A., & Schmidt, A. (2019). Performance anxiety in professional musicians: A systematic review on prevalence, risk factors, and clinical treatment effects. *Psychological Medicine*, *49*(14), 2287–2306.

Fishbein, M., Middlestadt, S., Ottati, V., Straus, S., & Ellis, A. (1988). Medical problems among ICSOM musicians: Overview of a national survey. *Medical Problems of Performing Artists*, *3*, 1–8.

Frost, J., Walton, C. C., Purcell, R., Fisher, K., Gwyther, K., Kocherginsky, M., & Rice, S. M. (2024). The mental health of elite-level coaches: A systematic scoping review. *Sports Medicine - Open*, *10*, 16. https://doi.org/10.1186/s40798-023-00655-8

Furuya, S., & Altenmüller, E. (2015). Acquisition and reacquisition of motor coordination in musicians. *Annals of the New York Academy of Sciences*, *1337*, 118–124.

Gembris, H., Menze, J., Heye, A., & Bullerjahn, C. (2020). High-performing young musicians' playing-related pain: Results of a large-scale study. *Frontiers in Psychology*, *11*, 564736. https://doi.org/10.3389/fpsyg.2020.564736

Gómez-López, B., & Sánchez-Cabrero, R. (2023). Current trends in music performance anxiety intervention. *Behavioral Sciences*, *13*, 720. https://doi.org/10.3390/bs13090720

Hambrick, D. Z., Macnamara, B. N., & Oswald, F. L. (2020). Is the deliberate practice view defensible? A review of evidence and discussion of issues. *Frontiers in Psychology*, *11*, 1134. https://doi.org/10.3389/fpsyg.2020.01134

Ioannou, C. I., Hafer, J., Lee, A., & Altenmüller, E. (2018). Epidemiology, treatment efficacy, and anxiety aspects of music students affected by playing-related pain: A retrospective evaluation with follow-up. *Medical Problems of Performing Artists*, *33*, 26–38.

Kallus, K. W. (2016). Stress and recovery: An overview. In K. W. Kallus & M. Kellmann (Eds.), *The Recovery-Stress Questionnaires: User manual* (pp. 27–48). Pearson Assessment.

Kenny, D. T. (2011). *The psychology of music performance anxiety*. Oxford University Press.

Kenny, D. T. (2023). The Kenny music performance anxiety inventory (K-MPAI): Scale construction, cross-cultural validation, theoretical underpinnings, and diagnostic and therapeutic utility. *Frontiers in Psychology*, *14*, 1143359. https://doi.org/10.3389/fpsyg.2023.1143359

Kenny, D. T., Driscoll, T., & Ackermann, B. J. (2018). Effects of aging on musical performance in professional orchestral musicians. *Medical Problems of Performing Artists*, *33*(1), 39–46.

Lee, A., Eich, C., Ioannou, C. I., & Altenmüller, E. (2015). Life satisfaction of musicians with focal dystonia. *Occupational Medicine*, *65*, 380–385.

Lubert, V. J., Nordin-Bates, S. M., & Gröpel, P. (2023). Effects of tailored interventions for anxiety management in choking-susceptible performing artists: A mixed-methods collective case study. *Frontiers in Psychology*, *14*, 1164273. https://doi.org/10.3389/fpsyg.2023.1164273

Norris, R. N. (1993). Applied ergonomics: Adaptive equipment and instrument modification for musicians. *Maryland Medical Journal*, *42*, 271–275.

Passarotto, E., Worschech, F., & Altenmüller, E. (2023). The effect of anxiety on practice behaviours and performance quality in expert pianists. *Frontiers in Psychology*, *14*, 1152900. https://doi.org/10.3389/fpsyg.2023.1152900

Sataloff, R. T., Brandfonbremer, A. G., & Lederman, R. (2010). *Performing arts medicine* (3rd ed.). Science & Medicine Inc.

Sickert, C., Klein, J. P., Altenmüller, E., & Scholz, D. S. (2022). Low self-esteem and music performance anxiety can predict depression in musicians. *Medical Problems of Performing Artists*, *37*(4), 213–220.

Spahn, C., Richter, B., & Zschocke, I. (2002). Health attitudes, preventive behavior, and playing-related health problems among music students. *Medical Problems of Performing Artists*, *17*, 22–28.

Spahn, C., Walther, J. C., & Nusseck, M. (2016). The effectiveness of a multimodal concept of audition training for music students in coping with music performance anxiety. *Psychology of Music*, *44*, 893–909.

Stanhope, J., Pisaniello, D., & Weinstein, P. (2022). The effect of strategies to prevent and manage musicians' musculoskeletal symptoms: A systematic review. *Archives of Environmental & Occupational Health*, *77*(3), 185–208.

Stanhope, J., & Weinstein, P. (2020). Why do we need to investigate non-classical musicians to reduce the burden of musicians' musculoskeletal symptoms? *Industrial Health*, *58*, 212–223.

Steinmetz, A., Scheffer, I., Esmer, E., Delank, K. S., & Peroz, I. (2015). Frequency, severity and predictors of playing-related musculoskeletal pain in professional orchestral musicians in Germany. *Clinical Rheumatology*, *34*, 965–973.

Türk-Espitalier, A. (2016). *Musicians in motion: 100 exercises with and without instrument*. Musikverlag Zimmermann.

Williams, S. (2017). *Quality practice: A musician's guide*. Retrieved March 04, 2025 from https://quality-practice.com/

Zalpour, C., Ballenberger, N., & Avermann, F. A. (2021). Physiotherapeutic approach to musicians' health: Data from 614 patients from a physiotherapy clinic for musicians (INAP/O). *Frontiers in Psychology*, *12*, 568684. https://doi.org/10.3389/fpsyg.2021.568684

Zamorano, A. M., Riquelme, I., Kleber, B., Altenmüller, E., Hatem, S. M., & Montoya, P. (2015). Pain sensitivity and tactile spatial acuity are altered in healthy musicians as in chronic pain patients. *Frontiers in Human Neuroscience*, *8*, 1016. https://doi.org/10.3389/fnhum.2014.01016

Zão, A., Altenmüller, E., & Azevedo, L. (2025). Factors associated with performance-related pain among musicians: A multicenter study using validated tools. *Journal of Occupational Rehabilitation*, *35*, 556–577.

7

DANCE INJURY

Psychological and psychosocial factors in prevention, recovery, and return to performance

Lynda Mainwaring

Introduction

Intrapersonal, interpersonal, and sociocultural factors influence the onset of injury (Tranaeus et al., 2022) as well as recovery from injury. How dancers think, behave, feel, and interact with others affect the entire injury and recovery process often without regard to the psychological and psychosocial factors. Psychological factors comprise the perception and interpretation of injury. Thus, psychological processes influence injury occurrence, healing, rehabilitation, recovery, and re-injury (Christakou et al., 2020).

According to modern understanding (World Health Organisation, 2019), recovery encompasses more than healing physical injury. The more comprehensive concept of recovery presented in this book conceptualises the recovery process as providing resources that promote ongoing health and well-being. It involves restoring a systemic balance and gaining or recapturing meaning, purpose in life and self-determination, resulting in personal empowerment and resilience (Beckmann et al., 2023). Aligned with this holistic conceptualisation of recovery, the purpose of this chapter is twofold: (1) to review theories and empirical research relevant to psychology of dance injury, and (2) to outline strategies for recovery including the prevention of injuries and re-injuries and a salubrious return to performance. Before reviewing relevant and dance-specific research, the terms prevention, recovery, and rehabilitation are defined.

Mainwaring, L. (2026). Dance injury: Psychological and psychosocial factors in prevention, recovery and return to performance. In E. Altenmüller, M. Kellmann, J. Beckmann, & G. M. Moyle (Eds.), *Recovery and well-being in the performing arts* (pp. 115–133). Routledge.

DOI: 10.4324/9781003566885-9

TABLE 7.1 Levels of prevention and examples in dance.

Construct	*Definition and focus*	*Example*	*Dance example*
Primordial prevention	To address determinants of and prevent risk factors for disease at the earliest possible point of intervention.	Public health or youth-based initiatives that promote, for example, physical activity, reduced sedentary activity, minimal or no tobacco and alcohol use. Socioeconomic policies.	Physical fitness training for strength and stamina and limiting overtraining.
Primary prevention	Initiatives to prevent the onset of illness, injury, disease or adverse events in healthy susceptible individuals before they occur.	Flu vaccinations to limit exposure risk. Health education related to diet, physical activity, or hypermobility.	Health education related to nutrition, workload, health behaviours, hypermobility and stress management.
Secondary prevention	Early disease or injury detection in healthy individuals with subclinical asymptomatic forms of a disease in the service of disease/injury prevention.	Screening for athletes with a history of repetitive hits to the head.	Screening dancers who have joint laxity or have a history of multiple hits to the head.
Tertiary prevention	Rehabilitation pursuits in individuals with illness, injury or disease to reduce the severity of illness and associated outcomes and restoring function through physical, psychological and social restoration.	Managing hypertension or diabetes through lifestyle changes, or medical management. Physical therapy to restore strength and function after a fracture.	Physical therapy to manage and restore strength and function after an ankle sprain or fracture. Pain management for chronic pain and overuse injuries.

(*Continued*)

TABLE 7.1 (Continued)

Construct	*Definition and focus*	*Example*	*Dance example*
Quaternary prevention	Initiatives taken to protect patients at risk of medical intervention that may not be needed or may cause more harm than benefit (iatrogenic) (Martins et al., 2019).	Reducing or avoiding unnecessary interventions that will lead to limited benefit.	Education (e.g., anatomy structure and function) or actions to protect dancers from medical interventions that will cause dancers more harm than good.

Prevention levels are outlined in Table 7.1 with general and dance-specific examples. Prevention ranges from the earliest way possible to limit risk of harm, injury or disease, through to managing the restorative process. The latter is tertiary prevention, also known as rehabilitation. Recovery is used here according to Kallus (2016), who described a "multilevel process in time for the re-establishment of personal resources and their full functional capacity" (p. 42).

Psychological and psychosocial risk factors for injury

The context in which dancers train, rehearse, and perform is fraught with high standards, comparisons with others, body objectification, *performance perfection* (Mainwaring, 2009), judgement, and criticism from self, significant others, teachers, and the audience (Hamilton et al., 1989; Hays, 2012, 2017; Moyle, 2019). The dance milieu is highly demanding, critical, intense, unyielding, and exerts tremendous pressure on the dancer.

The physical requirements of dance activity itself (high impact, intensity, and repetitive work), choreographic demands, and extreme workload set the stage for over exertion, fatigue, and risk of injury (Liederbach, 2000; Liederbach et al., 2013). Kadel et al. (1992) found increased injury rates among dancers exposed to more than five hours of dance per day, while Liederbach et al. (1992, 1994) reported injury was associated with fatigue, and elevated urinary catecholamine levels. Increases in injury are also associated with return to dance (RTD) after transition periods from holidays (Fuller et al., 2020) and during the end of the day or late in the performance season (De Wet, 2022; Liederbach, 2000). Recent research in sport demonstrated that athletes had a higher risk of overuse injuries when they were engaged in excessive training, training while tired, or when they perceived a decrease in personal accomplishments over three weeks of training (Tranaeus et al., 2024).

Bolling et al. (2021) reported that an imbalance between workload and capacity to cope with load was perceived by dancers as the main cause of dance injury. Workload (overload specifically) was described as complex involving dance demands, repertoire, schedules, training, and travel, all of which required a dynamic balance for injury prevention. In a review of dance research 'hot topics', high-intensity training and performance leading to fatigue was considered a primary cause of injury (Li et al., 2025). In the context of competitional sports, this has been described as an imbalance of stress (through training and competitions, and overtraining) and recovery or replenishment of resources (Kenttä & Hassmén, 1998). Lack of recovery, referred to as underrecovery has been identified as a major risk for physical and mental health problems in the sport context (Podlog et al., 2023).

There is a long history of examining the relationship between injury and fatigue in both sport (Bestwick-Stevenson et al., 2022) and dance (Dang et al., 2021; Liederbach & Compagno, 2001; Liederbach et al., 1992, 1994). Fatigue is not merely a physiological result of training; it spans psychological and behavioural aspects of training, performance, rehearsing, resting and managing workload, and has been identified as a modifiable risk factor in ballet (Campbell et al., 2019). In his book, *Conditioning for Dancers*, Welsh (2009) states "Fatigue of the whole body or of a specific muscle group can also lead dancers to engage in injurious movement patterns" (p. 26). Self-monitoring and interoception of fatigue and the body's response to load are self-regulation strategies that may benefit dancers, considering van der Sluis et al. (2019) reported that high self-monitoring protected girls from overuse injury in tennis. Similarly, Balk and Englert (2020) suggested that self-regulation skills (self-monitoring, regulation of thoughts and emotions, and engaging in self-control) are important in athletic recovery. Self-regulation skills are beneficial in both prevention of and recovery from injury, especially in terms of monitoring training and competition to avoid fatigue, inadequate recovery and risk of injury or recurrent injury.

Kenttä and Hassmén (1998) suggested that a lack of total recovery was a risk factor for athletic injury and presented a comprehensive conceptual model of overtraining and recovery that emphasised the interaction of socio-physiopsychological variables. The model specified that physiological, psychological and social stressors interact with an individual's overall capacity for stress and the overall recovery and restoration of homeostasis across systems. Brink et al. (2010) and Laux et al. (2015) identified stress and poor recovery prior to and at the time of sport injury. More specifically, van der Does et al. (2017) reported that reduced general recovery and well-being were related to a higher risk for traumatic injuries and that six weeks before injury occurred, sport-specific stress was elevated. Brink and Lemmink (2022) concluded that physical load, psychosocial stress and recovery need to be monitored over time in order to understand the complexity of the injury, stress, and recovery dynamic. Knowing the mechanisms of injury including psychological determinants may help with prevention and management.

Not only are fatigue and lack of recovery risks for injury, an athlete's history of injury, personality, life stressors and 'fewer' coping resources are also risk factors according to the most influential theoretical model in the sport psychology literature, the *Stress-Injury Model* (Williams & Andersen, 1998). High negative life stress is positively related to injury occurrence in sport (Cryan & Alles, 1983; Galambos et al., 2005; Ivarsson et al., 2017; van Mechelen et al., 1996; Wadey et al., 2019; Williams & Andersen, 1998) and dance (Adam et al., 2004; Air, 2013; Solomon & Micheli, 1986; van Winden et al., 2020, 2021). Furthermore, negative life events and dance-specific negative stress have been identified as risk factors for dance injury (Krasnow et al., 1999; Mainwaring et al., 1993; Patterson et al., 1998).

History of injury is a risk factor for musculoskeletal injury in both sport and dance (Fulton et al., 2014; Kenny et al., 2016; Toohey et al., 2017), with sport-related concussion identified as a risk factor for subsequent concussion as well as musculoskeletal injury (McCann et al., 2022; Roach et al., 2023; Wasserman et al., 2024). Despite theoretical speculation in the sport literature, personality has not been established as a risk factor for sport injury. Conversely, in dance, perfectionism (Krasnow et al., 1999), overachieving (Hamilton et al., 1989), performance identity (Bursik et al., in press) and oppressive passion for dance (Rip et al., 2006) have been related to injury and performing while hurt (Bursik et al., in press; Mayer & Thiel, 2018). Striving for perfection, meeting performance demands, and continuing to dance with injury may be part of a behavioural repertoire, or personality, that predisposes dancers to injury, protracted recovery, reinjury or exacerbation of injury.

The mosaic of personality requires understanding its nuance and complexity. Cumming and Duda (2012) determined that dancers who scored higher on concerns over mistakes and doubts about actions (two aspects of perfectionism) reported greater distress. In a replication of that work exploring different profiles of perfectionism, Nordin-Bates et al. (2017) reported that dancers with higher scores on *pure evaluative concerns perfectionism* and those with *mixed perfectionism* had greater physical and emotional exhaustion scores or more burnout symptoms than dancers with *pure person standards perfectionism* profiles. In a prospective study of athletes, those with high personal standards/striving and personal concerns were shown to have a six times higher risk of injury (De Maria et al., 2024).

In addition to the association between injury risk and perfectionism, there is a high association between perfectionism, preoccupation with bodily concerns, body image, drive for thinness, body perfectionism and dissatisfaction and eating disorders (Fittig & Jacobi, 2024; Liederbach & Compagno, 2001). Thomas et al. (2011) observed a positive relationship with reports of self-induced vomiting and a lifetime history of injury. Liederbach and Compagno (2001) reported bulimic tendencies were associated with more than one injury in university and professional ballet dancers. For adolescent ballet dancers, a greater number of lifetime disordered eating behaviours were associated with an increase of lifetime injuries (Thomas et al., 2011).

Dancers, and in particular ballet dancers and dance students, are susceptible to disordered eating (patterns of eating that do not meet the criteria for a diagnosable eating disorder) and eating disorders (Arcelus et al., 2013). In terms of eating disorders, Arcelus et al. (2013) reported that dancers had greater than three times the risk than non-dancers for developing anorexia and eating disorder not otherwise specified (i.e., atypical presentation of symptoms). The focus on the body, drive for thinness, pressure to conform to the aesthetic ideal, and the constant comparison to others make dancers vulnerable to restricted eating patterns and feeding disorders. Reel et al. (2018) reported that dancers made several eating modifications (primarily calorie restrictions) after injury, noted bodily changes during their recovery, had many concerns about relapse of a past eating disorder/s, and exhibited increased awareness of eating patterns and nutritional needs to promote recovery and healing. Reel et al. (2018) concluded that the consequences of diet restrictions, prolonged disordered eating, or eating disorders on the body (e.g., fatigue, energy deficits, menstrual dysfunction and osteoporosis) created opportunity for injuries. For example, Lambert et al. (2020) studied 112 professional ballet dancers and determined that those who self-reported meeting the criteria for disordered eating had reduced regional bone mineral density (spine and pelvis) and a higher frequency of stress fractures.

A lack of coping resources or poor ability to cope with life stress or stressors associated with dance training and performance puts dancers at risk for other maladaptive behaviours and heightened risk of injury. For example, alcohol and cigarette smoking in dancers has been related to injury (Novosel et al., 2019), while Wadey et al. (2019) reported a dose-response relationship between pre-injury adversity and coping with sport injury. Barrell et al. (2003) reported that professional and student dancers who endorsed high trait anxiety used more maladaptive or emotional-focused coping skills than those who reported low trait anxiety. Consequently, dancers who experience high levels of anxiety related to performance may not have the coping strategies to navigate performance stress, which may increase the possibility of stress-related injury.

In conjunction with personal factors, interrelated social, historical and economic factors, or external factors, may also influence injury. For example, the coronavirus pandemic (COVID-19) was a major stressor for the world's population, and dancers, in particular, experienced unprecedented stressors and deviations from their normal routines, heightened stress reactions, and reduced opportunities to dance, train, and perform (Valenzuela-Moss et al.,

2025). Consequently, during the COVID-19 pandemic there was a decrease in the prevalence of dance injuries (Barreau et al., 2025; Dang et al., 2021; Kishon & Sarig Bahat, 2023; Mattiussi et al., 2021) but there was an increase in eating disorders (Treasure, 2023). The general sense of uncertainty and threat orchestrated a high-risk environment during COVID-19, especially for those with a predisposition for anxiety (Treasure, 2023). For many dancers, the global COVID-19 pandemic resulted in social isolation, alternative and inadequate dance space (Valenzuala-Moss et al., 2025), financial worries and time to reflect on rest and recovery from injury, reduced fitness, reduced training, and restricted opportunities for dance (Kishon & Sarig Bahat, 2023; Kolitsida et al., 2023). Upon RTD post-COVID-19, injuries increased (Mattiussi et al., 2021). Harris (2021) suggested that the COVID-19 pandemic forced the dance community to re-think dance training and education and develop in-person training to reduce the risk of injury upon re-entry into dance.

Public health concerns are not the only events that impact dancers. Geopolitical unrest, uncertainty, and change itself are stressful. In particular, the tragedy, trauma, devastation, and displacement of war create multiple stressors for dancers living in war-torn zones and their families and colleagues around the world. Stressors associated with war have enormous and far-reaching implications physically and psychologically. In response to such concerns, the International Association for Dance Medicine and Science (n.d.) published an international statement of support and a resource list for dancers who may be in distress. In one of the few current studies related to war and its impact on creative artists, Ober et al. (2026) reported that despite the devastation of war in Ukraine and the reported need for financial assistance, artists were resilient, and their creative initiatives were not quelled, which highlights the devotion and passion of performing artists. It is also reminiscent of dancers' "perseverance and courageous spirit" (Eliot, 2008, p. 182) and dance in the service of 'public morale', 'respite' and 'delicate relief' and 'diversion' (Eliot, 2008) from the disruption and tragedies of World War II.

Psychological and psychosocial factors and recovery from injury

Reactions to, and recovery from, injury vary according to personal (internal) and situation (external) factors (Mainwaring et al., 2001). Following injury, dancers may experience negative thoughts and feelings such as anxiety, feelings of loss, shame, guilt (McEwan & Young, 2011), tension, confusion and bewilderment (Liederbach & Compagno, 2001), psychological distress and depression (Air, 2013), negative mood (Adam et al., 2004), intense negative emotions including frustration, sadness, reduced self-worth, and feelings of isolation and lost identity (Reel et al., 2018) or *fractured identities* and grief (Moore & Emmerich, 2024; Wainwright et al., 2005). Cahalan et al. (2015) reported that anxiety, depression, difficulty concentrating, and catastrophising were related to being severely injured, while Reel et al. (2018) reported that dancers were concerned about decreased physical prowess, weight gain, future opportunities, and social perceptions. They blamed themselves for their injuries and for separating themselves from their bodies in relation to pain. Dancers believe that they need to push themselves and that pain is a part of that process, given it was found that dancers identified injury with the limits of the body, rather than pain itself (Thomas & Tarr, 2009; Turner & Wainright, 2003).

Fernandez et al. (2023) focused specifically on modern dancers' psychological experiences of severe musculoskeletal injury and reported loss, grief, and uncertainty, which is consistent with the vast research on athletes' post-injury negative emotional reaction to injury. Also consistent with what we know about athletes, modern dancers reported seeking social support and growth experiences after injury.

Dancers continue to dance while injured are reluctant to disclose injuries (Harrison & Ruddock-Hudson, 2017) and rarely seek medical advice as they do not feel that the medical community appreciates their unique work environment nor their health care needs (Bowling, 1989; Kerr et al., 1992; Krasnow et al., 1994; Wang & Russell, 2018). Novosel et al. (2019) reported that less experienced dancers were more likely to be absent from dance post-injury than more experienced dancers. Fernandez et al. (2023) noted that 75% of the twelve dancers interviewed reported either a delayed or inaccurate diagnosis. Dancers require specialised care, and their perceptions of the healthcare system affect their decisions to access services (Keeler, 2020).

Both recovery and RTD are influenced by dynamic interactions among varied personal, social, historical, and economic factors. Biopsychosocial factors such as age; type, location, and severity of injury; dance level and genre; type of intervention; and access to dance or sport medicine specialists influence recovery as well as the onset of injury. Socio-historic contexts and factors influence dancers in many ways; for example, the world's public health outbreak COVID-19 affected dancers and injury rates both during and after the pandemic, with dancers experiencing a loss of purpose during lockdown (Moore & Emmerich, 2024), social isolation, financial concerns, physical deconditioning and persistent severe acute respiratory syndrome coronavirus 2 (SARS-CoV-2) symptoms (Barreau et al., 2025; Dang et al., 2021; Kishon & Sarig Bahat, 2023; Mattiussi et al., 2021). In short, a wide variety of factors influence recovery and RTD. The factors that lead to injury, the consequences of injury, and the interactions of extrinsic and intrinsic factors affecting recovery and RTD can be overwhelming to dancers. Helping dancers through these situations with psychological intervention can be beneficial.

Psychological considerations for returning to dance after injury

Twelve recommendations for psychological intervention to facilitate RTD and prevent, or mitigate, injury or psychological distress are described in Table 7.2. The interventions are evidence-based and related to the risk factors identified in the evidence reviewed here as well as practitioner experience and wisdom in returning dancers and athletes to elite performance.

TABLE 7.2 Psychological interventions for injured dancers and dancers returning to dance (RTD) performance.

Psychological intervention	*Brief description*	*Benefits*
Therapy referral	Referral to psychologist, psychiatrist, or treatment facility.	Appropriate treatment when justified for mental disorders.
Counselling referral	Referral to psychologist, psychiatrist, or mental health consultant for supportive counselling.	Support during or after the injury process and RTD.
Screening for psychological distress or psychiatric disorder	Brief assessment to screen for issues, such as anxiety, depression or eating disorder.	Identification of a condition for intervention or prevention.
Energy/stress management	Managing stress, improving coping, relaxation, and promotion of optimal health behaviours.	Balancing sympathetic and parasympathetic nervous system responses.
Mental skills	Sport and performance psychology skill training.	Skill retraining, confidence building and enhancing recovery, RTD and injury prevention.
Mindfulness	Focused attention on the present task and experience.	Facilitation of relaxation and focus to help manage or mitigate distractions.
Cognitive Behavioural Therapy (CBT)	A structured, time-limited intervention that promotes identification and management of negative thoughts and behaviours that cause emotional distress.	Improving coping and well-being.
Acceptance-based therapy	CBT-based therapy that promotes acceptance of aversive internal experiences and facilitates coping.	Strategies to accept and manage distressing thoughts and feelings and improve coping and well-being.

(Continued)

TABLE 7.2 (Continued)

Psychological intervention	*Brief description*	*Benefits*
Social support	Strategies to enhance relatedness to others.	Connections to others, comfort and perceived social support.
Education	Informational support and knowledge development.	Empowerment and prevention facilitation at all levels, especially primary, secondary and tertiary.
Performance planning	Re-establishing performance excellence through graduated practice and re-entry tasks and simulations.	Management of performance demands, expectations, anxiety and fear.
Integrated mind-body training.	Proprioception, neuromuscular retraining, self-regulation and somatic awareness training.	Fluid execution of skills and confidence. Enhanced self-regulation and interoception.

Seeking help from a psychologist, psychiatrist or mental health practitioner is recommended if there are psychological or psychiatric concerns or if supportive counselling is warranted. Referrals from clinic staff or physicians are beneficial in facilitating early intervention and follow-up after injury. For example, concerns about disordered eating or eating disorders should be addressed promptly with referrals to qualified practitioners. Often, there are waiting lists for programmes and mental health professionals. As Liederbach (2000) stated, "dance rehabilitation is a dynamic process" (p. 54) that requires clear communication between medical professionals and dancers. Supportive counselling through rehabilitation and RTD is best addressed by a practitioner who is knowledgeable about dance and performance psychology. Helping dancers transition and cope with career loss is especially important in the face of career-ending injuries, and when identity is intimately tied to dance.

Biopsychosocial screening may identify *at-risk* dancers (Cahalan et al., 2015) and dancers who fear re-injury and repercussions from injury (Vassallo et al., 2019). Liederbach (2000) reported that residual deficits in balance and proprioception or difficulties from earlier injuries or illnesses were found during screenings of dancers. Also, screening dancers for feeding and eating disorders and investing in educational initiatives (Piran, 1999) can reveal covert indicators of psychological distress and prevent injuries (Thomas et al., 2011). Russel (2013) suggested that screening dancers' physical and psychological attributes, prior injuries and dance activity may reduce injury.

Wang and Russell (2018) suggested that medical RTD guidelines would also benefit from incorporating psychological and psychosocial considerations. Hrubes and Janowski (2021) recommended a multifactorial, team-based approach to rehabilitation for dancers with dance-specific goals to return dancers to their pre-injury level of function. Mainwaring and Mor (2019) outlined guidelines for psychological intervention for injured dancers.

Van Winden et al. (2021) recommended post-injury stress management for dance students after identifying elevated stress levels. Mindfulness meditation and adaptive health behaviour practices (e.g., nutrition, sleep hygiene, and adaptive coping) and managing workload and rest schedules (Kenny et al., 2021) are ways to encourage healthy energy management. "Finding the right balance – learning to push hard enough to expand abilities, but not so hard as to invite injury – is the solution" (Berardi, 2005, as cited in Welsh, 2009, p. 26.).

Cultivating a positive mindset can be beneficial for reduced risk of injury (Williams et al., 1993) and promoting adaptive coping and well-being (Tranaeus et al., 2024). Teaching broad-based coping strategies was effective in helping to manage stress and injury in Korean dancers (Noh et al., 2005, 2007), whereas Cognitive Behavioural Therapy (CBT) and acceptance-based practices have been shown to be helpful for improving coping and well-being following sport injury (Tranaeus et al., 2024).

The benefits of psychological interventions to enhance rehabilitation experiences of injured athletes have been established through meta-analysis (Ivarsson et al., 2017; Li et al., 2020) and systematic review of the literature (Gledhill et al., 2018). Li et al. (2020) reported that psychological interventions that were most effective had six 60-minute sessions over seven to twelve weeks and focused on CBT. Using visualisation during recovery can promote relaxation, well-being and recovery from injury (Christakou et al., 2007; Cupal & Brewer, 2001). A recent review of motor imagery and action observation in the rehabilitation of lower limb injuries suggested that those cortical training techniques improved rehabilitation outcomes such as range of motion, muscle strength, activities of daily living and quality of life (Nanbancha et al., 2022). Mental practice activates perceptual-motor organisation, and motor cognition (Savaki & Raos, 2019). The use of image-based teaching cues (e.g., conditioning with imagery by Krasnow, 1997; Krasnow et al., 2011) can enhance sensory-motor awareness and integration and help with learning or re-learning dance movements after injury.

Social support for injured dancers can provide informational, emotional and tangible or practical support. Whether the injured dancer is integrated back into the studio early to observe or to assist with modified activities depends on the injury and the individual. If dancers, their medical team and support network work together to align RTD expectations and timelines, dancers will feel supported and confident in the recovery path. Patterson et al. (1998) reported that social support buffered the stress-injury relationship for ballet dancers.

Various educational endeavours are beneficial in RTD and can be implemented as primary, secondary or tertiary prevention initiatives. Bowling (1989) reported that 50% of the dancers surveyed suggested that the availability of good technique classes from teachers with an awareness of anatomy and the limitations of the body was critical. Information for dancers about pain and its management would help dancers distinguish between *good pain* or *performance pain* (Harrison et al., 2017) and pain that signals injury. Other educational interventions might include proprioception re-training, stretching for healing and recovery, coping skills, and mental skills for recovery and re-entry into performance.

Performance preparation and re-integration can be beneficial and might include simulation or actual re-immersion into performance settings before actual performances. Gradual re-introduction to bright lights, loud music and dancing on inclined floors, for example, can facilitate return to the theatre, which is especially important in the case of concussion. Also, communication among stakeholders helps dancers re-integrate without fear of repercussions to their well-being, employment or position in the company.

Conclusions and recommendations for practice

This chapter outlines important considerations to facilitate a holistic multifaceted recovery process for injured dancers. Empirical and theoretical work related to psychological and psychosocial aspects of sport and dance injury, in particular, is reviewed. Intrinsic and extrinsic factors contributing to injury onset and the recovery process were identified including personality, the stress-response, history of injury, the dance milieu, workload, social dynamics, and the socio-historic-economic context. Presented are twelve psychological interventions for injury management based on their efficacy and effectiveness for dance injury prevention and management. Also presented are self-regulation skills that play a crucial role in recovery and re-entry into performance (Beckmann, 2023). Providing dancers with active recovery strategies encourages empowerment and enhanced self-awareness throughout the recovery process and across multiple interrelated systems (physiological, psychological, and social).

Practitioners generally (including psychologists, psychiatrists, mental skills consultants, counsellors, and physical therapists) might benefit from incorporating these strategies and sport psychology techniques (e.g., goal setting, energy management, imagery training, and attentional training; Andersen, 2009) into their work with dancers. By doing so, they provide dancers with tools to navigate the challenges of recovery and salubrious return to the stage. Moreover, practitioners will find it rewarding to work with highly skilled and motivated clients eager to return to mastering their craft. Those unfamiliar with working with dancers or performing artists could benefit from continuing education to learn how to use these approaches. The reader is referred to Moyle (2019) that summarises the key roles and responsibilities of practitioners within the unique *landscape* of the performance world. Specialised knowledge in dance-related science, art and practice is required to shepherd dancers through the disruptive dance of injury. Not only does an holistic recovery process aid in the optimal RTD, but it also affords dancers with a reservoir of resources to draw upon throughout the ebbs and flows of daily life. From those resources, dancers gain actionable information, useful skills, a better appreciation of risk, and the means to balance stress with recovery and performance.

References

Adam, M. U., Brassington, G. S., & Matheson, G. O. (2004). Psychological factors associated with performance-limiting injuries in professional ballet dancers. *Journal of Dance Medicine & Science*, *8*(2), 43–46.

Air, M. E. (2013). Psychological distress among dancers seeking outpatient treatment for musculoskeletal injury. *Journal of Dance Medicine & Science*, *17*(3), 115–125.

Andersen, M. B. (2009). The 'canon' of psychological skills training for enhancing performance. In K. F. Hays (Ed.), *Performance psychology in action: A casebook for working with athletes, performing artists, business leaders, and professionals in high-risk occupations* (pp. 11–34). American Psychological Association.

Arcelus, J., Witcomb, G. L., & Mitchell, A. (2013). Prevalence of eating disorders amongst dancers: A systemic review and meta-analysis. *European Eating Disorders Review*, *22*(2), 92–101.

Balk, Y. A., & Englert, C. (2020). Recovery self-regulation in sport: Theory, research, and practice. *International Journal of Sports Science & Coaching*, *15*, 273–281.

Barreau, X., Courtin, C., Ramos-Pascual, S., Kumble, A., Saffarini, M., & Nogier, A. (2025). Epidemiology of musculoskeletal injuries in professional ballet dancers at the Opéra de Paris. *Clinical Journal of Sport Medicine*, 35(4), 489–449.

Barrell, G. M., & Terry, P. C. (2003). Trait anxiety and coping strategies among ballet dancers. *Medical Problems of Performing Artists, 18*(2), 59–64.

Beckmann, J. (2023). Self-regulation of recovery. In M. Kellmann, S. Jakowski, & J. Beckmann (Eds.), *The importance of recovery for physical and mental health. Negotiating the effects of underrecovery* (pp. 53–69). Routledge.

Beckmann, J., Kellmann, M., & Jakowski, S. (2023). Recovery is more than just healing: Advocating a broader perspective on recovery in physical and mental health. In M. Kellmann, S. Jakowski, & J. Beckmann (Eds.), *The importance of recovery for physical and mental health: Negotiating the effects of underrecovery* (pp. 266–270). Routledge.

Bestwick-Stevenson, T., Toone, R., Neupert, E., Edwards, K., & Kluzek, S. (2022). Assessment of fatigue and recovery in sport: Narrative review. *International Journal of Sports Medicine*, *43*(14), 1151–1162.

Bolling, C., van Rijn, R. M., Pasman, H. R., van Mechelen, W., & Stubbe, J. H. (2021). In your shoes: A qualitative study on the perspectives of professional dancers and staff regarding dance injury and its prevention. *Translational Sports Medicine*, *4*(3), 386–394.

Bowling, A. (1989). Injuries to dancers: Prevalence, treatment, and perceptions of causes. *British Medical Journal*, *298*(6675), 731–734.

Brink, M., & Lemmink, K. (2022). Recovery-stress balance and injury risk in team sports. In M. Kellmann & J. Beckmann (Eds.), *Recovery and well-being in sport and exercise* (pp. 87–97). Routledge.

Brink, M. S., Visscher, C., Arends, S., Zwerver, J., Post, W. J., & Lemmink, K. A. (2010). Monitoring stress and recovery: New insights for the prevention of injuries and illnesses in elite youth soccer players. *British Journal of Sports Medicine, 44*(11), 809–815.

Bursik, J., Thiel, A., Mayer, J., & John, J. M. (in press). The role of psychosocial factors in performing hurt: A systematic review covering the high-performance domains of sport, music, and dance. *International Review of Sport and Exercise Psychology*. https://doi.org/10.1080/1750984X.2025.2450791

Cahalan, R., Purtill, H., O'Sullivan, P., & O'Sullivan, K. (2015). A cross-sectional study of elite adult Irish dancers: Biopsychosocial traits, pain, and injury. *Journal of Dance Medicine & Science, 19*(1), 31–43.

Campbell, R. S., Lehr, M. E., Livingston, A., McCurdy, M., & Ware, J. K. (2019). Intrinsic modifiable risk factors in ballet dancers: Applying evidence-based practice principles to enhance clinical applications. *Physical Therapy in Sport, 38*, 106–114.

Christakou, A., Stavrou, N. A., Psychountaki, M., & Zervas, Y. (2020). Re-injury worry, confidence and attention as predictors of a sport re-injury during a competitive season. *Research in Sports Medicine, 30*(1), 19–29.

Christakou, A., Zervas, Y., & Lavallee, D. (2007). The adjunctive role of imagery on the functional rehabilitation of a grade II ankle sprain. *Human Movement Science, 26*(1), 141–154.

Cryan, P. D., & Alles, W. F. (1983). The relationship between stress and college football injuries. *The Journal of Sports Medicine and Physical Fitness, 23*(1), 52–58.

Cumming, J., & Duda, J. L. (2012). Profiles of perfectionism, body-related concerns, and indicators of psychological health in vocational dance students: An investigation of the 2 × 2 model of perfectionism. *Psychology of Sport and Exercise, 13*(6), 729–738.

Cupal, D. D., & Brewer, B. W. (2001). Effects of relaxation and guided imagery on knee strength, reinjury anxiety, and pain following anterior cruciate ligament reconstruction. *Rehabilitation Psychology, 46*(1), 28–43.

Dang, Y., Koutedakis, Y., Chen, R., & Wyon, M. A. (2021). Prevalence and risk factors of dance injury during COVID-19: A cross-sectional study from university students in China. *Frontiers in Psychology, 12*, 759413. https://doi.org/10.3389/fpsyg.2021.759413

De Maria, A., Galli, F., Zelli, A., & Mallia, L. (2024). A multi-design investigation of perfectionism risk profiles for traumatic injury in sport. *Psychology of Sport and Exercise*, 72, 102603. https://doi.org/10.1016/j.psychsport.2024.102603

De Wet, J. S., Africa, E., & Venter, R. (2022). Recovery-stress states of professional ballet dancers during different phases of a ballet season. *Journal of Dance Medicine & Science, 26*(1), 8–15.

Eliot, K. (2008). Starved for beauty: British ballet and public morale during the second World War. *Dance Chronicle, 31*(2), 175–210.

Fernandez, M. K. R., Keeler, L. A., Arthur-Cameselle, J. N., & Kuntz, P. (2023). Qualitative analysis of modern dancers' post-injury psychological experiences. *Journal for Advancing Sport Psychology in Research, 3*(2), 4–18.

Fittig, E., & Jacobi, C. (2024). Psychosocial risk factors. In S. Herpertz, M. de Zwaan, & S. Zipfel (Eds.), *Handbook of eating disorders and obesity* (pp. 147–157). Springer.

Fuller, M., Moyle, G. M., Hunt, A. P., & Minett, G. M. (2020). Injuries during transition periods across the year in pre-professional and professional ballet and contemporary dancers: A systematic review and meta-analysis. *Physical Therapy in Sport*, *44*, 14–23.

Fulton, J., Wright, K., Kelly, M., Zebrosky, B., Zanis, M., Drvol, C., & Butler, R. (2014). Injury risk is altered by previous injury: A systematic review of the literature and presentation of causative neuromuscular factors. *International Journal of Sports Physical Therapy*, *9*(5), 583–595.

Galambos, S. A., Terry, P. C., Moyle, G. M., & Locke, S. A. (2005). Psychological predictors of injury among elite athletes. *British Journal of Sports Medicine*, 39(6), 351–354.

Gledhill, A., Forsdyke, D., & Murray, E. (2018). Psychological interventions used to reduce sports injuries: A systematic review of real-world effectiveness. *British Journal of Sports Medicine*, *52*(15), 967–971.

Hamilton, L. H., Hamilton, W. G., Meltzer, J. D., Marshall, P., & Molnar, M. (1989). Personality, stress, and injuries in professional ballet dancers. *The American Journal of Sports Medicine*, *17*(2), 263–267.

Harris, D. (2021). Returning to the dance studio safely after a pandemic. *National Dance Society Journal*, *6*(1), 26.

Harrison, C., & Ruddock-Hudson, M. (2017). Perceptions of pain, injury, and transition-retirement: The experiences of professional dancers. *Journal of Dance Medicine & Science*, *21*(2), 43–52.

Hays, K. F. (2012). The psychology of performance in sport and other domains. In S. M. Murphy (Ed.), *The Oxford handbook of sport and performance psychology* (pp. 24–45). Oxford University Press.

Hays, K. F. (2017). Performance psychology with performing artists. *Oxford Research Encyclopedia of Psychology*. Retrieved April 24, 2025 from https://oxfordre.com/psychology/view/10.1093/acrefore/9780190236557.001.0001/acrefore-9780190236557-e-191

Hrubes, M., & Janowski, J. (2021). Rehabilitation of the dancer. *Physical Medicine and Rehabilitation Clinics of North America*, *32*(1), 1–20. https://doi.org/10.1016/j.pmr.2020.08.003

International Association for Dance Medicine & Science. (n.d.). *IADMS refugee dance and mental health statement*. Retrieved April 24, 2025 from https://iadms.org/media/6378/iadms-refugee-dance-and-mental-health-statement.pdf

Ivarsson, A., Johnson, U., Andersen, M. B., Tranaeus, U., Stenling, A., & Lindwall, M. (2017). Psychosocial factors and sport injuries: Meta-analyses for prediction and prevention. *Sports Medicine*, *47*(2), 353–365.

Kadel, N. J., Teitz, C. C., & Kronmal, R. A. (1992). Stress fractures in ballet dancers. *The American Journal of Sports Medicine*, *20*(4), 445–449.

Kallus, K. W. (2016). Stress and recovery: An overview. In K. W. Kallus & M. Kellmann (Eds.), *The Recovery-Stress Questionnaires: User manual* (pp. 27–48). Pearson.

Keeler, C. E. (2020). Access to health care among dancers. *Physical Medicine and Rehabilitation Clinics of North America*, *32*(1), 21–33.

Kenny, S. J., Critchley, M. L., Whittaker, J. L., Kodalore Vijayan, V. W., & Emery, C. A. (2021). Association between pre-participation characteristics and risk of injury amongst pre-professional dancers. *Physical Therapy in Sport*, *52*, 239–247.

Kenny, S. J., Whittaker, J. L., & Emery, C. A. (2016). Risk factors for musculoskeletal injury in preprofessional dancers: A systematic review. *British Journal of Sports Medicine*, *50*(16), 997–1003.

Kenttä, G., & Hassmén, P. (1998). Overtraining and recovery: A conceptual model. *Sports Medicine*, *26*(1), 1–16.

Kerr, G., Krasnow, D., & Mainwaring, L. M. (1992). The nature of dance injuries. *Medical Problems of Performing Artists*, *7*(1), 25–29.

Kishon, L., & Sarig Bahat, H. (2023). Factors associated with musculoskeletal injuries in pre-professional modern dancers before and after the COVID-19 pandemic. *Applied Sciences*, *13*(5), 3018. https://doi.org/10.3390/app13053018

Kolitsida, M., Cumming, J., Lavis, A., & Sanchez, E. (2023). The impact of the COVID-19 pandemic on the mental health and wellbeing of dance freelancers in the United Kingdom. *Journal of Dance Education*, *23*(3), 190–199.

Krasnow, D. (1997). C-I Training: The merger of conditioning and imagery as an alternative training methodology for dance. *Medical Problems of Performing Artists*, *12*(1), 3–8.

Krasnow, D., & Deaveau, J. (2011). *Conditioning with imagery for dancers*. Thompson Educational Publishers.

Krasnow, D., Kerr, G., & Mainwaring, L. M. (1994). Psychology of dealing with the injured dancer. *Medical Problems of Performing Artists*, *9*(1), 7–9.

Krasnow, D., Mainwaring, L. M., & Kerr, G. (1999). Injury, stress, and perfectionism in young dancers and gymnasts. *Journal of Dance Medicine & Science*, *3*(2), 51–58.

Lambert, B. S., Cain, M. T., Heimdal, T., Harris, J. D., Jotwani, V., Petak, S., & McCulloch, P. C. (2020). Physiological parameters of bone health in elite ballet dancers. *Medicine & Science in Sports and Exercise*, *52*(8), 1668–1678.

Laux, P., Krumm, B., Diers, M., & Flor, H. (2015). Recovery-stress balance and injury risk in professional football players: A prospective study. *Journal of Sports Sciences*, *33*(20), 2140–2148.

Li, H., Li, B., Wu, X., Qiu, X., Kim, S., & Tang, X. (2025). A systematic review and hot topic analysis of ballet injury research: CiteSpace visualization atlas. *Molecular & Cellular Biomechanics*, *22*(2), 1117. https://doi.org/10.62617/mcb1117

Li, S., Wu, Q., & Chen, Z. (2020). Effects of psychological interventions on the prevention of sports injuries: A meta-analysis. *Orthopaedic Journal of Sports Medicine*, *8*(8), 232596712092832. https://doi.org/10.1177/2325967120928325

Liederbach, M. (2000). General considerations for guiding dance injury rehabilitation. *Journal of Dance Medicine & Science*, *4*(2), 54–65.

Liederbach, M., & Compagno, J. M. (2001). Psychological aspects of fatigue-related injuries in dancers. *Journal of Dance Medicine & Science*, *5*(4), 116–120.

Liederbach, M., Gleim, G. W., & Nicholas, J. A. (1992). Monitoring training status in professional ballet dancers. *The Journal of Sports Medicine and Physical Fitness*, *32*(2), 187–195.

Liederbach, M., Gleim, G. W., & Nicholas, J. A. (1994). Physiologic and psychological measurements of performance stress and onset of injuries in professional ballet dancers. *Medical Problems of Performing Artists*, *9*(1), 10–14.

Liederbach, M., Schanfein, L., & Kremenic, I. J. (2013). What is known about the effect of fatigue on injury occurrence among dancers? *Journal of Dance Medicine & Science*, *17*(3), 101–108.

Mainwaring, L. M. (2009). Working with perfection. In K. F. Hays (Ed.), *Performance psychology in action: A casebook for working with athletes, performing artists, business leaders, and professionals in high-risk occupations* (pp. 139–159). American Psychological Association.

Mainwaring, L. M., Kerr, G., & Krasnow, D. (1993). Psychological correlates of dance injuries. *Medical Problems of Performing Artists*, *8*(1), 3–6.

Mainwaring, L. M., Krasnow, D., & Kerr, G. (2001). And the dance goes on: Psychological impact of injury. *Journal of Dance Medicine & Science*, *5*(4), 105–115.

Mainwaring, L. M., & Mor, S. (2019). Managing psychological disturbances in performing artists. In L. E. Elson (Ed.), *Performing arts medicine* (pp. 151–162). Elsevier.

Martins, C., Godycki-Cwirko, M., Heleno, B., & Brodersen, J. (2019). Quaternary prevention: An evidence-based concept aiming to protect patients from medical harm. *British Journal of General Practice*, *69*(689), 614–615.

Mattiussi, A. M., Shaw, J. W., Williams, S., Price, P. D., Brown, D. D., Cohen, D. D., Clark, R., Kelly, S., Retter, G., Pedlar, C., & Tallent, J. (2021). Injury epidemiology in professional ballet: A five-season prospective study of 1596 medical attention injuries and 543 time-loss injuries. *British Journal of Sports Medicine*, *55*(15), 843–850.

Mayer, J., & Thiel, A. (2018). Presenteeism in the elite sports workplace: The willingness to compete hurt among German elite handball and track and field athletes. *International Review for the Sociology of Sport*, *53*(1), 49–68.

McCann, R., Schussler, E., Martinez, J., & Ramirez, V. (2022). The effect of concussion history on lower extremity injury risk in college athletes: A systematic review and meta-analysis. *International Journal of Sports Physical Therapy*, *17*(5), 753–765.

McEwen, K., & Young, K. (2011). Ballet and pain: Reflections on a risk-dance culture. *Qualitative Research in Sport, Exercise and Health*, *3*(2), 152–173.

Moore, C. A., & Emmerich, N. (2024). Balletic bodies under lockdown: The consequences of a pandemic for highly disciplined habitus. *Sociology of Health & Illness*, *46*(1), 95–113.

Moyle, G. M. (2019). Supervision in performance settings (dance, music, acting). *Oxford research encyclopedia of psychology*. Retrieved April 24, 2025 from https://oxfordre.com/psychology/view/10.1093/acrefore/9780190236557.001.0001/acrefore-9780190236557-e-325

Nanbancha, A., Mawhinney, C., & Sinsurin, K. (2022). The effect of motor imagery and action observation in the rehabilitation of lower limb injuries: A scoping review. *Clinical Rehabilitation*, *37*(2), 145–161.

Noh, Y.-E., Morris, T., & Andersen, M. B. (2005). Psychosocial factors and ballet injuries. *International Journal of Sport and Exercise Psychology*, *3*(1), 79–90.

Noh, Y.-E., Morris, T., & Andersen, M. B. (2007). Psychological intervention programs for reduction of injury in ballet dancers. *Research in Sports Medicine*, *15*(1), 13–32.

Nordin-Bates, S. M., Raedeke, T. D., & Madigan, D. J. (2017). Perfectionism, burnout, and motivation in dance: A replication and test of the 2x2 model of perfectionism. *Journal of Dance Medicine & Science*, *21*(3), 115–122.

Novosel, B., Sekulic, D., Peric, M., Kondric, M., & Zaletel, P. (2019). Injury occurrence and return to dance in professional ballet: Prospective analysis of specific correlates. *International Journal of Environmental Research and Public Health*, *16*(5), 765. https://doi.org/10.3390/ijerph16050765

Ober, J., Rusakov, S., & Matusevych, T. (2026). The effects of the war in Ukraine on the environment of Ukrainian artists: An evaluation by a diagnostic survey. *Media, War & Conflict, 19*(1), 3–26.

Patterson, E. L., Smith, R. E., Everett, J. J., & Ptacek, J. T. (1998). Psychosocial factors as predictors of ballet injuries: Interactive effects of life stress and social support. *Journal of Sport Behavior, 21*, 101–112.

Piran, N. (1999). Eating disorders: A trial of prevention in a high-risk school setting. *Journal of Primary Prevention, 20*(1), 75–90.

Podlog, L., Conti, C., Di Fronso, S., & Bertollo, M. (2023). Underrecovery in elite athletes: Antecedents, implications, and prevention strategies. In M. Kellmann, S. Jakowski, & J. Beckmann (Eds.), *The importance of recovery for physical and mental health: Negotiating the effects of underrecovery* (pp. 70–83). Routledge.

Reel, J. J., Podlog, L., Hamilton, L., Greviskes, L., Voelker, D. K., & Gray, C. (2018). Injury and disordered eating behaviors: What is the connection for female professional dancers? *Journal of Clinical Sport Psychology, 12*(3), 365–381.

Rip, B., Fortin, S., & Vallerand, R. J. (2006). The relationship between passion and injury in dance students. *Journal of Dance Medicine & Science, 10*(1–2), 14–20.

Roach, M. H., Aderman, M. J., Ross, J. D., Kelly, T. F., Malvasi, S. R., Posner, M. A., Svoboda, S. J., Pasquina, P. F., & Cameron, K. L. (2023). Risk of upper extremity musculoskeletal injury within the first year after a concussion. *Orthopaedic Journal of Sports Medicine, 11*(5). https://doi.org/10.1177/23259671231163570

Russell, J. (2013). Preventing dance injuries: Current perspectives. *Open Access Journal of Sports Medicine, 4*, 199–210.

Savaki, H. E., & Raos, V. (2019). Action perception and motor imagery: Mental practice of action. *Progress in Neurobiology, 175*, 107–125.

Solomon, R., & Micheli, L. (1986). Concepts in the prevention of dance injuries: A survey and analysis. In C. G. Shell (Ed.), *The dancer as athlete: The 1984 Olympic scientific congress proceedings* (Vol. 8, pp. 201–212). Human Kinetics.

Thomas, H., & Tarr, J. (2009). Dancers' perceptions of pain and injury: Positive and negative effects. *Journal of Dance Medicine & Science, 13*(2), 51–59.

Thomas, J. J., Keel, P. K., & Heatherton, T. F. (2011). Disordered eating and injuries among adolescent ballet dancers. *Eating and Weight Disorders – Studies on Anorexia, Bulimia and Obesity, 16*(3), e216–e222.

Toohey, L. A., Drew, M. K., Cook, J. L., Finch, C. F., & Gaida, J. E. (2017). Is subsequent lower limb injury associated with previous injury? A systematic review and meta-analysis. *British Journal of Sports Medicine, 51*(23), 1670–1678.

Tranaeus, U., Gledhill, A., Johnson, U., Podlog, L., Wadey, R., Bjornstal, D. W., & Ivarsson, A. (2024). 50 years of research on the psychology of sport injury: A consensus statement. *Sports Medicine, 54*(7), 1733–1748.

Tranaeus, U., Martin, S., & Ivarsson, A. (2022). Psychosocial risk factors for overuse injuries in competitive athletes: A mixed-studies systematic review. *Sports Medicine, 52*(4), 773–788.

Treasure, J. (2023). Eating disorders overview. In E. McNaught, J. Treasure, & J. Griffiths (Eds.), *Eating disorders: The basics* (pp. 136–152). Routledge.

Turner, B. S., & Wainwright, S. P. (2003). Corps de ballet: The case of the injured ballet dancer. *Sociology of Health & Illness, 25*(4), 269–288.

Valenzuela-Moss, J., Shah, S., Sheng, D., Zaslow, T., Wren, T., & Edison, B. (2025). Effects of COVID-19 quarantine restrictions on training and injury in ballet dancers. *Medical Research Archives*, *13*(1), 1–14. https://doi.org/10.18103/mra.v13i1.6218

van der Does, H. T. D., Brink, M. S., Otter, R. T. A., Visscher, C., & Lemmink, K. A. P. M. (2017). Injury risk is increased by changes in perceived recovery of team sport players. *Clinical Journal of Sport Medicine*, *27*(1), 46–51.

van der Sluis, A., Brink, M. S., Pluim, B. M., Verhagen, E. A. L. M., Elferink-Gemser, M. T., & Visscher, C. (2019). Self-regulatory skills: Are they helpful in the prevention of overuse injuries in talented tennis players? *Scandinavian Journal of Medicine & Science in Sports*, *29*(7), 1050–1058.

van Mechelen, W., Twisk, J., Molendijk, A., Blom, B., Snel, J., & Kemper, H. C. G. (1996). Subject-related risk factors for sports injuries: A 1-yr prospective study in young adults. *Medicine & Science in Sports & Exercise*, *28*(9), 1171–1179.

van Winden, D., van Rijn, R. M., Savelsbergh, G. J. P., Oudejans, R. R. D., & Stubbe, J. H. (2020). Limited coping skills, young age, and high BMI are risk factors for injuries in contemporary dance: A 1-year prospective study. *Frontiers in Psychology*, *11*, 1452. https://doi.org/10.3389/fpsyg.2020.01452

van Winden, D., van Rijn, R. M., Savelsbergh, G. J. P., Oudejans, R. R. D., & Stubbe, J. H. (2021). The association between stress and injury: A prospective cohort study among 186 first-year contemporary dance students. *Frontiers in Psychology*, *12*, 770494. https://doi.org/10.3389/fpsyg.2021.770494

Vassallo, A. J., Pappas, E., Stamatakis, E., & Hiller, C. E. (2019). Injury fear, stigma, and reporting in professional dancers. *Safety and Health at Work*, *10*(3), 260–264.

Wadey, R., Evans, L., Hanton, S., Sarkar, M., & Oliver, H. (2019). Can preinjury adversity affect postinjury responses? A 5-year prospective, multi-study analysis. *Frontiers in Psychology*, *10*, 1411. https://doi.org/10.3389/fpsyg.2019.01411

Wainwright, S. P., Williams, C., & Turner, B. S. (2005). Fractured identities: Injury and the balletic body. *Health*, *9*(1), 49–66.

Wang, T. J., & Russell, J. A. (2018). A tenuous pas de deux: Examining university dancers' access to and satisfaction with healthcare delivery. *Medical Problems of Performing Artists*, *33*(2), 111–117.

Wasserman, E. B., Chretien, A., Harmon, K. G., Putukian, M., Okonkwo, D., Solomon, G. S., Cardenas, J., Herzog, M. M., Sills, A., & Mack, C. D. (2024). Subsequent musculoskeletal injury after concussion in national football league players. *British Journal of Sports Medicine*, *58*(18), 1068–1074.

Welsh, T. (2009). *Conditioning for dancers*. University of Florida Press.

Williams, J. M., & Andersen, M. B. (1998). Psychosocial antecedents of sport injury: Review and critique of the stress and injury model'. *Journal of Applied Sport Psychology*, *10*(1), 5–25.

Williams, J. M., Hogan, T. D., & Andersen, M. B. (1993). Positive states of mind and athletic injury risk. *Psychosomatic Medicine*, *55*(5), 468–472.

World Health Organisation. (2019). *Recovery practices for mental health and well-being. WHO QualityRights Specialized training*. Retrieved March 04, 2025 from https://iris.who.int/handle/10665/329646

8

RECOVERY OF THE SINGER'S VOICE

Bernhard Richter

Anatomical and physiological basics of the voice

The vocal apparatus is usually made up of three main parts: the respiratory system, the larynx, and the vocal tract. The human voice is the result of a highly coordinated interaction between breathing, vocal fold vibration, and articulation movements. The movement patterns underlying this process are among the most complex neuromuscular activities the human body is capable of. It is not only the synchronous activation of certain muscle groups that is crucial for healthy and efficient voice production. Rather, the voice must be understood as a holistic expression of the human being, embodying physiological, psychological, and psychosocial dimensions. The voice is not just a biomechanical phenomenon, but a psychobiological achievement that reflects the integration of bodily functions and individual personality structure.

Vocal physiology, as a specialised branch of physiology, investigates the complex interplay of respiratory mechanisms, laryngeal function, and the dynamics of the vocal tract. Breathing provides the airflow necessary for voice production. During exhalation, pressure builds up under the closed vocal folds, which acts as the driving force for the initiation of vocal fold vibrations. The space between the vocal folds – the glottis – can be modulated to open and close. As soon as the subglottic pressure exceeds the medial pressure of the adducted folds, a discrete burst of air can escape.

Richter, B. (2026). Recovery of the singer's voice. In E. Altenmüller, M. Kellmann, J. Beckmann, & G. M. Moyle (Eds.), *Recovery and well-being in the performing arts* (pp. 134–152). Routledge.

DOI: 10.4324/9781003566885-10

When this cycle repeats periodically, the vocal folds vibrate according to the *Myoelastic-Aerodynamic Theory* (van den Berg, 1958). The periodic interruption of the transglottal airflow leads to the production of the so-called primary sound source or voice source. The subglottal pressure is modulated by both the pitch and the intensity: higher fundamental frequencies and higher sound pressure levels require proportionally higher subglottal pressures (Sundberg, 2018). The primary signal produced at the level of the larynx consists of a fundamental frequency and its overtones. This signal undergoes complex spectral shaping in the vocal tract, particularly in the resonance chambers of the throat and oral cavity. These anatomical spaces serve as acoustic filters that have a decisive influence on the timbre and projection of the human voice (Sundberg, 1995).

Voice production works according to mechanical principles that occur at high speed. In humans, the frequency of vocal fold vibrations ranges from just over 50 Hz to over 1,500 Hz. In classical singing, Mozart's operas illustrate this wide range clearly: for example, the bass role of Osmin in *Die Entführung aus dem Serail* reaches D2 (73 Hz), while the Queen of the Night in *Die Zauberflöte* reaches F6 (1,397 Hz). Even higher frequencies are achieved in non-classical singing styles. According to the Guinness Book of Records (2025), voice frequencies of over 5,000 Hz have been documented. This frequency range corresponds to that of a modern concert grand piano: the lowest string vibrates at 27.5 Hz, while the highest reaches 4,186 Hz.

The frequencies of vocal fold vibrations during singing and speaking are far above the temporal resolution of the human eye. Therefore, special technological methods are required to adequately visualise and analyse the rapid vibration sequences of the vocal folds. Currently, laryngostroboscopy is the primary tool used for the qualitative characterisation of phonatory mucosal movements and, increasingly, for quantitative assessment (Woo, 2020). For specific questions such as the investigation of vocal onset, stroboscopy can be supplemented by high-speed video laryngoscopy (Richter et al., 2024). Stroboscopic examinations of professional singers have repeatedly revealed morphological irregularities that do not consistently correlate with subjective or functional voice impairments. The research group led by Sataloff has described such findings in several studies, pointing to the frequent dissociation between structural abnormalities and clinical symptoms (Elias et al., 1997; Myint et al., 2016; Sataloff et al., 2012). These observations have been confirmed by data from our own research group. In a cohort of 36 professional sopranos, stroboscopic analysis revealed visible structural changes in 24 singers. However, of these 24, only 9 reported symptoms of hoarseness, while 15 remained completely symptom-free. Conversely, three singers with normal stroboscopic laryngeal profiles still reported hoarseness (Traser et al., 2012).

The human voice as an endurance system

The human voice is fundamentally designed to perform continuous, long-lasting tasks (Titze et al., 2003). In this respect, functional analogies can be drawn to the musculoskeletal system, which has also evolved to enable daily locomotion and sustained physical activity (Thurber et al., 2019). While this basic functionality supports routine vocal behaviour, professional singing places exceptionally high demands on both the performer and the medical and therapeutic environment. This is in many ways comparable to high-performance sports, especially in endurance sports, such as running or long-distance cycling. On the other hand, endurance training may benefit vocal functions in professional singers (Yilmaz et al., 2025).

Among all occupational groups that rely heavily on their voice, singers are consistently identified as the group at highest risk for developing voice disorders (Verdolini & Ramig, 2001; Williams, 2003). This observation is confirmed by epidemiological findings. A comprehensive meta-analysis by Pestana and colleagues (2017) found a strikingly high prevalence of voice disorders among singers, with 46% reporting symptoms of dysphonia. These findings underscore the vulnerability of voice professionals to chronic voice strain and point to the need for preventive care strategies and evidence-based voice health measures specifically tailored to demanding performance contexts. Therefore, appropriate strategies for recovery are important. As throughout this volume, a broader perspective on recovery is adopted, which goes beyond regeneration and resilience. However, in the field of vocal care of the professional voice, such comprehensive recovery strategies still need to be implemented in many institutions and scientifically evaluated.

Kellmann and Kallus (2001) have postulated a broader perspective on recovery that goes beyond regeneration or 'being cured' or 'being normal again' (Beckmann et al., 2023). This broader perspective addresses recovery as a resource that enables individuals not only to recover from stress but also to develop resilience to health-threatening stress. Kallus (2016, p. 42) defined recovery as "an inter- and intraindividual multilevel (e.g., psychological, physiological, social) process in time for the re-establishment of personal resources and their full functional capacity".

As elaborated by Altenmüller (this volume, Chapter 1), a key requirement for recovery is to take and to make time for it. This is specifically important in the world of professional singing, since economic constraints and performance pressures are prevalent. Furthermore, as in all performing arts, daily exercise is required to maintain vocal, general physical and performative skills (Wiegert et al., in press). The first step therefore is to interrupt or stop a stressful activity to terminate or at least reduce the stress. Since there are different types of stress, such as physical and mental stress, recovery can involve switching between these types of stress, for example, ending or interrupting practicing, moving to teaching activities, and again returning to mental practice of an opera libretto. In teaching and mental practice, special care must be taken, because simply listening to the singing voice of a student or the mental imagination of arias or songs may subliminally activate the vocal apparatus and produce additional physical stress (Prebil et al., 2020; Tanaka, 2021). It is believed that the human mirror neuron system based on brain circuits of the frontal and parietal lobe constitutes the physiological basis of this effect (Belyk et al., 2016).

As in all performing professions, there exist large individual differences in the type of recovery that singers prefer. For successful recovery, it is therefore crucial that an individual recovery strategy is implemented. In addition, singers must pro-actively plan or schedule self-initiated recovery strategies, including social activities that are chosen by the person themselves and tailored to their needs (Kellmann, 2002; Kellmann et al., 2023). A central aspect of the recovery model postulated by Kellmann and Kallus (2001) is the idea of a balance between stress and recovery. Increasing stress must be accompanied by an increase in corresponding recovery to maintain a balance between the two and thereby avoid negative consequences of underrecovery (Beckmann et al., 2023).

Requirements for the training of professional singers

A historical review of voice pedagogy shows that the traditional model was predominantly based on imitation and reproduction. Teaching often focused on didactic instruction, with reflective or self-regulated learning playing only a minor role. In this educational environment, the teacher's personal educational philosophy plays a decisive role. Teaching approaches range from the classical master-apprentice model to contemporary models based on scientific findings, modern learning theory, and evidence-based practices (Meyer & Helding, 2021; Ragan, 2018).

Empirical data suggests that traditional training paths are not necessarily associated with high professional performance. According to Gembris and Langner (2005), the success rate of professional vocal training for solo singers in Germany remains critically low. In their study of 100 graduates of German music academies, only 12% of those who originally aspired to a solo career were ultimately able to obtain a soloist contract. This remarkable discrepancy between original ambitions and professional outcomes underscores the need for curriculum and structural reforms, particularly regarding employability and sustainable performance development.

To address these shortcomings and promote a more holistic educational framework, a model curriculum for vocal training at German universities was introduced (Richter & Mürbe, 2020; Richter et al., 2013). This curriculum explicitly includes skills in recovery, reflecting the growing recognition of the recovery-stress balance as a crucial factor in maintaining high performance over a longer period of time (Kellmann & Kallus, 2001; Kellmann et al., 2018). However, a comprehensive recovery concept as proposed in this book needs to be further developed and implemented in all training institutions (Altenmüller & Moyle, this volume, Chapter 18).

Significant parts of preventive-oriented programmes have already been implemented into the regular curriculum at various universities of music in Germany. At the University of Music in Freiburg, in addition to the above-mentioned content tailored to singers, music physiology is offered as a minor and as a separate master's degree for all instrumentalists and singers alike. This means that one of the demands set out by Altenmüller et al. (this volume, Chapter 1) namely to offer performers health promotion programmes tailored to their specific needs and to reduce the number of work-related complaints among performers in the long term through prevention programmes and courses has already been fulfilled.

Most professional singers begin intensive vocal practice much later than instrumentalists who start around the age of seven with their instrumental training (Jørgensen, 1997). In singers, professional training usually needs the completion of pubertal voice development, which occurs in females at the age of 13–14, and somewhat later in males at the age of 15–16 (Blatt, 1983). This developmental discrepancy has important implications for the design of the curriculum in vocal pedagogy. Since the time window for acquiring motor and cognitive skills in singing is shorter compared to instrumental instruction, it is essential to systematically teach basic voice-related knowledge early in the training process.

Including the basics of voice physiology in the curriculum at the beginning of formal training therefore not only promotes vocal performance and health but also lays the foundation for a sustainable and resilient singing career. This approach is in line with current frameworks for performance development, which emphasise early psychoeducation, individual stress management, and long-term recovery strategies to optimise performance development and prevent maladaptation (Kellmann & Beckmann, 2022; Kellmann & Kallus, 2001).

The curriculum includes content from established programmes, such as those of the Studio for Voice Research at the Dresden University of Music and the Institute for Music Medicine at the Freiburg University of Music. In addition to voice physiology, students are introduced to evidence-based voice hygiene practices, including hydration strategies that have been shown to have a positive effect on voice function and the health of the vocal apparatus (Saeedi et al., 2026; Sivasankar & Leydon, 2010; Vermeulen et al., 2021). Emphasis is also placed on teaching meaningful strategies and time intervals for practice.

In the medium and long term, every professional singer should be supported by a reliable, interdisciplinary team, usually consisting of a voice teacher and a

TABLE 8.1 Voice hygiene recommendations (dos and don'ts).

Dos	*Don'ts*
• Ensure adequate individual hydration (approximately 2.5 l per day) • Ensure sufficient sleep	• Avoid nicotine use • Refrain from unnecessary medication use, especially non-steroidal anti-inflammatory drugs (e.g., aspirin) • Avoid inhaled corticosteroids if not medically essential • Do not take medications prior to performances unless tested during rehearsal conditions
Warm-up and practice: • Always warm up before singing • Allow at least two hours of wakefulness and physical activity before starting vocal exercises • Begin warm-ups with humming and gentle pitch transitions • Beginners should practice in intervals of 5 × 5 minutes daily; professionals in 10 × 10 minute segments	• Never sing without warming up properly • Practice should never result in hoarseness. If hoarseness occurs, discontinue practice immediately
Rehearsals and performances: • Avoid vocal fatigue during rehearsals – performance takes priority • Undergo regular assessments by both a vocal coach and a voice-specialised physician • Know and respect the physiological limits of your voice	• Never rehearse silently when hoarse • Do not begin a performance unless you are confident in your vocal readiness • Avoid singing beyond your vocal range or endurance

phoniatric specialist, who together monitor and accompany vocal and artistic development throughout their career. This long-term support enables individual decisions and timely interventions, especially at critical transition points. As a brief guide to vocal hygiene, the following recommendations, summarised in Table 8.1, can serve as a practical framework. These 'dos and don'ts' are based on systematic studies, empirical findings and clinical experience and aim to promote sustainable vocal function, reduce stress-related risks, and improve regeneration processes (Achey et al., 2016; Timmermans et al., 2005). Such an approach is particularly important in the early stages of a professional career. Premature engagement with demanding repertoire, such as dramatic roles, from the late Romantic period, such as Wagner's Tristan (tenor) and Isolde (soprano), Verdi's Otello (tenor) and Jago (baritone), or Puccini's Turandot (soprano), or singing beyond one's current vocal capabilities carries a significant risk of long-term vocal damage. If not managed, these stress factors can lead to maladaptive vocal behaviour, impaired performance, and increased recovery needs (Richter & Echternach, 2011).

The integration of structured, continuous support systems is therefore in line with current perspectives in performance science, which emphasise individual stress monitoring, preventive strategies, and the promotion of regeneration competence to maintain long-term artistic and vocal health (Kellmann & Beckmann, 2022; Kellmann & Kallus, 2001).

The human voice throughout life: Endocrine influences and age-related changes

The human undergoes constant change throughout life (Spahn & Richter, 2006). This developmental plasticity is clear in everyday life – for example, in the ability to estimate the age of a conversation partner on the telephone without visual cues (Caruso et al., 1994; Hunter et al., 2016). This perceptual ability is based on subtle, acoustically encoded cues that reflect biologically determined changes that occur universally over time (Mueller, 1997).

The main reason for these voice changes is the dynamic hormonal balance, which fluctuates greatly during the different stages of life. The most influential hormones include the sex hormones testosterone, estrogen, and progestogens. Although these hormones are present in all humans, their concentration and biological effects vary considerably depending on the stage of development and reproductive phase. Their influence is not limited to reproductive function, but also extends to a variety of anatomical and physiological areas relevant to voice production and regulation (Zamponi et al., 2021).

During puberty, these hormones trigger rapid growth of the larynx, leading to audible changes in the fundamental frequency of speech and singing characteristics, especially during and after voice change. In addition to structural changes, sex hormones influence:

- The flexibility of the throat muscles that support the laryngeal skeleton and influence the position of the larynx in the vocal tract;
- the tension of the vocal fold muscles (vocalis muscle) and, indirectly, the elasticity and flexibility of the mucous membrane layer above them;
- saliva and mucus secretion, which is crucial for maintaining moisture and lubrication of the larynx and supraglottic tract.

Other hormone-sensitive factors include ossification processes in the laryngeal cartilage (Jurik, 1984) and respiratory flexibility, especially the expansion and control of the chest (Triebner et al., 2017). With age, hormone levels decrease, as does biomechanical flexibility, which affects voice production, resonance control, and respiratory coordination.

In postmenopausal women, hormone withdrawal typically leads to a decrease in fundamental frequency and an increase in voice hoarseness in the speaking voice (Lã & Ardura, 2022). The transition between chest and head voice becomes more difficult, and overall voice capacity tends to decrease, especially in terms of phonation duration. These changes may be accompanied by increased dry mouth and a globus sensation, both of which are often hormone-related. In ageing men, the fundamental frequency of the speaking voice often increases, occasionally leading to an atypically high voice profile. In addition, a reduction in vocal range is frequently observed. In both sexes, age-related vibrato instability and impaired neuromuscular coordination are common phenomena (Torre & Barlow, 2009).

Furthermore, exogenous health-related stress factors such as tobacco use, alcohol abuse, and systemic diseases, which become more common with age, have harmful effects on vocal health in both men and women (Ayoub et al., 2019). Interestingly, professional singers may even compensate for these noxious influences for a certain time (Gehling et al., 2014).

Short-term strategy for recovery from functional voice overuse in professional singers

Compared to instrumentalists, singers have the unique characteristic that even minor impairments in vocal function have an immediate impact on their performance. Therefore, singers seek the advice of a voice doctor at the first signs of slight voice fatigue or hoarseness. Since vocal performance on a professional level needs a holistic approach for recovery – as outlined above – specialised health care professionals, vocal teachers and voice trainers need to support an individual approach to develop resilience to health-threatening stress, including psychological, physiological, and social aspects. Thus, the re-establishment of personal resources and their full functional capacity is warranted. In a recent consensus meeting in London, coproduced across a range of disciplines within voice care, a consensus statement on voice care and recovery was given (Flock et al., 2025). It aimed at offering practical advice to those working in voice care. Consensus was reached regarding multidisciplinary and biopsychosocial recommendations for voice care assessment and treatment. Furthermore, consensus was reached on practitioner approach to health care, psychosocial considerations, and service design. However, no consensus was reached for recovery of the voice. The need for greater expert-by-experience involvement and prospective scientific studies including randomised controlled trials was emphasised (Flock et al., 2025).

In cases of functional voice overload, commonly referred to as dysodia (Seidner & Wendler, 1989), targeted short-term interventions can facilitate effective recovery and prevent long-term voice dysfunction. One such intervention, which is particularly relevant in the treatment of professional singers, is a temporary interruption of all vocal commitments, including rehearsals and stage performances. This method has been operationalised by the '3-minute/4-day rule' (Richter, 2011), which has proven useful in clinical practice for restoring voice function while minimising the risk of overuse consequences. According to this protocol, the singer is prescribed four days of vocal rest, during which all vocal strain is strictly minimised. This includes refraining from rehearsals, not rehearsing new roles (even silently or by memorisation), avoiding music, and speaking as little as possible.

Despite the general vocal rest, structured vocal stimulation is carried out three times a day with humming exercises using the voiced nasal consonant /m/ (Richter & Echternach, 2011). Each session consists of tone sequences in semitone steps, rising from a comfortable starting pitch – defined individually within the singer's 'comfort zone'. Extreme pitches, both in the low and high registers, should be avoided. All tones should be produced with a dynamic of mezzopiano and without physical effort.

This protocol is conceptually and methodologically consistent with the principles of Semi-Occluded Vocal Tract Exercises, which have been developed and substantiated over the past two decades by researchers such as Titze and colleagues (Apfelbach & Guzmán, 2024; Heller-Starck et al., 2024; Savareh et al., 2023; Titze, 2006).

Each exercise session follows a structured pattern: three minutes of humming, followed by three minutes of silence, during which small sips of water are taken. A complete session lasts 30 minutes, with a strict alternation between vocalisation and silence/hydration.

From a physiological point of view, this exercise routine aims to achieve several specific effects:

- Activation of the mucosal wave: humming is intended to stimulate the vibration of the vocal folds, thereby gently 'massaging' the vocal fold epithelium.
- Controlled stretching of the vocal folds: the increase in pitch in semitone steps causes a slight lengthening of the vocal folds, which contributes to a controlled stretching of the intrinsic laryngeal muscles.
- Maximum concentration with minimum effort: the limited duration of three minutes per vocal exercise promotes optimal concentration, while the breaks allow for cognitive and physical recovery before the next round.
- Hydration and muscle relaxation: water intake serves to moisten the mucous membrane and facilitates relaxation of the laryngeal muscles via the swallowing mechanism.

After application of this strategy, most singers report a significant reduction in vocal fatigue within two to three days. Clinical self-reports and laboratory vocal-loading studies indicate that perceptual and acoustic signs of vocal fatigue can improve substantially within the first 24–72 hours after rest and load reduction (Hunter et al., 2009). Nevertheless, principles of tissue recovery argue for maintaining a multiday rest window: experimental animal models show that the early inflammatory and re-epithelialisation phases of vocal-fold wound healing cluster across ~three to five days post-injury, a period during which premature vibration may disrupt regenerative processes (Branski et al., 2005). Contemporary clinical guidance for dysphonia also emphasises time-limited but meaningful voice conservation and early evaluation if symptoms persist, while randomised data taken after surgery of vocal nodes suggest that short, complete rest for around three to four days, followed by guided, gradual phonation outperforms prolonged absolute rest (Kaneko et al., 2017). In accordance with the principles of recovery, especially those aimed at preventing insufficient recovery, it is essential that the entire four-day break is observed. Premature resumption of vocal activity can negate the recovery gains achieved during the initial rest period and increase the risk of relapse or chronic overload (Carroll et al., 2006).

When the duration and reasons for voice rest are clearly communicated and agreed upon between the singer and the theatre management, a high level of acceptance for this structured intervention is generally observed in the treatment of singers. The singer experiences a subjective improvement in vocal function, while the theatre benefits from minimal disruption to the rehearsal schedule, allowing for efficient contingency planning if necessary.

In addition to the humming programme, straw phonation with water resistance therapy can also be used. The effectiveness of this method has been confirmed by the results of various research groups (Echternach et al., 2020, 2021; Titze et al., 2025), further substantiating its relevance for voice restoration protocols.

Structured voice rest and psychosocial considerations in the treatment of hoarseness in professional singers

In cases of hoarseness (dysphonia) that leads to a temporary inability to sing, complete voice rest may be indicated (Stachler et al., 2018). However, this approach must be handled with care: complete voice rest can be psychologically stressful for professional singers whose identity and routine are closely linked to the use of their voice. Therefore, this aspect must be pro-actively addressed in clinical counselling. A transparent discussion can lead to better compliance and support constructive coping strategies that are consistent with the principles of recovery orientation (Richter, 2011).

Under normal circumstances, complete voice rest should not exceed three days. Within this period, most acute symptoms usually show significant improvement, especially when anti-inflammatory or antibiotic medication is taken at the same time (Hunter et al., 2009). It is important that singers are explicitly instructed not to whisper with effort, as tense whispering can strain the vocal folds (Echternach et al., 2024). A gradual return to controlled voice training should usually begin on the fourth day, if symptoms improve. Only in justified exceptional cases should complete voice rest be extended beyond five days. It is unlikely that voice impairments that do not improve significantly within this period can be improved by further voice rest alone, so alternative or additional therapeutic measures should be considered (Kaneko et al., 2017).

Working conditions on stage

Since the 17th century, the art of opera has been the centre of attention, and singers have been surrounded by an aura of celebrity not unlike the cultural status of today's rock stars. Opera works were composed with deliberate consideration of the vocal abilities of individual performers, with roles tailored to showcase their particular strengths and maximise audience admiration (Rosselli, 1992). However, from the early 19th century onwards, a clear paradigm shift in the demands placed on the voice can be observed: the opera moved from the 'bel canto' aesthetic of lyrical beauty and agility towards a more dramatic vocal style designed to project over increasingly large orchestras. This shift demanded greater vocal power, darker timbres, and often a sacrifice of the florid agility that had characterised earlier styles (Stark, 2003). This development also gave rise to first attempts to provide opera singers with professional health care. However, as Watt (2023) states in his retrospective analysis of health behaviours of professional singers in the 19th century, health regimes for singers often blended medical advice with superstition. Generally, in this time, practices around voice care were part of broader public health discourses including hygiene, clean air, bathing, or diet (Watt, 2023).

The development in musical aesthetics coincided with several structural and technological changes. Venues became larger, orchestras grew in both size and complexity, and innovations in instrument making altered the soundscape of opera houses. Parallel to these developments, there was a change in the cultural and artistic status of singers. No longer unchallenged at the centre of opera production, the conceptual and musical ambitions of the composer and the work of art itself increasingly took centre stage. This change is particularly evident in the works of Richard Wagner, who strove to create a 'Gesamtkunstwerk', or 'total work of art', in which the singers served the unity of the composition rather than displaying their personal virtuosity. Perhaps the most vivid example of this is the failed early attempts to stage *Tristan und Isolde*. After 77 rehearsals at the Vienna Court Opera in the early 1860s, the work was deemed unperformable and withdrawn, proof of the unprecedented vocal demands placed on the performers (Schick, 2017).

This phenomenon was not an isolated case. Richard Strauss' *Salome* is another instructive example. During the preparatory phase for the Dresden premiere in 1905, a considerable number of singers withdrew from their roles after the first piano rehearsal because they found the parts initially unsingable (Messmer, 1994).

These historical examples underscore an important point: as the demands on opera shifted towards more dramatic and vocally demanding compositions, reports of vocal crises and chronic overuse of the voice among singers increased. Thus, overuse of the voice is not a new or unusual phenomenon among professional singers. Rather, it is closely linked to the historical and structural development of opera performance itself.

Beyond musical demands: Environmental and global stressors in the modern career of professional singers

In addition to the significantly increased musical and technical demands, contemporary singers face a range of additional challenges that reflect the comprehensive changes in the structure of the performing arts. The life of high-performing professional singers is increasingly shaped by tour schedules, frequent travel and performance across multiple time zones, which impose environmental and logistical stressors. Everyday life for touring performers is patterned around travel times and performance schedules (Zendel, 2021). Sleep-disrupting travel, such as long-haul or overnight flights has been shown to reduce both sleep quality and quantity (Fowler et al., 2015). Such disturbances can alter vocal function and can take a significant toll on the voice, disrupting the recovery process under conditions of compromised rest (Bagnall, 2011).

Among these factors, indoor climatic conditions are a particularly critical and often underestimated stress factor. The microclimate on opera stages, especially in terms of humidity, can deviate significantly from the optimal conditions recommended for vocal performances (Richter et al., 2000). When travelling and performing on unfamiliar stages, singers are often exposed to suboptimal or fluctuating air quality, which can lead to increased susceptibility to vocal fatigue, irritation of the mucous membranes, or delayed vocal recovery. In addition, singers working in contemporary, director-driven opera productions are sometimes exposed to potentially hazardous stage materials and performance requirements. These may include the use of chemically treated props, artificial smoke, or physically demanding choreographic elements, all of which can pose significant health risks, particularly to the vocal apparatus and respiratory tract (Richter et al., 2002).

In particular, younger or less experienced performers may lack the confidence or authority to question such conditions, even if they endanger their health or vocal health (Uni-Europa, 2025). This dynamic points to an important psychosocial dimension of professional singing: the interplay of artistic vulnerability, professional hierarchy, and physical risks can impair both vocal well-being and psychological recovery (Allison, 2021). Therefore, in today's opera world, the ability to maintain vocal health is no longer just a matter of singing technique or training but depends equally on coping strategies that take into account the environmental, logistical, and psychological stress factors of a globally mobile artistic life.

Self-regulation and recovery in professional singing careers

In accordance with the recovery-stress model developed by Kellmann and Kallus (2001), professional singers must demonstrate a high degree of self-regulation skills. This includes the ability to manage one's own physical and psychological resources effectively, often without access to protected recovery environments or institutionalised support systems.

A professional singer must develop an increased awareness of their physical and psychological states, possess robust self-management skills, and maintain the flexibility to respond adaptively to performance-related and professional stressors (Blevis et al., this volume, Chapter 5). Such skills are not only essential for maintaining artistic performance, but also play a central role in preventing cumulative overload and vocal dysfunction. In this context, recovery is not a passive state, but an active regulatory process that requires continuous assessment of stressors and individual coping strategies, as described by Beckmann (2023).

Singers must plan their careers well and carefully and view the profession from a lifelong perspective (Altenmüller et al., this volume, Chapter 1; Spahn & Richter, 2006). This means that they must be aware that a singing career is usually of limited duration (Mathmann et al., 2024). It is precisely in this respect that the concept of rest plays an important role in the context of a lifelong perspective. Consciously maintaining vocal health by incorporating rest breaks into a singer's daily routine can thus lead to robust vocal function that is maintained over many years.

Conclusion and recommendations for practice

For singers it can be helpful to teach knowledge about the physiology of the voice during university studies, including meaningful career planning that takes vocal hygiene into account. In this context recovery is an active regulatory process that requires continuous assessment of stressors and individual coping strategies. These should be learned at an early stage of training.

Every professional singer should be supported by a reliable, interdisciplinary team, usually consisting of a voice teacher and a phoniatric specialist, who together monitor and accompany vocal and artistic development throughout their career. This long-term support enables individual decisions and timely interventions, especially at critical transition points. Moreover, singers are advised not to perform vocal repertoire with great vocal demands too early in their careers.

Humming exercises are recommended, which are intended 'massaging' and 'stretching' the vocal folds. Vocal rest plays an important therapeutic role, especially in cases of voice impairment. Recovery as an overarching concept that also includes dealing with psychological and professional stress factors can enable long-term positive vocal function and a long career as a singer.

Acknowledgement

I thank Eckart Altenmüller for his suggestions regarding the deepening of the scientific discussion with respect to the holistic concept of recovery as elaborated in this book.

References

Achey, M. A., He, M. Z., & Akst, L. M. (2016). Vocal hygiene habits and vocal handicap among conservatory students of classical singing. *Journal of Voice*, *30*, 192–197.

Allison, J. (2021). *An exploration of mid-career opera singers' non-performance work and its impact on their professional identities* [Doctoral dissertation, University of Toronto]. University of Toronto Research Repository. https://utoronto.scholaris.ca/server/api/core/bitstreams/56738b02-4d29-400e-b573-8cc650d19cd2/content

Apfelbach, C. S., & Guzmán, M. (2024). Acoustic, aerodynamic, morphometric, and perceptual changes during and after semi-occluded vocal tract exercise: An integrative review. *Journal of Voice*, *38*(2), 404–425.

Ayoub, M. R., Larrouy-Maestri, P., & Morsomme, D. (2019). The effect of smoking on the fundamental frequency of the speaking voice. *Journal of Voice*, *33*(5), 802–802.

Bagnall, A. D. (2011). Some vocal consequences of sleep deprivation. *Journal of Voice*, *25*(1), 57–65.

Beckmann, J. (2023). Self-regulation of recovery. In M. Kellmann, S. Jakowski, & J. Beckmann (Eds), *The importance of recovery for physical and mental health: Negotiating the effects of underrecovery* (pp. 53–69). Routledge

Beckmann, J., Kellmann, M., & Jakowski, S. (2023). Recovery is more than just healing: Advocating a broader perspective on recovery in physical and mental health. In M. Kellmann, S. Jakowski, & J. Beckmann (Eds.), *The importance of recovery for physical and mental health: Negotiating the effects of underrecovery* (pp. 266–270). Routledge.

Belyk, M., Pfordresher, P. Q., Liotti, M., & Brown, S. (2016). The neural basis of vocal pitch imitation in humans. *Journal of Cognitive Neuroscience*, *28*(4), 621–635.

Blatt, I. M. (1983). Training singing children during the phases of voice mutation. *Annals of Otolology, Rhinology & Laryngology*, *92*(5), 462–468.

Branski, R. C., Rosen, C. A., Verdolini, K., Hebda, P. A., & Kaganov, I. (2005). Acute vocal fold wound healing in a rabbit model. *Annals of Otology, Rhinology & Laryngology*, *114*(1), 19–24.

Carroll, T. L., Nix, J. H., Hunter, E. J., Emerich, K., & Titze, I. R. (2006). Objective measurement of vocal fatigue in classically trained singers. *Journal of Voice*, *20*(3), 443–450.

Caruso, A. J., Mueller, P. B., & Xue, A. (1994). Relative contributions of voice and articulation to listener judgements of age and gender: Preliminary data and implications. *Voice*, *3*, 1–9.

Echternach, M., Köberlein, M., Döllinger, M., Kirsch, J., & Pilsl, T. (2024). Does forced whisper have an impact on voice parameters? *European Archives of Otorhinolaryngology*, *281*(9), 4873–4880.

Echternach, M., Köberlein, M., Gellrich, D., Guzman, M., Laukkanen, A. M., Burk, F., Döllinger, M., Richter, B., & Kainz, M. A. (2021). Duration of biodynamic changes associated with water resistance therapy. *Logopedics, Phoniatrics, Vocology*, *46*(3), 126–133.

Echternach, M., Raschka, J., Kuranova, L., Köberlein, M., Richter, B., Döllinger, M., & Kainz, M. A. (2020). Immediate effects of water resistance therapy on patients with vocal fold mass lesions. *European Archives of Otorhinolaryngology*, *277*(7), 1995–2003.

Elias, M. E., Sataloff, R. T., Rosen, D. C., Heuer, R. J., & Spiegel, J. R. (1997). Normal strobovideolaryngoscopy: Variability in healthy singers. *Journal of Voice*, *11*(1), 104–107.

Flock, L., King, S. R., Williams, J., Finlay, E., Smikle, H., Benito, M., Benton-Stace, F., Brown, J, Mann-Daraz, A. J., Hart, L., Mclean, K., Prucnal, Z., Barry, L., Lynes, R., Toy, M., Valentine, K., Slattery, S., & Aldridge-Waddon, L. (2025). Working together to find a voice: Recommendations for voice healthcare based on expert-by-experience and practitioner consensus. *Journal of Voice*, *39*(4), 1137.e9–1137.e17. https://doi.org/10.1016/j.jvoice.2023.02.023.

Fowler, P. M., Duffield, R., Vaile, J., & Minett, G. M. (2015). Effects of sleep hygiene and artificial bright light interventions on recovery from simulated international air travel. *European Journal of Applied Physiology*, *115*(6), 123–134.

Gehling, D., Sridharan, S., Fritz, M., Friedmann, D. R., Fang, Y., Amin, M. R., & Branski, R. C. (2014). Backstage at Broadway: A demographic study. *Journal of Voice*, *28*(3), 311–315.

Gembris, H., & Langner, D. (2005). *Von der Musikhochschule auf den Arbeitsmarkt. Erfahrungen von Absolventen, Arbeitsmarktexperten und Hochschullehrern* [From music college to the job market. Experiences of graduates, job market experts and university lecturers]. Wißner.

Guinness World of Records. (2025). *Highest vocal note by a male*. Retrieved June 26, 2025 from https://www.guinnessworldrecords.com/world-records/79003-highest-vocal-note-by-a-male

Heller-Stark, A., Maxfield, L., Herrick, J., Smith, M., & Titze, I. (2024). Comparative study of two semi-occluded vocal tract protocols: A randomized clinical trial. *Journal of Speech, Language, and Hearing Research*, *67*(11), 4275–4287.

Hunter, E. J., Ferguson, S. H., & Newman, C. A. (2016). Listener estimations of talker age: A meta-analysis of the literature. *Logopedics, Phoniatrics, Vocology*, *41*(3), 101–105.

Hunter, E. J., Titze, I. R., & Chan, R. W. (2009). Quantifying vocal fatigue recovery: Dynamic vocal recovery trajectories after a vocal loading exercise. *Annals of Otology, Rhinology & Laryngology*, *118*(6), 449–460.

Jørgensen, H. (1997). Time for practicing? Higher level music students' use of time for instrumental practicing. In H. Jørgensen & A. C. Lehmann (Eds.), *Does practice make perfect? Current theory and research on instrumental music practice* (pp. 123–139). Norges musikkhogskole.

Jurik, A. G. (1984). Ossification and calcification of the laryngeal skeleton. *Acta Radiologica: Diagnosis*, *25*(1), 17–22.

Kallus, K. W. (2016). Stress and recovery: An overview. In K. W. Kallus & M. Kellmann (Eds.), *The Recovery-Stress Questionnaires: User manual* (pp. 27–48). Pearson Assessment.

Kaneko, M., Shiromoto, O., Fuji-Kurachi, R., Kishimoto, Y., Tateya, I., & Hirano, S. (2017). Optimal duration for voice rest after vocal fold surgery: A randomized clinical study. *Journal of Voice*, *31*(3), 384–390.

Kellmann, M. (2002). Underrecovery and overtraining: Different concepts – Similar impact? In M. Kellmann (Ed.), *Enhancing recovery: Preventing underperformance in athletes* (pp. 3–24). Human Kinetics.

Kellmann, M., & Beckmann, J. (Eds.). (2022). *Recovery and well-being in sport and exercise*. Routledge.

Kellmann, M., Bertollo, M., Bosquet, L., Brink, M., Coutts, A. J., Duffield, R., Erlacher, D., Halson, S. L., Hecksteden, A., Heidari, J., Kallus, K. W., Meeusen, R., Mujika, I., Robazza, C., Skorski, S., Venter, R., & Beckmann, J. (2018). Recovery and performance in sport: Consensus statement. *International Journal of Sports Physiology and Performance*, *13*(2), 240–245.

Kellmann, M., Jakowski, S., & Beckmann, J. (Eds.). (2023). *The importance of recovery for physical and mental health: Negotiating the effects of underrecovery*. Routledge.

Kellmann, M., & Kallus, K. W. (2001). *The Recovery-Stress Questionnaire for Athletes: User manual*. Human Kinetics.

Lã, F. M. B., & Ardura, D. (2022). What voice-related metrics change with menopause? A systematic review and meta-analysis study. *Journal of Voice*, *36*(3), 438.e1–438.e17. https://doi.org/10.1016/j.jvoice.2020.06.012

Mathmann, P., Konerding, U., Deuster, D., & Neumann, K. (2024). The influence of age, gender, health-related behaviors, and other factors on occupationally relevant health complaints of singers. *Journal of Voice*, *38*(1), 170–180.

Messmer, F. (1994). *Richard Strauss. Biographie eines Klangzauberers Richard Strauss*. [Biography of a sound magician Richard Strauss]. Atlantis-Verlag.

Meyer, D., & Helding, L. (2021). Practical science in the studio: "No-tech" strategies. *Journal of Singing*, *77*(3), 317–323.

Mueller, P. B. (1997). The aging voice. *Seminars in Speech and Language*, *18*(2), 159–169.

Myint, C., Moore, J. E., Hu, A., Jaworek, A. J., & Sataloff, R. T. (2016). A comparison of initial and subsequent follow-up strobovideolaryngoscopic examinations in singers. *Journal of Voice*, *30*(4), 472–477.

Pestana, P. M., Vaz-Freitas, S., & Manso, M. C. (2017). Prevalence of voice disorders in singers: Systematic review and meta-analysis. *Journal of Voice*, *31*(6), 722–727.

Prebil, N., Hočevar Boltežar, I., & Šereg Bahar, M. (2020). Risk factors for voice problems in professional actors and singers. *Zdravstveno Varstvo*, *59*(2), 92–98.

Ragan, K. (2018). Defining evidence-based voice pedagogy: A new framework. *Journal of Singing*, *74*(5), 541–550.

Richter, B. (2011). Phoniatrie [Phoniatrics]. In C. Spahn, B. Richter, & E. Altenmüller (Eds.), *MusikerMedizin. Diagnostik, Therapie und Prävention von musikerspezifischen Erkrankungen* (pp. 291–327). Schattauer.

Richter, B., & Echternach, M. (2011). Stimmärztliche Betreuung und Behandlung von Sängern [Medical treatment of singers' voices]. *HNO, 59*(6), 547–555.

Richter, B., Echternach, M., & Traser, L. (2024). Investigation methods for vocal onset – A historical perspective. *Bioengineering, 11*(10), 989. https://doi.org/10.3390/bioengineering11100989

Richter, B., Löhle, E., Knapp, B., Weikert, M., Schlömicher-Thier, J., & Verdolini, K. (2002). Harmful substances on the opera stage: Possible negative effects on singers' respiratory tracts. *Journal of Voice, 16*(1), 72–80.

Richter, B., Löhle, E., Maier, W., Kliemann, B., & Verdolini, K. (2000). Working conditions on stage: Climatic considerations. *Logopedics, Phoniatrics, Vocology, 25*(2), 80–86.

Richter, B., & Mürbe, D. (2020). Voice science and hygiene in singing education. In A. am Zehnhoff-Dinnesen, T. Nawka, B. Wiskirska-Woźnica, & K. Neumann (Eds.), *Phoniatrics I: Fundamentals – voice disorders – disorders of language and hearing development* (pp. 86–90). Springer.

Richter, B., Mürbe, D., Schmid, B., & Sandel, M. (2013). Stimmphysiologie in der Ausbildung von Sängern und Schauspielern [Vocal physiology in the training of singers and actors]. In B. Richter (Ed.), *Die Stimme* (pp. 114–160). Henschel.

Rosselli, J. (1992). *Singers of Italian opera: The history of a profession.* Cambridge University Press.

Saeedi, S., Baghban, K., Seifpanahi, M. S., Nazari, M. A., Moshtagh, A., Manoosi, M., & Ayubi, E. (2026). The vocal hygiene treatment programs for singers: A systematic review. *Journal of Voice, 40*(2), 376–385.

Sataloff, R. T., Hawkshaw, M. J., Johnson, J. L., Ruel, B., Wilhelm, A., & Lurie, D. (2012). Prevalence of abnormal laryngeal findings in healthy singing teachers. *Journal of Voice, 26*(5), 577–583.

Savareh, S., Moradi, N., Yazdi, M. J. S., Soltani, M., & Latifi, M. (2023). Immediate effects of semi-occluded vocal tract exercises as a vocal warm-up in singers. *Journal of Voice, 37*(6), 875–880.

Schick, H. (2017). *Zwischen Skandal und Triumph: Richard Wagners Wirken in München.* Retrieved September 6, 2025 from https://epub.ub.uni-muenchen.de/25457/1/Hartmut_Schick_Zwischen_Skandal_und_Triumph_Richard_Wagners_Wirken_in_Muenchen.pdf

Seidner, W., & Wendler, J. (1989). Der Dysodiebegriff – historische und aktuelle Aspekte [The concept of dysodia – Historical and current aspects]. *Sprache - Stimme - Gehör, 13*, 55–59.

Sivasankar, M., & Leydon, C. (2010). The role of hydration in vocal fold physiology. *Current Opinion in Otolaryngology & Head and Neck Surgery, 18*(3), 171–175.

Spahn, C., & Richter, B. (2006). The development of the singing voice across the lifespan. In H. Gembris (Ed.), *Musical development from a lifespan perspective* (pp. 119–130). Peter Lang.

Stachler, R. J., Francis, D. O., Schwartz, S. R., Damask, C. C., Digoy, G. P., Krouse, H. J., McCoy, S. J., Ouellette, D. R., Patel, R. R., Reavis, C. C. W., Smith, L. J., Smith, M., Strode, S. W., Woo, P., & Nnacheta, L. C. (2018). Clinical Practice Guidelines: Hoarseness (Dysphonia) (Update). *Otolaryngology - Head and Neck Surgery, 158*(Suppl. 1), S1–S42. https://doi.org/10.1177/0194599817751030. Erratum

in: *Otolaryngology - Head and Neck Surgery, 159*(2), 403. https://doi.org/ 10.1177/0194599818766900
Stark, J. (2003). *Bel canto: A history of vocal pedagogy*. University of Toronto Press.
Sundberg, J. (1995). The singer's formant revisited. *Voice, 4*, 106–119.
Sundberg, J. (2018). The singing voice. In S. Früholz & P. Belin (Eds.), *The Oxford handbook of voice perception* (pp. 117–142). Oxford University Press.
Tanaka, S. (2021). Mirror neuron activity during audiovisual appreciation of opera performance. *Frontiers of Psychology, 11*, 563031. https://doi.org/10.3389/fpsyg.2020.563031. Erratum in *Frontiers of Psychology, 14*, 1329662. https://doi.org/10.3389/fpsyg.2023.1329662
Thurber, C., Dugas, L. R., Ocobock, C., Carlson, B., Speakman, J. R., & Pontzer, H. (2019). Extreme events reveal an alimentary limit on sustained maximal human energy expenditure. *Science Advances, 5*(6), eaaw0341. https://doi.org/10.1126/sciadv.aaw0341
Timmermans, B., Vanderwegen, J., & De Bodt, M. S. (2005). Outcome of vocal hygiene in singers. *Current Opinion in Otolaryngology & Head and Neck Surgery, 13*(3), 138–142.
Titze, I. R. (2006). Voice training and therapy with a semi-occluded vocal tract: Rationale and scientific underpinnings. *Journal of Speech, Language, and Hearing Research, 49*(2), 448–459.
Titze, I. R., Maxfield, L., & Cox, K. T. (2025). Optimizing diameter, length, and water immersion in flow resistant tube vocalization. *Journal of Voice, 39*(2), 403–409.
Titze, I. R., Svec, J. G., & Popolo, P. S. (2003). Vocal dose measures: Quantifying accumulated vibration exposure in vocal fold tissues. *Journal of Speech, Language, and Hearing Research, 46*(4), 919–932.
Torre, P. 3rd, & Barlow, J. A. (2009). Age-related changes in acoustic characteristics of adult speech. *Journal of Communication Disorders, 42(5)*, 324–333.
Traser, L., Richter, B., Nusseck, M., & Echternach, M. (2012). Standardisierte Stimmdiagnostik bei professionellen Sopranistinnen in der musikermedizinischen Sängersprechstunde [Standardised voice diagnostics for professional sopranos in the medical consultation for singers]. *Musikphysiologie und Musikermedizin, 19*(2), 140–147.
Triebner, K., Matulonga, B., Johannessen, A., Suske, S., Benediktsdóttir, B., Demoly, P., Dharmage, S. C., Franklin, K. A., Garcia-Aymerich, J., Gullón Blanco, J. A., Heinrich, J., Holm, M., Jarvis, D., Jõgi, R., Lindberg, E., Moratalla Rovira, J. M., Muniozguren Agirre, N., Pin, I., Probst-Hensch, N., Puggini, L., … Gómez Real, F. (2017). Menopause is associated with accelerated lung function decline. *American Journal of Respiratory and Critical Care Medicine, 195*(8), 1058–1065.
UNI Europa. (2025). *Health and safety in the live performance sector: The show must go on* (Version 2). UNI Europa. https://www.uni-europa.org/wp-content/uploads/sites/3/2025/07/HS_in_live_performance_ver2_June2025-2.pdf
van den Berg, J. (1958). Myoelastic-aerodynamic theory of voice production. *Journal of Speech and Hearing Research, 3*, 227–244.
Verdolini, K., & Ramig, L. O. (2001). Review: Occupational risks for voice problems. *Logopedics, Phoniatrics, Vocology, 26*(1), 37–46.
Vermeulen, R., van der Linde, J., Abdoola, S., van Lierde, K., & Graham, M. A. (2021). The effect of superficial hydration, with or without systemic hydration, on voice quality in future female professional singers. *Journal of Voice, 35*(5), 728–738.

Watt, P. (2023). How did nineteenth-century singers care for their voice? *Royal Musical Association Research Chronicle*, *54*, 65–93.

Wiegert, P., Rydell, R., Houmann, A., Johnson, D. T., & Åhlander, V. L. (in press). Heard but not seen: Swedish opera choristers' thoughts on occupational environment and vocal health, an explorative qualitative study. *Journal of Voice*. https://doi.org/10.1016/j.jvoice.2025.01.036

Williams, N. R. (2003). Occupational groups at risk of voice disorders: A review of the literature. *Occupational Medicine*, *53*(7), 456–460.

Woo, P. (2020). Objective measures of stroboscopy and high-speed video. *Advances in Oto-Rhino-Laryngology*, *85*, 25–44.

Yilmaz, C., Bostanci, Ö., Eken, Ö., Alkahtani, R., & Aldhahi, M. I. (2025). Maximizing phonation: Impact of inspiratory muscle strengthening on vocal durations and pitch range. *BMC Pulmonary Medicine*, *25*(1), 15. https://doi.org/10.1186/s12890-024-03471-2

Zamponi, V., Mazzilli, R., Mazzilli, F., & Fantini, M. (2021). Effect of sex hormones on human voice physiology: From childhood to senescence. *Hormones*, *20*(4), 691–696.

Zendel, A. (2021). Precarious mobilities in the touring music industry. *Popular Music History*, *14*(1–2), 3–24.

9

OPTIMISING RECOVERY

Supporting artists to flourish in circus, and in life

Melanie Stuckey, David Munro, Stephanie Greenspan, and Joanna Nicholas

Introduction

Circus arts could very well be described as embodied creativity combined with athleticism. At its core, circus regularly pushes the boundaries of human physical capabilities, exhibiting a unique blend of strength, flexibility, balance and endurance. Alongside the physical skills, circus artists must also develop psychological (cognitive and affective), social and creative capacities to optimise performance, connect with audiences in a meaningful way, and support flourishing[1] in life inside and outside of circus. Training to achieve such circus skills requires the experience of stress and fatigue through functional overreaching; yet rest and rejuvenation are necessary for recovery specific to circus practice, along with having time and energy for life outside of circus. A comprehensive recovery strategy is required to optimise the positive (e.g., performance gains, well-being) and mitigate the negative (e.g., injury, burnout) training adaptations (Kellmann et al., 2018).

Since circus training and performance require holistic development, recovery must avoid focusing exclusively on physical rest. The *Four Domains for Development for All* (4D4D4All) framework (Agans et al., 2024) expands on the *Circus for Development* framework, which was developed based on the unique holistic experience of circus practice (Stuckey et al., 2021). Both frameworks describe four developmental domains of movement (or circus) experiences (physical, psychological, social, and creative; Agans et al., 2024;

Stuckey, M., Munro, D., Greenspan, S., & Nicholas, J. (2026). Optimising recovery: Supporting artists to flourish in circus, and in life. In E. Altenmüller, M. Kellmann, J. Beckmann, & G. M. Moyle (Eds.), *Recovery and well-being in the performing arts* (pp. 153–174). Routledge.

DOI: 10.4324/9781003566885-11

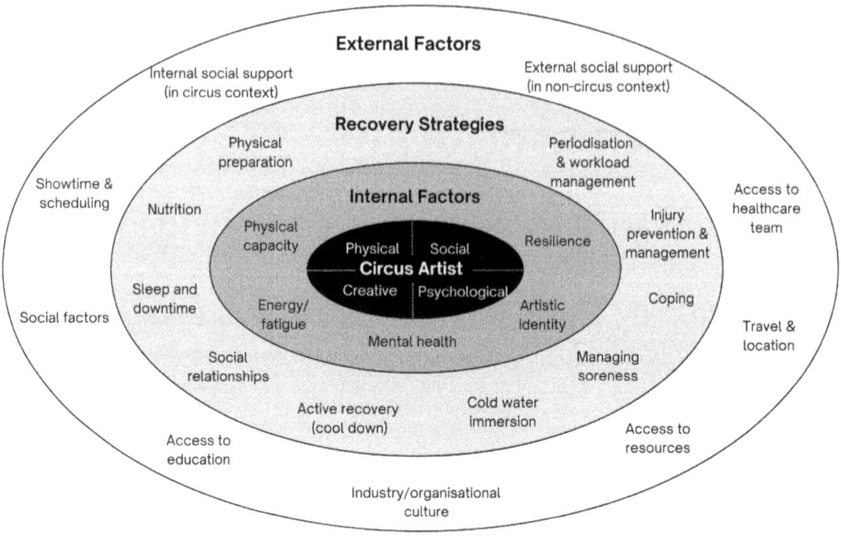

FIGURE 9.1 Holistic recovery approach to optimising performance and well-being in circus.

Stuckey et al., 2021). The 4D4D4All model more explicitly describes the importance of both individual (internal) and environmental (external) factors and how a systems approach to movement experiences leads to flourishing people and communities (Agans et al., 2024). Aligning with this, recovery should take a holistic perspective addressing internal and external aspects of all four domains (Figure 9.1), so the artist will not only be in optimal condition to perform, but also to experience a meaningful and fulfilling life.

External aspects are dependent on the greater social and specific circus contexts, which vary greatly. Recreational circus is available as youth or adult programmes at circus training or community facilities, or within dance or physical education curriculum. They often offer performance opportunities in showcases or recitals. Pre-professional and professional intensive training programmes may co-exist with recreational programmes, but typically include an audition process, more hours of training, and performances across the year. Professionalising circus programmes are diploma or degree programmes from an accredited post-secondary institution and typically include around 20–30 hours of physical training per week alongside an academic courseload. The professional context ranges from freelance performers who train independently and perform in various settings including nightclubs, corporate events, and seasonal shows, to artists employed by companies to perform in resident or travelling shows with eight or more performances per week, year-round with two to four weeks of vacation leave per year.

Experiences within each context will depend on the combination of circus disciplines practised. The unique physical and psychosocial skills required for each of the discipline subgroups (aerial acrobatics, ground acrobatics, manipulation, character, music; Greenspan et al., 2022) are further differentiated by the specific apparatus, the style of the act, and the artists' personal characteristics and preferences. Furthermore, individuals may perform more than one role at a given time. For example, many artists have additional responsibilities including creation, set-up, costume production, or coaching (Cayrol et al., 2019). Thus, circus artists require individualised approaches to recovery tailored to their unique participation.

Recovery in circus

Recovery serves multiple functions. Commonly, it is considered as having sufficient rest between training or performances to integrate training gains and re-energise. However, recovery is also important to prepare for and address the high mental and emotional demands of circus (Stuckey et al., 2025), support career/practice longevity, and ensure that artists are flourishing both within and outside of circus. Finally, recovery is important for creativity. In movement, such as circus, creativity is an embodied process (Richard et al., 2023) that can be supported through physical, psychological, and social elements (Agans et al., 2024). Embodied creativity is described as a 'messy process' that can often feel destabilising, confronting, and uncomfortable as new ideas are explored (Richard et al., 2023). An artist's physical abilities, psychological resilience, and openness to inspiration, feedback, and failure with others can impact creative outcomes. Thus, individual recovery, along with an environment that supports recovery, can optimise characteristics that foster creativity and bring new ideas and skills to the circus industry.

Historical context influencing recovery practices

Until 1927, when the first circus school was set up in Moscow, Russia, circus skills were considered to be 'secrets' taught only to members of a specific circus family (Burtt & Lavers, 2017). It was not until the mid-to-late 1900s that state and national training schools were implemented in China (Wang, 2024), Western Europe, Canada, and Australia (Burtt & Lavers, 2017). Circus pedagogy outside of familial upbringing has developed over a relatively short period of time. Originally developed from the Russian gymnastics programme, the overarching training models primarily followed a linear pathway (Burtt & Lavers, 2017), focused on repetition of skill training (Wang, 2024). While studies in sport sciences strongly support models that align with training cycles and performance goals (e.g., periodisation and workload management), circus has been slow to shift from its traditions. Adapting sport models to circus is further complicated by sometimes intensive performance schedules (up to ten shows per week; Faltus & Richard, 2022). Little research has focused on recovery in circus artists, though research in dance and sport can guide strategies for this population.

Factors affecting recovery in circus artists

Currently, recovery from circus training and performance is impacted by a multitude of factors including scheduling and implementation, as well as non-circus lifestyle practices that may support or hinder recovery. Most factors impact more than one domain of the 4D4D4All model, and considerations need to be made for both individual and environmental influences.

Sleep

Sleep impacts all domains of the 4D4D4All model with positive effects on several performance metrics, training gains, well-being, and physical and mental health (Reardon et al., 2019). Consequently, it is considered the foundation of recovery. Healthy adults usually require a minimum of seven hours, while adolescents and younger adults require nine to ten hours of sleep per night (Reardon et al., 2019). The only study examining sleep in circus reported that on average, sleep duration, latency, and quality were sufficient in professionalising students (Decker et al., 2019). However, many still felt fatigued, especially during the mid-term exam period (Decker et al., 2022). Fatigue was lower in artists working in a professional company (Donohue et al., 2020), suggesting that age and lifestyle, not simply circus training or performance, may be contributing factors. Artists in touring companies may face sleep challenges, including the impacts of disturbed circadian rhythm from frequently changing time zones (Reardon et al., 2019). Freelance or part-time artists working multiple jobs or those with caregiving responsibilities may have different sleep and fatigue characteristics. Establishing sleep routines can be challenging around performance schedules and lifestyles. Naps may be effective in the short-term, though long-term solutions are preferred (Kellmann et al., 2018). Circus artists may choose to avoid sleep medications, as they are often associated with increased injury risk and impaired performance; however, non-pharmacological options, such as cognitive behavioural therapy, melatonin, and others may be suitable alternatives (Reardon et al., 2019).

Nutrition

Adequate energy intake is vital in providing the body with fuel to meet energy expended, repair and recover following training or performance, and maintain daily body and cognitive functioning. Nutrition primarily impacts the physical and psychological domains, though the social domain may be impacted if motivation for social interaction is impacted by underfuelling or difficulty with interpersonal relationships in instance of disordered eating or eating disorders (Mountjoy et al., 2023; Reece et al., 2023). Along with sleep, nutrition is a recovery priority due to its impact on performance and well-being. Circus artists can face difficulties in meeting nutritional requirements. Travelling circus artists may encounter different cultural cuisines and varying levels of access to nourishing foods and cooking facilities (Faltus & Richard, 2022). Students at professionalising circus schools may be preparing meals for themselves for the first time, while attempting to meet their high energy requirements. Performing artists may have outdated beliefs about carbohydrates and limited nutrition knowledge which could potentially lead to inadequate energy intake and malnourishment from eliminating food groups (Nicholas & Grafenauer, 2023). They may also feel pressured to conform to aesthetic ideals (van Rens, 2022; Walby & Stuart, 2021), which increases the risk of disordered eating behaviours and eating disorders.

Rates of disordered eating are higher in pre-professional and professional circus artists compared to the general population, and those considered at risk of an eating disorder are more likely to score higher on exercise addiction (van Rens, 2022). The combination of potentially insufficient energy intake with high energy expenditure can lead to low energy availability (LEA), which describes a state of inadequate energy to support functions required by the body to maintain optimal health and performance (Mountjoy et al., 2023). LEA can occur with or without disordered eating or exercise behaviours, and artists may be more susceptible during transitions in training or performance cycles, or periods of increased energy demands. Prolonged and/or severe LEA can lead to relative energy deficit in sport (REDs), which can impair physiological and/or psychological functioning (Mountjoy et al., 2023). It has been described in dance (Allen et al., 2024) and likely occurs in circus as well. Thus, assuring adequate energy intake should be a primary recovery goal for circus artists.

Since LEA and REDs impact hormones, monitoring reproductive hormone-related functions can be a simple self-monitoring strategy. Artists who are biologically female and not taking hormonal contraceptives or therapies can track their menstrual cycle length and frequency (Keay et al., 2022), with a monthly bleed being a sign of healthy hormone function. Those who are biologically male and not on hormonal therapy, can track morning erections as an indicator of testosterone status (Hackett & Kirby, 2023). Changes in these patterns, such as absence of menstruation or loss of morning erections, could indicate insufficient intake to meet energy demands.

Along with adequate overall energy intake, the consumption of carbohydrates, protein, and fluids plays an important role in performance and recovery. Strategies for dancers and athletes may be applicable to the circus artist with adjustments according to discipline, artistic style, and workload characteristics. The recommended daily intake for dancers and athletes ranges from 3 to 12 g of carbohydrate and 1 to 2 g of protein per kg body weight (Amawi et al., 2024; Challis & Stevens Edd, 2019). Carbohydrate intake before, during, and after exercise can ensure energy and cognitive function are sustained during training or performance (Brown & Wyon, 2014). Consumption of protein three to four hours before training and/or performance and combining protein (essential amino acids) and carbohydrates during training promotes peak rates of muscle protein synthesis, reduces muscle damage, and extends time to exhaustion during training (Amawi et al., 2024). Appropriate hydration is important for cognitive function, digestion, and muscle function to support optimal performance (Amawi et al., 2024). Ingesting 500–600 mL of water two to three hours and an additional 200–300 mL of water 10–20 minutes prior to training is recommended for athletes to commence training in a well-hydrated state. Fluid intake during and after exercise should align with fluid deficits (sweat and urine loss), ensuring body weight reduction does not exceed 2% (Amawi et al., 2024). This is particularly important in hot environments, such as performance in outdoor summer festivals or training in summer camps. Optimising dietary intake of nutrients necessary for physical and psychological functioning is integral to artists' performance and well-being.

Physical preparation

Physical preparation is a pro-active, long-term recovery strategy that focuses on building an appropriate capacity, confidence, and resilience to withstand the physical, technical, mental, and artistic demands of training. It addresses the physical, psychological and creative domains of the 4D4D4All model. Incorporating a well-designed physical preparation programme will assist an artist to better absorb shocks, support intricate movements, and recover more quickly from the physical stress of performances and training. Historically many artists relied solely on 'doing more' circus for physical preparation. However, it is now recognised that multi-training (or cross-training) can produce beneficial results when compared to single training techniques only (Jakiwa et al., 2023). For example, many aerial acts (e.g., trapeze, rope) require sufficient strength for the artist to pull up their own body weight. If a fundamental weakness exists in this area, the artist will find it challenging to acquire difficult and complex movements to successfully and safely complete an aerial act. Targeted training activities that strengthen the muscles required for such actions can better address the issue while mitigating injury risk. Symmetry and imbalances that often occur due to unilateral movements in acts performed repeatedly with dominant side tricks can also be addressed with strength and conditioning programmes. Two strategies to optimise physical preparation in circus are discussed next.

Periodisation

Periodisation is commonly implemented in elite sport and involves systematically planning training programmes to optimise performance and recovery

(Mujika et al., 2018). It can be difficult to implement in professional circus contexts where condensed or overlapping performance schedules can leave little time for distinct training cycles (Faltus & Richard, 2022; Wyon & Allard, 2021). In some instances, artists will spend more time in performance than training. Implementation in training programmes may be more feasible (Wyon & Allard, 2021) but periodisation of performance schedules is possible and may also be required (Richard et al., this volume, Chapter 12). Adaptable, discipline-specific planning should be used rather than a one-size-fits-all approach.

Integrated periodisation includes considerations for training, recovery, nutrition, psychology, and skill across different phases of training (Mujika et al., 2018). Skill periodisation is particularly crucial in circus, where skill demands may outweigh physical capacity requirements (i.e., motor skill/timing may be more crucial to execution than strength or endurance). Understanding these requirements in relation to artist skill level and physical capacity is needed to develop appropriate training plans. It has been proposed that the time spent in each periodised phase varies depending on a dancer's stage of training or career (Wyon & Allard, 2021). This translates well to circus, where, similar to pre-professional dance (Wyon & Allard, 2021), first-year students will often spend more time on general preparation and technical skill development, gradually shifting the focus more towards artistry and performance in the following years. Across the training programme, structured sub-phases can be divided from the macrocycle (entire training cycle; e.g., twelve months) to mesocycles (training blocks; e.g., twelve weeks) and microcycles (e.g., weeks within each training block) for detailed planning. Rest and recovery are prioritised in each cycle to optimise performance and prevent injury and burnout.

Tapering is a strategy used to reduce training-induced fatigue before major performances or competitions. It involves decreasing training volume while maintaining intensity in the days leading up to a performance, allowing artists to rest and regenerate without losing training adaptations (Wyon, 2010). Tapering adapted from team sports appears suitable for dance, as both are characterised by multiple performance or competition periods (Wyon & Allard, 2021). However, circus companies often have a more condensed performance schedule than sports teams (eight to ten shows per week and a nine to twelve-week period of touring; Faltus & Richard, 2022). Barriers within the circus context include rehearsals scheduled for a short, intensive block (e.g., several weeks or months) leading right up to show opening due to artistic director and venue costs and availability for rehearsals, as well as traditional training mindsets to work up to the last minute in an attempt to 'perfect' the show. Table 9.1 gives examples of how periodisation and tapering could be implemented in different circus contexts.

TABLE 9.1 Key training focus or characteristics for different phases of periodisation across team sport, dance, and circus (proposed).

Sport (Mujika et al., 2018) Scenario 1: Team sport. Scenario 2: Individual sport.	**Dance** (Wyon & Allard, 2021)	**Circus: Recreational** Often terms or blocks. Summer camps. Macrocycle one term e.g., ten weeks.	**Circus: Pre-professional/ professionalising training programme** Audition-based programmes usually over a year with a few months off over summer.	**Circus: Freelance, semi-pro/professional** Scenario 1: Professional artist, seasonal winter and summer shows, four-month macrocycle or twelve-month cycle with 2 × 4-mth blocks. Scenario 2: Freelance professional artist and coach. Coaches 12–20 hours per week, two competitions planned for second half of the year. 12-month macrocycle.
General preparation: Scenario 1: Aerobic conditioning, resistance training, and team-based activities supported by individual sessions. May include specialised training (e.g., altitude). Scenario 2: High volume, low to moderate intensity, low-specificity and mixed training modalities (e.g., resistance, cross-training).	**General preparation:** Focuses on enhancing students' technical abilities, including core techniques and specialist techniques based on the course and year of study. This phase may also include strength and conditioning sessions for specific skills like jumping or lifting.	**General preparation:** (Re)building physical capacity, controlled ramp up following time-off. First few weeks more focus on conditioning to building physical capacity, revising established skills, gradual increase in intensity.	**General preparation:** (Re) building physical capacity, controlled ramp up following time-off. First two months of year: Strength training, more cross training than skills training, moderate volume strength and conditioning e.g., 2 × 60-minute conditioning sessions at lower intensity. If extended break focus more on strenth and conditioning and foundational skills. If maintained capacity over break can move to specific prep earlier.	**General Preparation:** Scenario 1: Duration one month, as skills are very established focus is on new act creation, revisiting a previous act, individual strength and conditioning such as resistance training or cross training specific to building capacity for the show. Scenario 2: Focus on rebuilding physical capacity after holiday, increased focus on strength and conditioning, conditioning focused on building capacity for the demands of performance e.g., anaerobic training longer - lactate tolerance to build tolerance and ability to sustain high intensity routine, skills sessions focused on revisiting and developing new skills to include in competition routines. Normal coaching load and level of demonstration and spotting.

Specific preparation/ pre-competition: Scenario 1: Match play, sport-specific technical-tactical training. Scenario 2: Moderate and high volume, high intensity (e.g. race pace), high specificity, may include specialised training (e.g. altitude), may include competition.	**Specific preparation:** Aims to build on the technical skills developed in the previous phase by extending students' artistic skills through movement and non-movement principles, applied in structured rehearsals, improvisation, or self-generated choreography.	**Specific preparation:** Learning new specific skills, sequences of skills to build endurance, choreography, conditioning lower volume and higher intensity built into class. Working towards routine or acts for end-of-term showcase.	**Specific preparation:** Act creation, choreography, and sequences of skills. Duration could be two to three months. Some skill building and maintaining physical capacity through lower volume but higher intensity of conditioning. Microdosing conditioning e.g., 15-minute blocks, higher intensity, three to four days per week within other training sessions rather than distinct strength and conditioning sessions.	**Specific preparation**: Increased focus on choreography, finalising acts, and rehearsals. May include conditioning but as less of a focus. Scenario 1: Duration one month, rehearse specific acts, building up to rehearsing full show with multiple acts, final week in the venue. Scenario 2: Increased focus on choreography and routine training. Several conditioning sessions focused on demands of the performance (e.g., anaerobic or aerobic training, strength or flexibility for specific skills). As we get closer to competition run the entire routine (limit number of full runs in a session so as not to overload musculoskeletal system e.g., max two to three runs of four minute routine at full intensity).
Taper: Scenario 1: 2-3 week taper, including reduced sRPE, lower overall training volume with match-specific play.	**Taper:** Manipulate volume and intensity of the dancer's workloads thereby allowing them to rest and regenerate.	**Taper:** May rehearse acts in open training time or outside of class, minimising extensive rehearsals.	**Taper:** Rehearsing piece, dress rehearsal, reduce strength and conditioning several weeks prior and cease completely one week out from performance.	**Taper:** Reduce volume of training and rehearsals, dress rehearsal or full show at full intensity, reduce strength and conditioning several weeks prior and cease completely one week out from performance.

(Continued)

TABLE 9.1 (Continued)

Scenario 2: Low volume, high intensity, high specificity.	before performing, remove extraneous activities that can lead to fatigue and use free time to rest and recover. Reduce volume of supplementary (including strength and conditioning) training several weeks prior and cease the week of performance. Example in pre-prof setting for Saturday performance: Wednesday: Final day of full-day rehearsals, choreography finalised. Thurs/Fri: Class, full dress rehearsal and video analysis, and if required very specific, short-duration rehearsals.	e.g., once or twice the day before, use visualisation or video feedback to minimise physical workload.		Scenario 1: Marking acts in the performance space, running full show only once or twice per day, no strength and conditioning. Scenario 2: Marking acts in the performance space, running full act only once or twice (particularly the day prior and day of competition), no strength and conditioning. Use visualisation or video feedback to minimise physical workload. Reduce coaching physical workload load by using alternative coaching methods such as use of videos and student demonstrations rather than excessive physical demonstrations and spotting.

	Saturday: Opening night. Throughout season: Class and any required rehearsals scheduled in morning and early afternoon, break from 3 pm for food and rest prior to warm-up and evening show.			
Scenario 1: Main competition/regular season: Weekly/ twice-weekly match fixture, recovery from match, specific conditioning between matches to maintain fitness and peak for key matches, preparation for match. Scenario 2: Competition: Single or multiple-day competition events, may include multiple rounds e.g., semis, finals, etc.	**Performance:** Centres on actual dance performances, showings, auditions, and tours.	**Performance:** End-of-term recital or annual showcase, one or two acts, one to four shows.	**Performance:** Performance season at end of academic year. Multiple acts in multiple shows. Often two months towards end of year, could be over two to three weekends.	**Performance:** Multiple acts in multiple shows or one major competition. Scenario 1: Duration of one month of shows. Depending on length and number of performances may include maintaining strength and conditioning. Specific conditioning between performances to maintain fitness. Scheduled on light or one-show days. Scenario 2: One or two performances for each competition. If competitions are scheduled close in date and different acts/ routines are being performed, ensure both routines are considered in specific preparation phase, also incorporate rest days following first competition before rehearsing for second competition. Reduce

(Continued)

TABLE 9.1 (Continued)

				coaching physical workload load by using alternative coaching methods, such as use of videos and student demonstrations rather than excessive physical demonstrations and spotting.
Play-offs/finals: Scenario 1: As per main competition/ regular season phase with major fitness/ performance peak.	-	-	-	-
Transition/off-season/ injury: Scenario 1: Individual maintenance conditioning, corrective surgery and/or injury rehabilitation. Scenario 2: Rest, recover, and regenerate, may include some maintenance training (e.g., reduced training, cross-training).	**Transition:** Involves reflecting on the performance phase, assessing achieved and missed goals, planning rehabilitation and prehabilitation training for the summer break, and setting goals for the next year's preparation phase.	**Transition/ off-season/injury:** Holiday break, may maintain physical capacity through cross training or conditioning offered over holidays.	**Transition/off season/ injury:** Recovering from showtime, holiday break, also may maintain physical capacity and known skills and proficiency, sometimes summer camps.	**Transition/off season:** Recovering from showtime, holiday break, also may maintain physical capacity and known skills and proficiency, sometimes coaching or participating in summer camps. Scenario 1: One month rest period, complete break from training one-week, individual maintenance conditioning and injury rehabilitation. Scenario 2: Two-week holiday, commence coaching after holiday, may coach at international camps, cross-training and individual maintenance conditioning or injury rehabilitation.

Progressive overload and managing workload

Following any training involving a physical stimulus, sufficient time is required for tissues and body systems to recover and adapt before applying physical stimulus again. Tissue repairs leading to training gains occur during the period between trainings. The time required for recovery varies from 24 to 72 hours based on the type and intensity of training, as well as the targeted tissues and systems (Gabbett & Oetter, 2025). Training schedules should allow for sufficient recovery for positive rather than negative adaptations.

Monitoring training load, training response (e.g., fatigue, soreness, mood), and performance outcome are equally important for making informed decisions regarding subsequent training and recovery (Gabbett & Oetter, 2025; Wyon & Allard, 2021). Various methods are available for tracking external (e.g., accelerometers) and internal (e.g., heart rate, Rating of Perceived Exertion; Borg & Kaijser, 2006) load measures. Session Rating of Perceived Exertion (sRPE; Foster et al., 1996; Shaw et al., 2020) may be particularly useful in circus as it does not require the artist to wear a device that may interfere with performance. Combined with training volume (minutes/hours), sRPE can provide an estimate of daily and weekly training load, which can be used to develop training plans (Wyon & Clarke, 2021). Systematic increases in training load, also known as progressive overload, are important for gradually increasing physical capacity and building robust athletes and artists (Gabbett & Oetter, 2025; Wyon & Allard, 2021). For training gains, the training load must be sufficient to exceed an athlete's current capacity, without causing excessive fatigue or injury (Kellmann et al., 2018). In circus, there is a pattern of increased injury rates when artists return from a break and have a probable sudden workload spike (Stuckey et al., 2022). The recommended training load increase for dance of no more than 5–10% each week (Wyon & Clarke, 2021) may be applicable to circus.

While there are no studies examining workload management in circus, we suggest two example strategies that may apply. First, for artists who practice multiple disciplines with different physical demands, alternating training types across the week may allow adequate recovery between sessions. For example, a recreational artist practising multiple disciplines may train aerial silks on Monday and Friday, strength on Wednesday, and contortion on Tuesday and Saturday. For pre-professional or professional artists specialising in a single discipline, a potentially more relevant strategy is the polarised approach, which redistributes the same total amount of training load within a weekly microcycle such that days with high workloads are separated by days with low workloads or rest (Gabbett & Oetter, 2025). This type of cycle would support daily training of the same discipline. A polarised training approach may suit the nature of some circus training based on scheduling and facility access, or personal circumstances of artists. For example, an aerial artist may book training space two days per week (ideally separated by at least two days, e.g., Monday and Thursday) and schedule these as higher load days to train dynamic skills, strength, and choreography. The remainder of the week may include two days of focused light conditioning or mobility, a day of endurance exercise, and two days of complete rest. While polarised training has proved effective in sport, ideal implementation in circus needs to be studied as there may be complexities with days off related to technical slippage (Orlando et al., 2011). Furthermore, these training strategies would require overcoming socio-cultural conceptualisation, as artists may hold strong beliefs in the importance of training in their discipline daily.

Stress management

Circus artists face a number of psychological stressors, which vary by circus context and discipline (van Rens, 2022). While these fall within the psychological domain, they affect and interact with the other three domains. Intense schedules and finances are common stressors for professional artists (Cayrol et al., 2019) and professionalising students (Decker et al., 2022). Professional artists feel pressure from the audience to perform well (Filho et al., 2016) and from the task of memorising their own act as well as being attuned to the entire show (Ross & Shapiro, 2017). They may also need to develop multicultural sensitivity and deal with language barriers (Filho et al., 2016). Discipline-specific stressors include fear of failure for aerialists and jugglers, pain management for contortionists, and management of interpersonal relationships for duo/group acts (Filho et al., 2016). These stressors can be managed by a number of psychological (e.g., attention control strategies, emotion regulation, mental imagery/rehearsal), social (e.g., team building, communication exercises), physical (e.g., periodisation, workload management, mastery through repeated rehearsal, breathing techniques), and environmental strategies (e.g., pre-performance routines to check equipment/environmental conditions; cultural awareness; Filho et al., 2016; Ross & Shapiro, 2017).

Resilience and coping are important for the management of psychological stressors and overall well-being (Decker et al., 2022; van Rens, 2022). Resilience is associated with lower risk of developing disordered eating behaviours, lower levels of depression, anxiety and stress, and higher levels of flourishing (van Rens, 2022). In professionalising circus students, their perceptions of having sufficient mental and physical abilities to cope with challenges negatively relate to anxiety, fatigue, and psychological distress (Decker et al., 2022). Beyond internal resources, feelings of being supported by the school were also important to the management of stressors and mental health (Decker et al., 2022). The nature of circus training is well-suited to the development of resilience (van Rens, 2022); supportive environments can ensure artists are adequately resourced to manage the stressors of training and performance.

Identity development

Becoming a circus artist requires the development of an artistic identity, which involves learning how to express the self, emotions, and concepts through body movements (Filho et al., 2016). Skill and mastery are fundamental to the identity (Filho et al., 2016), which also may be based on a physically and emotionally taxing dedication to the artform (Martinez, 2024), as well as aspects of perfectionism (van Rens, 2022). The explorative process involved in developing an artistic identity is often very personal, and an artist's sense of self can become deeply rooted in a unidimensional identity. Like athletes (Purcell et al., 2022), circus artists may also struggle with transitions, especially the transition out of circus. As artists may consider circus to be their whole life, it can be important to encourage hobbies and relationships outside of circus (Cayrol et al., 2019) to support the development of a robust, multidimensional identity. A strong artistic identity may also contribute to artists' drive to train circus skills every day, thereby influencing recovery practices (or lack thereof), which may in turn lead to overtraining (Kellmann et al., 2018). Developing a multidimensional identity may assist with promoting downtime and time away from circus training, therefore optimising recovery.

Social support

Healthy social support is an important factor in mental well-being and contributes to psychosocial recovery by providing support for managing emotions and challenges, as well as having fun and meaningful experiences (Purcell et al., 2022). Social support can come from internal (i.e., circus) or external (i.e., non-circus) relationships (Purcell et al., 2022). Many circus communities see themselves as a family, and participants within these spaces create strong relationships that provide robust internal support. Circus artists may bond over shared identification with the 'circus freak' archetype, embracing their 'weirdness' together, while others may connect through shared experiences of pain (Martinez, 2024). Experiences of internal and external social support may vary by circus context. Touring circus artists may feel lonely and experience erosion of familial or other close relationships as they are away for extended periods of time, but may develop close bonds with their castmates (Walby & Spencer, 2020). Non-touring artists may experience less challenges with social isolation (Donohue et al., 2020). Freelance artists may have different experiences. Some may train alone and may experience isolation if they are in competition with other local freelance artists for gigs. Others may have strong relationships with other artists with whom they train or coach. While internal relationships are supportive and create a sense of belonging in circus, it is important that external relationships are also prioritised to develop a sense of meaning and belonging both inside and outside of circus.

Other recovery strategies

While a pro-active, long-term approach to recovery is ideal, schedules may limit rest times between bouts of intense work and disrupt routines. Resultantly, artists often rely on other strategies to help manage fatigue, soreness, and physical recovery. The following strategies have not been studied in circus artists, but may be applicable to this context.

Active recovery is submaximal exercise, such as jogging or active stretching, that, when done for six to ten minutes post-exercise, can have positive effects for maintaining or improving performance (Ortiz et al., 2019). This is inconsistently practised by circus artists, who tend to use passive stretching as a cool-down strategy. This does not, however, effectively decrease delayed-onset muscle soreness (DOMS) or enhance recovery of strength and range of motion (Afonso et al., 2021). Incorporating an active cool-down following training or performance may help optimise recovery in circus artists.

Cold water immersion for up to 15 minutes is generally more effective than other passive and active recovery methods for alleviating soreness and fatigue, as well as for recovery of power after high-intensity and eccentric exercise (Moore et al., 2022). Massage and self-massage with a device, such as foam rollers and massage guns are popular recovery modalities in circus. Despite perceived effectiveness, only small benefits have been demonstrated for reducing or preventing DOMS and improving flexibility, and no significant improvements have been demonstrated for fatigue, strength, sprint, or endurance performance (Davis et al., 2020). Foam rolling has some beneficial effects on DOMS and pressure pain threshold, and rolling 90–120s total (applied in bouts of 30–60s, interspersed with 10–30s of rest) reduces muscle stiffness and increases range of motion (Hendricks et al., 2020). Massage guns applied following exercise for >2 minutes per muscle group at frequencies less than 40 Hz can reduce muscle stiffness, improve range of motion and strength for up to 24 hours post-exercise, but have no impact on fatigue (Ferreira et al., 2023). Although these strategies may have only minor physical effects, they may be relevant when performing skills that require high physical demands. Individual responses and preferences should also be considered in a tailored recovery plan, as modalities may have positive psychological effects if they offer a familiar routine or feel good to an artist.

Creating a circus environment that supports recovery

Many barriers to optimal recovery exist in the circus environment. While some may be unavoidable, organisations can make adjustments to promote and better support recovery that is tailored to the organisation and context; for example, organisations focused primarily on performance (e.g., professional companies) versus those whose main purpose is the training of artists (e.g., recreational and pre-professional circus schools). Since Richard et al. (this volume, Chapter 12) describe in-depth recovery strategies used by Cirque du Soleil (a large company with touring and resident shows), we focus here primarily on strategies that could support trainees and artists who work freelance or in smaller companies.

Circus and organisational culture

As described above, institutionalised circus training developed over only a century and continues to be based in traditions of linear teachings and repetition (Burtt & Lavers, 2017; Wang, 2024). While circus practice tends to be very athletic, most circus artists identify strongly with their developed artist identity (Filho et al., 2016), which may cause resistance to aligning more closely with sport culture and the evidence-based training and recovery strategies employed therein. Injury masking and acceptance of pain are also common (Cayrol et al., 2019; Martinez, 2024; Walby & Stuart, 2021), which can hinder recovery and make it more likely that an artist will train or perform through pain. Understanding that the long-held tradition of 'the show must go on' may not be in the best interest of artist health and well-being should always be respected. Taking time off to recover from injury can be an especially challenging scenario for many artists whose sense of identity is closely entwined with their ability to perform on stage, who want to avoid letting down their castmates, or who feel pressured by their employer or their financial situation to continue performing (Cayrol et al., 2019; Walby & Stuart, 2021). While these personal factors cannot all be addressed at an organisational level, the 4D4D4All model can guide the creation of a culture that supports the whole artist by, for example, promoting strength and conditioning, a robust identity, and meaningful relationships that extend beyond circus. This can help artists realise the importance of recovery and see themselves beyond a unidimensional artist. Furthermore, providing access to recovery resources and support to address potential issues can not only improve artist performance and well-being, but can also mitigate negative outcomes, which can have organisational effects (e.g., disrupted shows, insurance claims). Adopting a holistic recovery-centred culture in circus can promote creativity and flourishing, which benefits the individual, the organisation, and the circus industry at large.

Multidisciplinary team

Since optimal performance is reliant on many factors, a multidisciplinary team is part of an ideal support system for artists. Considering the primary recovery factors, a team with expertise in sleep, nutrition, strength and conditioning, injury prevention and management, and psychology would ensure that artists are holistically supported. While the employment of such a team is not feasible for the majority of circus organisations, developing strong relationships and creating referral networks with trusted practitioners knowledgeable to the nuances and technical needs of circus, and supporting artists to navigate to these resources could help to overcome the resistance artists may have to care-seeking or access barriers they may face (Cayrol et al., 2019). Financial barriers are of significant concern for artists, as are wait times for healthcare appointments (which also have financial implications for professional performers; Cayrol et al., 2019). Organisations may be able to negotiate discounts or prioritisation for artists with trusted practitioners, which may alleviate artist burden. Cooperation between healthcare practitioners and the applicable stakeholders in the circus organisation (e.g., coach, artistic director, etc.) is important to ensure that the circus environment is able to adapt to the artist's needs. Positive challenges may be used to support artists to develop the skills needed to confidently carry out an individualised recovery practice (Agans et al., 2024). Clear communication, goal setting, transparent objective measures and the monitoring of the artists' physical and psychosocial needs are all important for best practice recovery.

Conclusions and recommendations for practice

Reconceptualising recovery in circus as a holistic practice that supports artist flourishing is vital to enhance the performance, creativity, and well-being of circus artists, while promoting fulfilment in life. The 4D4D4All model provides a structure to ensure that all aspects of the artist and environment are considered. Circus is far from a uniform practice. Ideally to support recovery, overall circus culture would shift from a focus on training through repetition and 'doing more' to adopting evidence-based recovery practices, though research is needed to learn how to best adapt these dance and sport recovery practices to the circus context. Organisations looking to better support recovery for their artists could build networks with healthcare and coaching professionals for knowledge sharing and referrals. To address artist recovery, tailored plans could be developed to support each individual's unique needs based on personal physical, psychological, social, and creative factors, as well as context-related factors, such as professional status and discipline(s) trained/performed. An ideal plan would focus on pro-active, long-term strategies to build a robust and resilient artist to withstand the challenging demands of training and performing, with short-term strategies that can be easily accessed for additional support when needed. Recovery practices in all of the four domains could be taught or promoted using the concept of positive challenges to support artists to build confidence in their recovery competencies. As described in the 4D4D4All model, individuals and their contexts are interrelated and co-develop each other (Agans et al., 2024). Thus, a shift in circus culture to one that better supports artist recovery and well-being will positively impact the environment, mutually enhancing the outcomes for artists and circus at large.

Note

1 Flourishing describes a state of subjective well-being achieved when an individual displays positive feeling and function in life. It is based on an individual's experience of development and success (Brown et al., 2017).

References

Afonso, J., Clemente, F. M., Nakamura, F. Y., Morouço, P., Sarmento, H., Inman, R. A., & Ramirez-Campillo, R. (2021). The effectiveness of post-exercise stretching in short-term and delayed recovery of strength, range of motion and delayed onset muscle soreness: A systematic review and meta-analysis of randomized controlled trials. *Frontiers in Physiology*, *12*, 677581. https://doi.org/10.3389/fphys.2021.677581

Agans, J. P., Stuckey, M. I., Cairney, J., & Kriellaars, D. (2024). Four domains for development for all (4D4D4All): A holistic, physical literacy framework. *Journal of Applied Sport Psychology*, *36*(6), 880–901.

Allen, N., Kelly, S., Lanfear, M., Reynolds, A., Clark, R., Mountjoy, M. L., Wyon, M., & Wolman, R. (2024). Relative energy deficiency in dance (RED-D): A consensus method approach to REDs in dance. *BMJ Open Sport & Exercise Medicine*, *10*(1), e001858. https://doi.org/10.1136/bmjsem-2023-001858

Amawi, A., AlKasasbeh, W., Jaradat, M., Almasri, A., Alobaidi, S., Hammad, A. A., Bishtawi, T., Fataftah, B., Turk, N., Al Saoud, H., Jarrar, A., & Ghazzawi, H. (2024). Athletes' nutritional demands: A narrative review of nutritional requirements. *Frontiers in Nutrition*, *10*, 1331854. https://doi.org/10.3389/fnut.2023.1331854

Borg, E., & Kaijser, L. (2006). A comparison between three rating scales for perceived exertion and two different work tests. *Scandinavian Journal of Medicine & Science in Sports*, *16*(1), 57–69.

Brown, D. J., Arnold, R., Fletcher, D., & Standage, M. (2017). Human thriving: A conceptual debate and literature review. *European Psychologist*, *22*(3), 167–170.

Brown, D., & Wyon, M. (2014). The effect of moderate glycemic energy bar consumption on blood glucose and mood in dancers. *Medical Problems of Performing Artists*, *29*(1), 27–31.

Burtt, J., & Lavers, K. (2017). Re-imagining the development of circus artists for the twenty-first century. *Theatre, Dance and Performance Training*, *8*(2), 143–155.

Cayrol, T., Godfrey, E., Draper-Rodi, J., & Bearne, L. (2019). Exploring professional circus artists' experience of performance-related injury and management: A qualitative study. *Medical Problems of Performing Artists*, *34*(1), 14–24.

Challis, J., Stevens Edd, A., & IADMS Dance Educators' Committee. (2019). *Resource for dancers and teachers: Nutrition resource paper*. International Association for

Dance Medicine & Science. Retrieved March 04, 2025 from https://iadms.org/media/3589/iadms-resource-paper-nutrition-resource-paper.pdf

Davis, H. L., Alabed, S., & Chico, T. J. A. (2020). Effect of sports massage on performance and recovery: A systematic review and meta-analysis. *BMJ Open Sport & Exercise Medicine*, 6(1), e000614. https://doi.org/10.1136/bmjsem-2019-000614

Decker, A., Aubertin, P., & Kriellaars, D. (2019). Sleep and fatigue of elite circus student-artists during one year of training. *Medical Problems of Performing Artists*, *34*(3), 125–131.

Decker, A., Richard, V., Cairney, J., Jefferies, P., Houser, N., Aubertin, P., & Kriellaars, D. (2022). Assessment of professional circus students' psychological characteristics at four strategic timepoints over the scholastic year: A longitudinal study using the Stress Process Model. *Medical Problems of Performing Artists*, *37*(4), 249–258.

Donohue, B., Gavrilova, Y., Galante, M., Burnstein, B., Aubertin, P., Gavrilova, E., Funk, A., Light, A., & Benning, S. D. (2020). Empirical development of a screening method for mental, social, and physical wellness in amateur and professional circus artists. *Psychology of Aesthetics, Creativity, and the Arts*, *14*(3), 313–324.

Faltus, J., & Richard, V. (2022). Considerations for the medical management of the circus performance artist and acrobat. *International Journal of Sports Physical Therapy*, *17*(2), 307–316.

Ferreira, R. M., Silva, R., Vigário, P., Martins, P. N., Casanova, F., Fernandes, R. J., & Sampaio, A. R. (2023). The effects of massage guns on performance and recovery: A systematic review. *Journal of Functional Morphology and Kinesiology*, *8*(3), 138. https://doi.org/10.3390/jfmk8030138

Filho, E., Aubertin, P., & Petiot, B. (2016). The making of expert performers at Cirque du Soleil and the National Circus School: A performance enhancement outlook. *Journal of Sport Psychology in Action*, *7*(2), 68–79.

Foster, C., Daines, E., Hector, L., Snyder, A. C., & Welsh, R. (1996). Athletic performance in relation to training load. *Wisconsin Medical Journal*, *95*(6), 370–374.

Gabbett, T. J., & Oetter, E. (2025). From tissue to system: What constitutes an appropriate response to loading? *Sports Medicine*, *55*, 17–35.

Greenspan, S., Munro, D., Nicholas, J., Stubbe, J., Stuckey, M. I., & van Rijn, R. M. (2022). Circus-specific extension of the International Olympic Committee 2020 consensus statement: Methods for recording and reporting of epidemiological data on injury and illness in sport. *BMJ Open Sport & Exercise Medicine*, *8*(3), e001394. https://doi.org/10.1136/bmjsem-2022-001394

Hackett, G., & Kirby, M. (2023). A practical guide to the assessment and management of testosterone deficiency in adult men. *Trends in Urology & Men's Health*, *14*(3), 21–25.

Hendricks, S., den Hollander, S., Lombard, W., & Parker, R. (2020). Effects of foam rolling on performance and recovery: A systematic review of the literature to guide practitioners on the use of foam rolling. *Journal of Bodywork and Movement Therapies*, *24*(2), 151–174.

Jakiwa, J., Rustam, S., Atan, S. A., Azli, M. S., Maliki, A. B. H. M., Nadzmi, A., Rahman, A. F. A., Samsir, S., Sun, Z., Kuo, P. T., & Bee, N. C. T. S. (2023). The effects of multi-sport intervention on agility performance among young athletes. *International Journal of Human Movement and Sports Sciences*, *11*(4), 864–871.

Keay, N., Lanfear, M., & Francis, G. (2022). Clinical application of monitoring indicators of female dancer health, including application of artificial intelligence in female hormone networks. *Internal Journal of Sports Medicine and Rehabilitation*, *5*, 24. https://doi.org/10.28933/ijsmr-2022-04-2205

Kellmann, M., Bertollo, M., Bosquet, L., Brink, M., Coutts, A. J., Duffield, R., Erlacher, D., Halson, S. L., Hecksteden, A., Heidari, J., Kallus, K. W., Meeusen, R., Mujika, I., Robazza, C., Skorski, S., Venter, R., & Beckmann, J. (2018). Recovery and performance in sport: Consensus statement. *International Journal of Sports Physiology and Performance*, *13*(2), 240–245.

Martinez, L. V. (2024). "That's what makes somebody circus": The collaborative process of transforming the meaning of pain through discourse in circus organizations. *Circus: Arts, Life, and Sciences*, *3*(1), 28–56. https://doi.org/10.3998/circus.3899

Moore, E., Fuller, J. T., Buckley, J. D., Saunders, S., Halson, S. L., Broatch, J. R., & Bellenger, C. R. (2022). Impact of cold-water immersion compared with passive recovery following a single bout of strenuous exercise on athletic performance in physically active participants: A systematic review with meta-analysis and meta-regression. *Sports Medicine*, *52*(7), 1667–1688.

Mountjoy, M., Ackerman, K. E., Bailey, D. M., Burke, L. M., Constantini, N., Hackney, A. C., Heikura, I. A., Melin, A., Pensgaard, A. M., Stellingwerff, T., Sundgot-Borgen, J. K., Torstveit, A. K., Jacobsen, A. U., Verhagen, E., Budgett, R., Engebretsen, L., & Erdener, U. (2023). 2023 International Olympic Committee's (IOC) consensus statement on relative energy deficiency in sport (REDs). *British Journal of Sports Medicine*, *57*(17), 1073–1098.

Mujika, I., Halson, S., Burke, L. M., Balagué, G., & Farrow, D. (2018). An integrated, multifactorial approach to periodization for optimal performance in individual and team sports. *International Journal of Sports Physiology and Performance*, *13*(5), 538–561.

Nicholas, J., & Grafenauer, S. (2023). Investigating pre-professional dancer health status and preventative health knowledge. *Frontiers in Nutrition*, *10*, 1271362. https://doi.org/10.3389/fnut.2023.1271362

Orlando, C., Levitan, E. B., Mittleman, M. A., Steele, R. J., & Shrier, I. (2011). The effect of rest days on injury rates. *Scandinavian Journal of Medicine & Science in Sports*, *21*(6), e64–e71.

Ortiz Jr, R. O., Elder, A. J. S., Elder, C. L., & Dawes, J. J. (2019). A systematic review on the effectiveness of active recovery interventions on athletic performance of professional-, collegiate-, and competitive-level adult athletes. *The Journal of Strength & Conditioning Research*, *33*(8), 2275–2287.

Purcell, R., Pilkington, V., Carberry, S., Reid, D., Gwyther, K., Hall, K., Deacon, A., Manon, R., Walton, C. C., & Rice, S. (2022). An evidence-informed framework to promote mental wellbeing in elite sport. *Frontiers in Psychology*, *13*, 780359. https://doi.org/10.3389/fpsyg.2022.780359

Reardon, C. L., Hainline, B., Aron, C. M., Baron, D., Baum, A. L., Bindra, A., Budgett, R., Campriani, N., Castaldelli-Maia, J. M., Currie, A., Derevensky, J. L., Glick, I. D., Gorczynski, P., Gouttebarge, V., Grandner, M. A., Han, D. H., McDuff, D., Mountjoy, M., Polat, A., ... Engebretsen, L. (2019). Mental health in elite athletes: International Olympic Committee consensus statement. *British Journal of Sports Medicine*, *53*(11), 667–699.

Reece, L., Farnsworth, N., Whitney, K. E., & Ackerman, K. A. (2023). Eating disorders and Relative Energy Deficiency in Sport (RED-S). In M. A. Christino, E. I. Pluhar, & J. M. Lyle (Eds.), *Psychological considerations in the young athlete* (pp. 59–79). Springer.

Richard, V., Glăveanu, V., & Aubertin, P. (2023). The embodied journey of an idea: An exploration of movement creativity in circus arts. *The Journal of Creative Behavior*, *57*(2), 221–236.

Ross, A., & Shapiro, J. (2017). Under the big top: An exploratory analysis of psychological factors influencing circus performers. *Performance Enhancement & Health*, *5*(3), 115–121.

Shaw, J. W., Springham, M., Brown, D. D., Mattiussi, A. M., Pedlar, C. R., & Tallent, J. (2020). The validity of the session rating of perceived exertion method for measuring internal training load in professional classical ballet dancers. *Frontiers in Physiology*, *11*, 480. https://doi.org/10.3389/fphys.2020.00480

Stuckey, M. I., Bruinooge, B., Aubertin, P., & Kriellaars, D. (2022). Clinical burden of injuries in students at a professional Circus College: A 7.5-year longitudinal study. *Medical Problems of Performing Artists*, *37*(2), 98–105.

Stuckey, M., Richard, V., Decker, A., Aubertin, P., & Kriellaars, D. (2021). Supporting holistic wellbeing for performing artists during the COVID-19 pandemic and recovery: Study protocol. *Frontiers in Psychology*, *12*, 577882. https://doi.org/10.3389/fpsyg.2021.577882

Stuckey, M. I., Greenspan, S., Nicholas, J., Richard, V., Stubbe, J. H., & van Rens, F. E. C. A. (2025). Mental health in pre-professional and professional circus artists: A narrative review. *Sport, Exercise, and Performance Psychology*, *14*(4), 587–601.

van Rens, F. (2022). *Circus psychology: An applied guide to thriving under the big top*. Routledge.

Walby, K., & Spencer, D. (2020). Circus aerialism and emotional labour. *Emotions and Society*, *2*(2), 215–232.

Walby, K., & Stuart, S. (2021). "You have to accept the pain": Body callusing and body capital in circus aerialism. *Qualitative Sociology Review*, *17*(4), 6–23.

Wang, V. (2024). The flip side. *Circus: Arts, Life, and Sciences*, *3*(1), 57–63.

Wyon, M. (2010). Preparing to perform: Periodization and dance. *Journal of Dance Medicine & Science*, *14*(2), 67–72.

Wyon, M., & Allard, G. (2021). *Periodization: A framework for dance training*. Bloomsbury Publishing.

Wyon, M., & Clarke, S. (2021). *Strength and conditioning for dancers*. The Crowood Press.

PART III

Inside an organisation

Complex challenges for recovery and well-being

10

MUSICIANS IN CLASSICAL ORCHESTRAS

Challenges and employer responsibilities

Eckart Altenmüller

Introduction

Musicians in classical orchestras are often regarded as having one of the most prestigious and fulfilling careers in the performing arts. However, behind the grandeur of concert halls and the enchantment of musical masterpieces lies a profession fraught with physical, mental, and social stressors. The demands of the job extend beyond artistic expression, requiring exceptional discipline, resilience, and a strong support system by employers, colleagues and the health system.

Orchestral musicians engage in continuous, highly precise movements, often leading to repetitive strain injuries. String players, for instance, may develop tendonitis due to the repetitive bowing motion, while brass players risk embouchure disorders from prolonged tension of facial muscles and/or pressure to the labial mucosa. Such injuries can threaten a musician's career if not managed properly (Vervainioti & Alexopoulos, 2015). Long hours of rehearsals and performances in fixed positions place significant strain on the body. Furthermore, a demanding repertoire must be prepared, adding hours of practice to the performance and rehearsal schedule. Continuous maintenance of professional playing abilities is taken for granted and requires mostly daily practice. This heavy workload may lead to bodily and mental overload and can have consequences for health and well-being (Kenny & Ackermann, 2015).

Altenmüller, E. (2026). Musicians in classical orchestras: Challenges and employer responsibilities. In E. Altenmüller, M. Kellmann, J. Beckmann, & G. M. Moyle (Eds.), *Recovery and well-being in the performing arts* (pp. 177–188). Routledge.

DOI: 10.4324/9781003566885-13

Violinists, for example, often suffer from shoulder and neck pain, while double bass players and harpists experience back pain due to the weight and positioning of their instruments. Poor ergonomics can exacerbate these conditions, making proper posture training and physiotherapy crucial (Chi et al., 2020). Furthermore, exposure to high sound pressure levels over time can result in noise-induced hearing loss or tinnitus. Brass and percussion players, who are often seated near loud instruments, are at particular risk (Schmidt et al., 2014). Protective measures such as earplugs and sound shields are essential, but their adoption varies widely and is frequently not well tolerated for several reasons: Communication within the orchestras may become difficult, especially during rehearsals, when the conductor speaks softly. Earplugs can muffle or distort sound, making it harder to hear nuances in dynamics, tone, and balance with the rest of the orchestra. Furthermore, earplugs can make it difficult to judge timing and ensemble coordination and alter how a musician perceives their own sound, leading to tuning difficulties. Some musicians find earplugs physically uncomfortable or distracting, especially during long rehearsals and performances (Zander et al., 2008). However, some musicians, especially those exposed to high sound levels (like brass and percussion players or those seated near them), do use specialised musician's earplugs that reduce volume while maintaining sound clarity. Some also use custom-moulded earplugs with adjustable filters to find a balance between protection and performance (Hake et al., 2024).

Not only bodily stressors, but also emotional stressors are frequent. Many orchestral musicians face immense pressure to perform flawlessly. The fear of making a mistake in a high-stakes concert can lead to performance anxiety, which, in severe cases, manifests in physical symptoms like tremors and arterial hypertension (Baadjou et al., 2016). The culture of perfectionism within classical music further compounds this stress (Cruder et al., 2023). A further challenge is that orchestral positions are limited and highly competitive. Many musicians are on short-term contracts, leading to financial instability. The fear of losing a position due to injury or declining performance can cause chronic stress and anxiety (Kenny et al., 2018).

Orchestra musicians often work when other people enjoy free time, in evenings, weekends, and during summer holiday at festivals. Such an erratic schedule, combined with extensive travel for tours and separation from families, may lead to social isolation and can cause exhaustion and burnout, if not a respective support system is established, allowing for recovery (Davison, 2022). This chapter explores these challenges and examines the role of the employer in facilitating recovery from heavy workloads and illness and maintaining overall well-being.

The German orchestral landscape: Historical roots and unique diversity

The German orchestral landscape is unique worldwide. With about 130 professional orchestras, Germany has the most dense and diverse orchestral structure in the world. In 2014, the German orchestral landscape was included in UNESCO's German Federal Inventory of the Intangible Cultural Heritage. The roots of German orchestras go back to the Renaissance and Baroque periods, when permanent court ensembles developed. Royal courts, such as those in Dresden, Munich, or Mannheim, maintained their own ensembles and promoted innovative musical developments, whereby the orchestras were in fierce competition with each other. The more brilliant the soloists and the larger the orchestra, the more prestige the respective sovereign possessed. The earliest root of still performing orchestras in Germany dates back to 1502 in Kassel, the capital of the Hessian Palatinate. In Hannover, the still existing 'Hofkapelle' – now 'State Orchestra of the State of Lower Saxony', was founded in 1636 and attracted outstanding musicians like Georg Friedrich Händel or Joseph Joachim, the latter a close friend to the romantic composers Brahms and Schumann.

With the enlightenment and the growing importance of the bourgeoisie in the 19th century, the orchestral landscape changed fundamentally. Music became increasingly accessible to a broader audience, and bourgeois concert societies and municipal orchestras emerged. The high value placed on classical music in Germany is also reflected in the extensive state funding. Public funding for German orchestras comes primarily from public sources (federal, state, and local governments). On average, public funding makes up about 80–90% of the orchestras' total income. Thus, orchestras receive significant public funding to ensure their artistic quality and cultural education work (German Music Information Centre, 2024).

In 1950, the Radio Philharmonic Orchestra of the NDR (North German Broadcasting) was founded. It has been managed by Matthias Ilkenhans for more than 20 years. In recent decades, both the self-image and the range of tasks of the orchestra have changed and expanded: today, the Radio Philharmonic Orchestra of the NDR is an internationally renowned ensemble that is in demand far beyond the broadcasting area focusing on concert formats that spark the audience's curiosity. Another focus for the orchestra is young audiences. The education programme offers children and young people specially designed, partly interactive concerts as well as a wide range of music education programmes. The orchestra gives a total of around 100 concerts per season, almost all of which are broadcast on NDR and are available online. Since 2020, cross-media formats, video productions, and concert livestream enriched the portfolio of the orchestra (NDR, 2024).

The home venue of the Radio Philharmonic Orchestra of the NDR is the large studio at the NDR-Konzerthaus in Hannover. The broad artistic spectrum is a hallmark of the orchestra; accordingly, the guest musicians are diverse. These include internationally acclaimed soloists like Andras Schiff, Ann-Sophie Mutter, or Anna Netrebko, and cross-over artists, like the King Singers. Concert tours have taken the orchestra to almost all prestigious concert venues in Europe, to Asia and South America, among other places.

The life and earning of a musician in a classical orchestra

Using the example of the Radio Philharmonic Orchestra of the NDR, the musicians' specific working conditions will be outlined. Orchestral musicians in Germany enjoy a high level of recognition and protection through various legal and contractual arrangements. Nevertheless, their working conditions are often characterised by long rehearsal periods, intensive concert schedules, and physical as well as mental stress. In Germany, orchestral musicians of some hundred opera and concert orchestras are publicly funded and are subject to special collective agreements for musicians, such as the 'collective agreement for cultural orchestras'. The exception to this are radio orchestras, which generally have better financial standing as they have their own collective agreements. These regulate working hours, remuneration, holiday entitlements, and social security. The regular weekly working days usually encompass six days and mostly more than 40 hours including rehearsing at home. Orchestral rehearsals and performances are scheduled precisely. Freelance musicians often have less protection because they work on a project-by-project basis and must negotiate their fees individually though there exist legal arrangements for appropriate remuneration. However, like musicians under permanent contract, most of them are organised in professional associations and Unions, such as the German Orchestra Association 'unisono' (former 'Deutsche Orchestervereinigung'), which advocates for fair working conditions and negotiates contracts.

At the Radio Philharmonic Orchestra of the NDR, the entire collective is allowed to work an average of 215 days a year. Each individual orchestra musician is allowed to work 200 days a year. However, this number of orchestra services is usually not reached in a year, as rehearsals and performances sometimes take place in smaller groups. A service lasts between two and a half to a maximum of three hours. A musician should not be required to work more than ten services in five days, which means that they should not work more than five hours a day on five days in a row. However, there are peak periods when musicians must play seven days a week. In addition, longer trips must also be taken into account. In such cases, longer breaks with several days of rest are planned. Solo instrumentalists, such as concertmasters and solo wind players, are privileged and only have to play 58% of the services the orchestra is scheduled to perform.

Orchestra musicians in permanent positions in orchestras receive a secure monthly salary of between € 3,000 and € 9,700 in Germany. This salary depends on the size, quality, and demands in repertoire of the orchestra. In Germany, orchestras are classified according to levels A to D, with A denoting larger orchestras with more than 100 excellently qualified musicians, such as the Gewandhaus Orchestra in Leipzig and D denoting smaller, mostly provincial orchestras with in between 25 and 40 musicians in smaller cities like

Lüneburg. Besides the size and quality of the orchestra also the musician's position in the orchestra hierarchy matters for salary. For example principal violinists (concert-masters) or solo woodwind players receive considerably more money than musicians in the tutti groups, with less exposure and no obligations to play solo passages in orchestral works. Academy students and temporary staff are even earning less and have no job security, since they are hired on the basis of contracts for one season or even only for one production. Student musicians, so-called academicians, who are generally still studying music in a conservatory or university, receive between € 800 and € 1,200 per month. Temporarily hired freelance musicians, who are needed when special instruments or very large ensembles are required, are paid by the service, with concert performances being better paid than rehearsals. Overall, the level of job satisfaction among the permanently employed orchestra musicians is very good, with 85% of employees being very satisfied. The sick leave rate is between 8% and 9%, which is slightly higher than in other occupations, where it is between 5% and 6% (Paternoga, 2005). This may be due to the fact that orchestra musicians only perform at their best when they feel completely healthy.

Everyday stressors for orchestra musicians

It is not the number of performances that musicians perceive as stressful, but rather the fact that they experience a lack of self-determination in many respects. From an early age, musicians in a top orchestra are prepared to deliver top performances. Disruptive factors that prevent them from achieving their personal best are perceived as stressful. It is therefore always important for the musicians to have optimal working conditions (Vastamäki et al., 2023). This includes the quality of seating, the lighting in the rehearsal room, the room temperature, the supply of fresh air, the space to move around, and above all, the room acoustics. Occasionally, working with inexperienced conductors can also be stressful, as they may not rehearse efficiently, talk too much, or even be impolite and overly authoritarian. Another important stress factor is social tension. A musician may have to sit next to the same person for 30 years and agree with them on many details, such as the division of services, the turning of pages during concerts, etc. It is this 'forced community', under pressure to deliver excellent results that is frequently perceived as very stressful. This is all the more true given that musicians generally have only marginal influence on who they will be playing and harmonising with over the next decades.

Two stress factors, frequently tabooed, are performance anxiety and dealing with ageing and the associated decline in physical and mental performance (Kenny et al., 2018). Both are strongly associated with shame and anxieties, and often musicians don't dare to seek support here. Generally, performance anxiety is more common in younger colleagues who have not yet developed sufficient routines (Fernholz et al., 2019). But many older musicians also painfully realise that the newcomers are better trained and play technically on a superior level. This may also lead to performance anxiety among older musicians. About 70% of orchestra musicians state in surveys that they occasionally suffer from performance anxiety (van Kemenade et al., 1995).

For orchestra members, concert tours are usually both enriching and a physical and mental burden. Getting to know a foreign country and making contacts with foreign colleagues is described as enriching, as is the deeper contact with colleagues from the orchestra. The strain comes from jet lag, long journeys between performance locations, a lack of opportunities to retreat, a lack of sleep, and an excessive number of concerts. The last tour of the Radio Philharmonic Orchestra of the NDR, 2024 in Japan comprised ten concerts in twelve days. This requires an enormous stamina and resilience from the orchestra members.

Recovery in the orchestra: Some definitions and applications

Clearly, recovery is important for members of the orchestra, and must be integrated in the management of the orchestra. Here, the definition of recovery of the World Health Organisation is adopted, which emphasises recovery in mental health as a journey towards regaining control of one's life, finding meaning and purpose, and achieving well-being despite mental health challenges. It's a personalised process of rebuilding and rediscovering strengths, rather than just the absence of symptoms. This involves self-determination, hope for the future, and a sense of connection with oneself and one's community (World Health Organisation, 2019). This holistic view on recovery is closely related to the approaches of Kellmann and Kallus (2001). They postulated such a broader perspective that goes beyond regeneration or 'being cured' or 'being normal again' (Beckmann et al., 2023). This broader perspective addresses recovery as a resource that enables individuals not only to recover from stress but also to develop resilience to health-threatening stress. Kallus (2016, p. 42) defined recovery as "an inter- and intraindividual multilevel (e.g., psychological, physiological, social) process in time for the re-establishment of personal resources and their full functional capacity" (for details, see, Altenmüller et al., this volume, Chapter 1).

For successful recovery in the orchestra, orchestra managers and employers must pro-actively plan or schedule appropriate recovery strategies which surmount the individual opportunities to recover from stress. The latter may be inadequate because strenuous and excessive orchestral activities leave little time for recovery. Furthermore, orchestra musicians often show a high level of perfectionism (Kenny & Ackermann, 2015). Perfectionism is associated with unrealistically high self-expectations, causing neglection of personal needs and time for rest (Alpheis & Altemüller, 2024). Given the high pressure to perform in orchestras, this frequently leads to a reduced self-esteem and an increased fear of failure. If the necessary conditions for recovery are not given, for example because of lack of time or opportunities, a vicious cycle can be initiated. This is specifically true for orchestra members in less well-paid smaller D orchestras, who tend to be heavily overcommitted during the 'season', because they play many more concerts and have more rehearsals than musicians working in prestigious ensembles like the Berlin Philharmonic Orchestra. If recovery is inadequate (underrecovery) for a longer period of time, stress can become chronic. Chronic stress can lead to a deterioration of the quality of playing, loss of motivation, and reluctance to prepare the concerts properly at home. If there is timely awareness of the need for recovery, pro-active strategies can be initiated by the responsible orchestra managers, and the vicious circle can be broken. A central aspect of the recovery model postulated by Kellmann and Kallus (2001) is the idea of a balance between stress and recovery. Increasing stress must be accompanied by an increase in corresponding recovery in order to maintain a balance between the two and thereby avoid negative consequences of underrecovery (Beckmann et al., 2024).

Support from the employer regarding recovery

Recovery, including increasing resilience and prevention of overuse and other stress-induced medical problems is extremely important for orchestral musicians. Here, it is advisable that initiatives come from the musicians themselves. For example, the Radio Philharmonic Orchestra of the NDR offers company sports, a voluntary offer that, typically for Germany, even includes a soccer team for musicians. Prevention also includes regular hearing tests and the provision of individually fitted hearing protection (Schurig et al., 2024). In addition, programmes are offered on how to deal with alcohol or nicotine or how to control obesity.

For the 'Academicians', i.e., the young orchestra musicians who are still in training, there are audition training, performance training, and courses in time management offered. For all musicians, courses in Yoga, Feldenkrais, or the Alexander technique, which are often organised by the musicians themselves, are free of charge for orchestra musicians. Unfortunately, these preventive measures are mostly used by musicians who are already stressed and suffer from performance anxiety or pain.

Although professional musicians are more health-conscious than members of other professional groups (Schoeb & Zosso, 2012), interest in measures supporting recovery is mostly restricted to musicians who are stressed and overcommitted. Healthy musicians are less interested (Ajidahun et al., 2019). Here, educational measures should be implemented, emphasising the importance of integrating recreational activities into everyday working life in the Orchestra right from the start of one's career. It is also important to prevent professional frustration arising from the lack of control over repertoire or conductor selection, as well as rigid working structures and working times. Chamber music concerts organised by the musicians themselves are very helpful, as they significantly increase motivation and job satisfaction (Vastamäki et al., 2017). It must be emphasised that according to existing concepts and research on an expanded understanding of recovery one measure does not fit all (Kallus, 2016). Rather, recovery is highly individual-specific and dependent on situational conditions. The realisation of effective recovery can also be understood as self-regulation, which requires self-determination. Prescribed recovery measures from the orchestral management thus could reinforce the perception of a lack of self-determination and interfere with the effectiveness of recovery measures (Beckmann, 2023).

Support from the employer regarding convalescence

Orchestra musicians on permanent contracts can benefit from company reintegration after long periods of illness. In this process, employers and health insurance companies support the musicians in gradually returning to work and prevent them from being unable to work again. A prescribed process within the company reintegration is the 'obligatory company integration management' according to the *Hamburger Modell.* This legally anchored measure is an instrument that helps employers to overcome the incapacity to work of musicians who have been ill for a longer time, usually several weeks. The procedure includes individual measures. In practice, musicians are initially allowed to enter the orchestra and participate only in a third or half of the orchestra's weekly services. Furthermore, they are allowed to select repertoire that does not exceed their physical or mental capacity limit at the given state of rehabilitation. In a process that can take several weeks or even a few months, the duration and difficulty of the repertoire are systematically increased. This is closely coordinated with the orchestra director and, above all, with colleagues in the sections. Payment is made through the sick pay of the statutory health insurance companies and amounts to 70% of the full salary.

Conclusion and recommendations for practice

In this chapter, health challenges, preventive measures, and support for recovery for musicians working in orchestras are exemplified in a German orchestra. Orchestra managers and responsible administrators must consider the following factors in order to lead an orchestra in a sustainable and creative way:

1 *Create health-promoting working conditions*

- Plan concerts and performances realistically and sustainably, with sufficient breaks. This is specifically important during stressful orchestra tours.

- Design rehearsal schedules in such a way as to avoid physical and mental exhaustion.
- Schedule prolonged rest periods after intensive concert phases.

2 *Support preventive measures*

- Offer physical and mental health services, for example, Alexander Technique, Feldenkrais, yoga, mental training.
- Offer workshops on stress management, resilience, and healthy lifestyles.

3 *Facilitate access to medical and therapeutic care*

- Collaborate with specialised doctors, physiotherapists, and psychologists, especially for musicians' illnesses (e.g., focal dystonia, tinnitus, burnout).
- Provide directories or partnerships with relevant specialists.

4 *Promote an open culture of communication*

- Reduce the stigma surrounding exhaustion or mental stress.
- Establish trusted individuals or contact points within the orchestra.

5 *Respect individual needs*

- Offer the possibility of individual arrangements, for example, for returning to work after illness, mental stress or family situations.
- Be flexible with regard to rehearsal commitments or tours if necessary for health reasons.

6 *Provide space for regeneration and retreat*

- Set up quiet rooms in rehearsal and performance venues.
- Ensure recovery time after tours.

7 *Strengthen social support and community*

- Promote team-building measures (joint activities, exchange formats).
- Actively create an inclusive and supportive working environment.

By implementing the above-mentioned structures and activities, through measures to increase resilience, meaningfulness, self-determination, hope for the future and a sense of connection with oneself and the orchestra, conditions are created that support holistic recovery, as we advocate in this book. Fostering such a positive workplace culture, orchestras can ensure that their musicians remain healthy, motivated, and able to perform at their best for years to come. Working conditions for musicians and the functionality of an excellently organised health system are excellent in Germany, and together with the Scandinavian countries among the top-leading in the world. German orchestral musicians are well protected by legal and collective bargaining frameworks, but challenges such as physical strain, psychological pressure and of course insecurity concerning future developments remain. Protection by the union 'unisono', health insurance funds and professional associations helps to overcome these challenges. The future will depend on how public funding and social appreciation of culture develop.

Acknowledgement

I thank Matthias Ilkenhans, the manager of the Radio Philharmonic Orchestra of the NDR, for sharing valuable insights and information on the 'life within an orchestra' with me. Parts of this article are based on an interview, which we conducted in late November 2024.

Note

The collective agreement for musicians in concert and theatre orchestras, dated from 1 October 2019 (TVK) specified for the Radio-Philharmonic Orchestra of the North German Broadcasting can be downloaded at https://www.ndr.de/der_ndr/zahlen_und_daten/klangkoerper142.pdf.

References

Ajidahun, A. T., Myezwa, H., Mudzi, W., & Wood, W. A. (2019). Barriers and facilitators in implementing an exercise-based injury prevention program for string players. *Work*, *64*(4), 713–720.

Alpheis, S., & Altenmüller, E. (2024). Comparison of perfectionism between music and medical students and its association with anxiety. *Medical Problems of Performing Artists*, *39*(2), 82–92.

Baadjou, V. A. E., Roussel, N. A., Verbunt, J. A. M. C. F., Smeets, R. J. E. M., & de Bie, R. A. (2016). Systematic review: Risk factors for musculoskeletal disorders in musicians. *Occupational Medicine*, *66*(8), 614–622.

Beckmann, J. (2023). Self-regulation of recovery. In M. Kellmann, S. Jakowski, & J. Beckmann (Eds.), *The importance of recovery for physical and mental health: Negotiating the effects of underrecovery* (pp. 53–69). Routledge.

Beckmann, J., Huber, M., & Andonian-Dierks, C. S. (2024). Chronic illness and well-being: Promoting quality of life with a broadened concept of recovery. In M. Kellmann & J. Beckmann (Eds.), *Fostering recovery and well-being in a healthy lifestyle: Psychological, somatic, and organizational prevention approaches* (pp. 3–23). Routledge.

Beckmann, J., Kellmann, M., & Jakowski, S. (2023). Recovery is more than just healing: Advocating a broader perspective on recovery in physical and mental health. In M. Kellmann, S. Jakowski, & J. Beckmann (Eds.), *The importance of recovery for physical and mental health: Negotiating the effects of underrecovery* (pp. 266–270). Routledge.

Chi, J. Y., Halaki, M., & Ackermann, B. J. (2020). Ergonomics in violin and piano playing: A systematic review. *Applied Ergonomics*, *88*, 103143. https://doi.org/10.1016/j.apergo.2020.103143

Cruder, C., Soldini, E., Gleeson, N., & Barbero, M. (2023). Factors associated with increased risk of playing-related disorders among classical music students within the risk of music students (RISMUS) longitudinal study. *Scientific Reports*, *13*(1), 22939. https://doi.org/10.1038/s41598-023-49965-7

Davison, D. (2022). Sources of occupational stress among the military musicians of the Royal Air Force. *BMJ Military Health*, *168*(3), 181–185.

Fernholz, I., Mumm, J. L. M., Plag, J., Noeres, K., Rotter, G., Willich, S. N., Ströhle, A., Berghöfer, A., & Schmidt, A. (2019). Performance anxiety in professional musicians: A systematic review on prevalence, risk factors and clinical treatment effects. *Psychological Medicine*, *49*(14), 2287–2306.

German Music Information Centre. (2024). *Orchestras, radio ensembles and opera choruses*. Retrieved March 04, 2025 from https://miz.org/en/articles/orchestras-radio-ensembles-and-opera-choruses/version/2024

Hake, R., Kreutz, G., Frischen, U., Schlender, M., Rois-Merz, E., Meis, M., Wagener, K. C., & Siedenburg, K. (2024). A survey on hearing health of musicians in professional and amateur orchestras. *Trends in Hearing*, *28*, 23312165241293762. https://doi.org/10.1177/23312165241293762

Kallus, K. W. (2016). Stress and recovery: An overview. In K. W. Kallus & M. Kellmann (Eds.), *The Recovery-Stress Questionnaires: User manual* (pp. 27–48). Pearson Assessment.

Kellmann, M., & Kallus, K. W. (2001). *The Recovery-Stress Questionnaire for Athletes: User manual*. Human Kinetics.

Kenny, D. T., & Ackermann, B. J. (2015). Performance-related musculoskeletal pain, depression and music performance anxiety in professional orchestral musicians: A population study. *Psychology of Music*, *43*(1), 43–60.

Kenny, D. T., Driscoll, T., & Ackermann, B. J. (2018). Effects of aging on musical performance in professional orchestral musicians. *Medical Problems of Performing Artists*, *33*(1), 39–46.

North German Broadcasting. (2024). *Webpage*. Retrieved March 04, 2025 from https://www.ndr.de/orchester_chor/radiophilharmonie/index.html

Paternoga, S. (2005). *Arbeits- und Berufszufriedenheit im Orchestermusikerberuf* [Job and career satisfaction in the profession of orchestral musician]. Rhombos.

Schmidt, J. H., Pedersen, E. R., Paarup, H. M., Christensen-Dalsgaard, J., Andersen, T., Poulsen, T., & Bælum, J. (2014). Hearing loss in relation to sound exposure of professional symphony orchestra musicians. *Ear and Hearing*, *35*(4), 448–460.

Schoeb, V., & Zosso, A. (2012). "You cannot perform music without taking care of your body": A qualitative study on musicians' representation of body and health. *Medical Problems of Performing Artists*, *27*(3), 129–136.

Schurig, E., Hake, R., Birke, M., Derks, D., Siedenburg, K., & Kreutz, G. (2024). Hearing health literacy among professional and amateur musicians. *Scientific Reports*, *14*(1), 28441. https://doi.org/10.1038/s41598-024-79875-1

van Kemenade, J. F., van Son, M. J., & van Heesch, N. C. (1995). Performance anxiety among professional musicians in symphonic orchestras: A self-report study. *Psychological Reports*, *77*(2), 555–562.

Vastamäki, M., Heliövaara, M., Vastamäki, H., & Ristolainen, L. (2023). Orchestra musicians' work environment and health versus general workforce. *Journal of Occupational and Environmental Medicine*, *65*(4), 344–348.

Vastamäki, H., Vastamäki, M., Laimi, K., & Saltychev, M. (2017). Confirmatory factor analysis of the Finnish Job Content Questionnaire (JCQ) in 590 professional musicians. *International Journal of Occupational and Environmental Medicine*, *8*(3), 174–180.

Vervainioti, A., & Alexopoulos, E. C. (2015). Job-related stressors of classical instrumental musicians: A systematic qualitative review. *Medical Problems of Performing Artists*, *30*(4), 197–202.

World Health Organisation. (2019). *Recovery practices for mental health and well-being. WHO quality rights specialized training.* Retrieved March 04, 2025 from https://iris.who.int/handle/10665/329646

Zander, M. F., Spahn, C., & Richter, B. (2008). Employment and acceptance of hearing protectors in classical symphony and opera orchestras. *Noise and Health*, *10*(38), 14–26.

11

WHAT WORKS AND WHAT DOESN'T

Managing mental and physical fatigue in a professional ballet company

Matthew Wirdnam, Aoife McDonnell, Dimity Azoury, and Susan Mayes

Introduction

Given recovery can be defined as more than a 'return to normal' but also encompasses increasing resilience to potential stressors and ensuring there is time to replenish mental resources (Altenmüller et al., this volume, Chapter 1), recovery strategies have been an integral part of The Australian Ballet's multidisciplinary strategy to attenuate fatigue, optimise performance and reduce the risk of injury (De Wet et al., 2022; The Australian Ballet, 2020). At the Australian Ballet, dancers participate in class and rehearsal for six to eight hours per day, six days per week and can perform 200 shows annually (The Australian Ballet, 2025a). Incomplete recovery from a single class, rehearsal or a performance has the potential to induce physical and mental fatigue and may place dancers at an increased risk of injury or impact their ability to learn new choreography (Wirdnam et al., 2024). The following chapter aims to address how physical fatigue and injury is managed, what mental fatigue is and how dancers currently perceive it, the role of integrated support systems within The Australian Ballet, and incorporates the perspective of a current professional ballet dancer.

Physical fatigue and recovery

Professional ballet involves physically demanding activities such as leaping, jumping, sprinting, overhead lifting and pointe work. Both the flat- and

Wirdnam, M., McDonnell, A., Azoury, D., & Mayes, S. (2026). What works and what doesn't: Managing mental and physical fatigue in a professional ballet company. In E. Altenmüller, M. Kellmann, J. Beckmann, & G. M. Moyle (Eds.), *Recovery and well-being in the performing arts* (pp. 189–204). Routledge

DOI: 10.4324/9781003566885-14

pointe-based[1] dancers require strength, power and poise (Maloney et al., 2024; McCormack et al., 2019; Schantz et al., 1984). Classes, rehearsal, and performing have the potential to lead to physical fatigue that may be linked to changes in cortical drive, muscle damage, dehydration, and glycogen depletion (Tornero-Aguilera et al., 2022). The potential for these activities to lead to fatigue and injury is further compounded by the sheer volume of physical work that dancers are required to complete (Shaw et al., 2021). Additionally, and somewhat different to many sports, dancers are required to complete their performances with 'grace' and with what looks like relative ease (i.e., lack of observed physical effort). Dancers at The Australian Ballet (TAB) have an extended four-week break over the December Christmas holidays, with the return to work period in January following the holidays targeted towards a gradual increase in load to prepare them for the year ahead.

Graduated return to work

The two weeks following the dancers' four-week holiday are busy with activities to promote injury prevention and optimise performance. The 'graduated return to work policy' (The Australian Ballet, 2020) was introduced in 1994 to address a high rate of stress fractures that followed a sudden increase in bone loading, such as jumping and pointe work at the start of the year. To counteract this spike in load, the intensity and hours of joint, tendon and bone loading are progressively built over a two-week period after a de-load or holiday to prevent muscle fatigue and injury. Modified ballet classes are offered to the dancers daily, and the physical demands are gradually increased over the initial two weeks. Acute injuries such as ankle sprains commonly occur at the end of an eight-hour day due to fatigue (Wirdnam et al., 2024), and therefore, afternoons during the first few days are used for administrative tasks, such as presentations to the dancers from various company departments, and education sessions from the health team. The hours and intensity of training are increased gradually over the first two weeks to allow adaptation to the high loading required to reach peak performance by their first performance in five weeks. Stress fracture rates have been observed to decline significantly once dancers were supported to gradually increase their workload.

Muscular fatigue and early signs of injury

Muscle fatigue and cramping can be an early sign of stress fracture or could be a warning sign that the joints and tendons may be vulnerable to injury (Warden et al., 2014). Dancers have been educated and are reminded at the start of their year not to ignore muscle cramping and to report to the physiotherapists for assessment. If caught early, only minor modifications to a dancer's workload would be required with no interruption to performances.

Early reporting of these minor symptoms has been key to injury prevention, especially bone stress injury.

Building rapport and trust between the dancers and the health team (made up of physiotherapists, a myotherapist, a strength and conditioning coach, a dietician, a general practitioner and sports and exercise medicine physician) is vital to ensure dancers feel comfortable reporting early symptoms of fatigue (Leach, 2005). This is one important aim of the extensive profiling or screening of all new dancers in the first weeks of the year (Bahr, 2016). Dancers are examined by the doctors and physiotherapists to ensure that any physical issues that may place them at risk of injury can be addressed prior to the first performance season (i.e., in week 5). History of past or current injury, joint range of movement, balance and other orthopaedic test results can inform the development of injury prevention and management plans. Inadequate muscle capacity to cope with a professional ballet career can lead to physical fatigue, and therefore, at the start of the dancer's employment with the company, muscle strength and endurance are tested, benchmarks and goals are agreed on, and the dancers are prescribed individualised programmes that support injury prevention and also support a dancer's ballet performance goals. Ongoing testing, such as strength, power, and balance is performed throughout the dancer's employment to ensure they are achieving their strength and ballet performance goals, such as more fluid movement through their hips or improved partnership skills. Finding the time to screen at regular intervals throughout the year is a challenge in a ballet company with a busy schedule, but dancers are encouraged to attend individual assessments every six to twelve weeks.

Shared decision making

TAB's health team is a multidisciplinary group consisting of doctors, physiotherapists, myotherapists, a strength and conditioning coach, a performance lifestyle advisor, psychologists, a dietitian, rehabilitation coaches and an administrator that has built in size and expertise over many years (The Australian Ballet, 2020). The team of dance medicine and science specialists supports the health and well-being needs of 80 company dancers and works closely with the company director and ballet staff. The vision of the team is to support dancers' health and well-being as well as optimising dancers' performance, and leadership and support from the artistic director, executive director and the board of directors is vital in establishing the resources to achieve the team's goals (The Australian Ballet, 2020).

The health team involve dancers in shared decision-making when devising an exercise programme to achieve their dance performance goals. A dancer's goal may be to improve the height of their allegro (jumps), and therefore, the exercise programme would target the muscles that support jumping. A connection between the exercises prescribed in the gym and ballet training in the studio is critical and can be facilitated by ballet staff. Empowering the dancer to communicate their ballet performance goals and supporting strategies with all support staff (director, ballet staff and health staff) has been most effective.

Preventing fatigue

Muscle fatigue is usually due to inadequate capacity of the muscles to cope with a particular workload (Tornero-Aguilera et al., 2022). Exercises are prescribed that strengthen the muscles required for safe participation in ballet training and muscles that have been found to be relatively weak when tested during the screening sessions (Bahr, 2016). There are usually two five-week rehearsal periods each year in preparation for the performances. Dancers gradually progress the strength-building exercises, especially during the rehearsal periods, but may then maintain a level of exercise once they start the performance season. Timing of these exercises needs to be considered to prevent muscle fatigue during rehearsals or a performance. To build strength and resilience, the muscle needs to be exercised to near-maximal fatigue (Schoenfeld et al., 2021), therefore, an ideal time for these exercises may be at the end of the day or on a non-performance day.

Certain repertoire may impose unusual loads that cause physical fatigue. At least six weeks prior to a new ballet or repertoire, the health team evaluates the risks of each role in a ballet and designs an injury prevention programme that includes advice on recovery strategies that are shared with the dancers (The Australian Ballet, 2025b). These documents remain on file to be reused when the repertoire is repeated at any time in the future or shared with other ballet companies.

Soft-tissue massage and release are encouraged to reduce muscle tension due to physical fatigue throughout the year, but particularly during busy rehearsal or performance seasons. Massage, dry needling, self-release with foam rollers and massage devices can be effective in reducing tension and promoting effective muscle recovery (Kużdżał et al., 2025). Stretching, particularly in ballet, is a commonly used recovery strategy. Caution is required with dancers who are hypermobile, as their soft-tissue structures lack the tissue recoil that allows the body to efficiently move with minimal muscle activity. Excessive soft-tissue release or stretching can reduce the spring-like tissue recoil, resulting in over-recruitment of muscles, muscle fatigue and an increased risk of injury. There is no evidence that stretching prevents injury or physical fatigue, and in fact stretching can have the opposite effect (Jamdvedt et al., 2010). Prevention of muscle tightness or fatigue by building better soft-tissue capacity through strengthening should be the priority (The Australian Ballet, 2018). Other popular strategies in this ballet company that can promote muscle recovery are ice and/or hot baths, garment compression, and gentle exercise such as swimming or yoga (Wirdnam et al., 2024).

Adequate, good-quality sleep is essential for recovery and injury prevention (Charest & Grandner, 2020; Jakowski et al., 2023). Athletes who sleep on average less than eight hours per night have 1.7 times greater risk of being injured than those who sleep more than eight hours (Charest & Grandner, 2020). Maintaining consistent sleep cycles and having enough sleep is a challenge for performing artists due to the late finish times of performances. Going to sleep is typically delayed for dancers after a performance (i.e., show) that can run from 7.30 pm to 10.30 pm, due to eating a late dinner and 'winding down'. Dancers in ballet companies usually sleep in late, therefore start their daily ballet class mid-morning, often fitting in an exercise programme prior to class. The dancers have been provided with ongoing education on strategies to improve the hours and quality of sleep, such as how consumption of caffeine and the composition of a late-night meal can reduce and/or negatively impact sleep total and sleep quality (Gardiner et al., 2023; Noguiera et al., 2021).

Barriers to preventing fatigue

A range of barriers have been observed to exist when encouraging dancers to engage in strategies that assist in preventing fatigue. For example, dancers may avoid muscle-strengthening exercises due to the myth that they will develop bulky muscles that may interfere with their graceful movement or ballet aesthetic (Farmer & Brouner, 2021; Long et al., 2021). Furthermore, body image concerns may prevent dancers from engaging in a strengthening programme and can lead to disordered eating and eating disorders, which are common in this aesthetic artform (Dantas et al., 2018). Under fuelling and poor nutrition have serious health consequences (Mountjoy et al., 2023), and have the potential to lead to fatigue, and the inability to recover effectively and cope with a professional ballet career. In response to these observations, The Australian Ballet (2024) has designed 'Body Image and Disordered Eating Guidelines' that aim to support dancers to reach their full potential as a professional ballet dancer by providing guidance for preventing and addressing concerns related to body image, disordered eating, or eating disorders.

Monitoring wellness

Monitoring of factors including fatigue, sleep quality, and overall wellness was tested in a pilot study using a wellness app with professional ballet dancers (Harrison et al., 2025). Wellness monitoring with an app aims to evaluate issues such as injury, pain, muscle soreness, fatigue, sleep hours and quality, and anxiety levels, and allow interventions to promote effective recovery. Though the use of a wellness app appears feasible, some dancers found this task to be a burden when completed daily, and this has not been adopted at TAB. Further, health staff need to have the capacity to respond in a timely manner if there are issues. Monitoring fatigue can also be achieved by observation from other support staff. Ballet coaches are often the initial people to observe dancer fatigue with signs such as difficulty picking up new choreography or a lack of power and endurance in movement. Drawing attention to these observations with the dancer and/or support staff can lead to appropriate interventions to enhance recovery.

Mental fatigue and perceptions of mental fatigue in professional ballet

Dancers at TAB are required to learn new and complex repertoire, which can include both contemporary and classical dance 'pieces' on an almost daily basis. Depending on the work, the repertoire can often be taught by different choreographers and repetiteurs, who bring their own style and approach to teaching. Furthermore, the company will often perform one show in the evening, while learning up to two new pieces of choreography during that same day. These activities may increase mental workload, which has the potential to result in mental fatigue (Borghini et al., 2014; Loch et al., 2022). Mental fatigue is a psychobiological state that is characterised by "feelings of tiredness" (Marcora et al., 2009, p. 857) and often precedes periods of cognitively demanding activities.

Perceptions of mental fatigue in professional ballet

Due to the unique mental demands of professional ballet, TAB sought to investigate the perceptions and experiences of mental fatigue in dancers and dance staff. The aim of this research was to increase our awareness of the burden that mental fatigue may or may not have on the experience of being a professional ballet dancer. Using focus groups and semi-structured interviews, four key themes identified by Wirdnam et al. (2024) were: (1) the perceived causes of mental fatigue, (2) the perceived symptoms of mental fatigue, (3) the perceived impacts of mental fatigue, and (4) commonly used strategies to combat mental fatigue. Dancers perceived that learning new choreography was a cause of mental fatigue, reporting that this was exacerbated when the learning was prolonged and when little opportunity for rest or recovery was provided (Wirdnam et al., 2024).

Bi-directional changes in mood and emotion were perceived to be a key symptom of mental fatigue and were often associated with an increase in perception of effort and a reduction in motivation (Wirdnam et al., 2024). The research identified that dancers perceived that mental fatigue had the potential to negatively impact physical and cognitive performance, and that mental fatigue increased their perceived risk of injury. Dancers attributed the increase in risk of an acute injury to a momentary loss of focus or attention, while chronic injuries were reported to be due to difficulty remembering newly learned steps and the need to repeat the same step. Caffeine and exposure to nature were both reported to be a common strategy to combat mental fatigue in dancers, aligning with previous findings in athletes particularly where nature exposure was found to assist with directed attention (Sun et al., 2024). These findings have boosted awareness of the impact that mental fatigue has on professional ballet dancers specifically and will be used to inform future research in this context.

Performance lifestyle advisor

The Performance Lifestyle Advisor (PLA) is responsible for delivering strategies to ensure that TAB dancers are supported to strive for success in their art form and life. This role provides the highest level of career, education, lifestyle management and advice to improve and enhance their performance capabilities and well-being (The Australian Ballet, 2025b). A dancer screening process is conducted during the initial meeting with the PLA. This is recorded using an online athlete management system (Fair Play AMS, 2025) and covers goals, physical and mental health, career development, well-being and education. The PLA plans education and key target areas for the year, for example, mindset and behaviours, emotional intelligence and stress management. One-on-one sessions are held weekly or fortnightly with dancers who are engaging in ongoing support or working through personal or career development topics. The PLA is available for dancers who are facing 'in the moment' challenges, and includes, but is not limited to, dancers who are feeling overwhelmed due to personal and/or environmental demands. This may present as struggles with time management, load management, performance anxiety, issues relating to comparison, and maladaptive perfectionism. Dwarika and Haraldsen (2023) identified that stressors included: physical stressors related to dance training, such as a high physical workload, and requirements concerning technical skill and choreographic demands; and psychosocial stressors related to the environment, such as managing finances and obligations, interrelations, and major life events.

If dancers require additional support, they may self-refer to the PLA to access a psychologist. The psychologists are based in both Melbourne (where the company is based) and Sydney (where the company undertakes extended tours), therefore if an in-person appointment is not possible, dancers use telehealth services. Each individual dancer has access to AUD$ 1,000 per year that can be used to support access to services from a psychologist or dietician. Furthermore, dancers have access to an onsite GP one day per week, who can create a Mental Health Care Plan for those dancers who qualify.

Touring

Touring can be a challenging time for dancers. It is a time of heightened stress, due to being in an unfamiliar environment, long days and a high workload. Pre-tour, dancers are encouraged to spend time planning and strategising around their pillars of well-being (i.e., physical health, mental health and social well-being), to optimise their well-being and recovery in a new environment (Du, 2024). Dancers can work one-on-one with the PLA to create SMART goals (Bailey, 2017) and plan the structure of their days. This includes optimising sleep, nutrition, physical, mental, and emotional recovery. Furthermore, consideration of both domestic and international travel is incorporated into the planning, given the demonstrated impacts upon performance and recovery that have been found in athletes (Botonis et al., 2025).

Well-being and stress

The World Health Organization (2025) defines mental health as 'a state of well-being in which the individual realises his or her own abilities, can cope with the normal stresses of life, can work productively and fruitfully, and is able to make a contribution to his or her community'. Mental health therefore is not just the absence of mental illness; it is also the promotion of mental well-being (Dwarika & Haraldsen, 2023), which aligns with the broader definition of recovery by Beckmann et al. (2023) that includes increasing resilience to potential stressors and ensuring there is time to replenish mental resources.

Dealing with stress and environmental demands is a key area of dancer mental health and well-being (Blevins et al., 2019; this volume, Chapter 5). Dancing stressors can be broken down into three categories:

1. Situational stressors include time management issues, career uncertainty, and injuries.
2. Interpersonal stressors – perceived pressure and expectations, body image issues.
3. Cultural stressors – describe factors inherent in dance culture. Cultural hegemony, physical ideals and narrow-minded identity ideals (Dwarika & Haraldsen, 2023).

Assessing well-being

The PLA uses Spotlight [a psychometric tool developed by Mindflick® (Mindflick, 2025)] to enhance performance capabilities and facilitate well-being. It is a contemporary personality profiling tool accredited by the British Psychological Society (Burnell et al., 2023), designed to help individuals maximise their strengths and perform at their best. It is a support tool that is utilised to help individuals understand and explore different ways of viewing challenges to optimise performance and well-being. The report is broken down into performance chapters which include strengths, take cares, building confidence, developing resilience, maintaining energy, managing stressors, coping under pressure and dealing with problems. The PLA focuses on the most relevant chapters, depending on the specific challenge(s) a dancer is experiencing. Examples include working on managing stressors to attenuate mental fatigue and developing strategies to maintain energy during times of touring and high physical/mental load. The aim of the PLA support is to facilitate positive mental health outcomes for dancers including flourishing mental health, increased life quality, positive emotional states, increased confidence and self-efficacy (Dwarika & Haraldsen, 2023). Additional recovery strategies for promoting well-being and positive mental health include relaxation methods (e.g., meditation, Progressive Muscle Relaxation; Kellmann et al., 2024), the Psychological Skills Training strategies of self-talk and emotional control, and mindfulness (Wang et al., 2025).

Mindfulness has been described as 'paying attention on purpose, in the present moment, and without judgment'. Engaging in a mindfulness programme may alleviate a range of physical and mental health challenges (Birnkraut et al., 2025; Kaufman et al., 2009; Moyle, 2016). Davidson et al. (2003) suggest that an eight-week programme of mindfulness meditation significantly increases the left-sided anterior activation of the brain, associated with significant positive affect on trait anxiety and positive increase in immune function in athletes. Dancers at TAB have reported positive benefits of meditation including attenuation of anxiety levels, reduction in feeling overwhelmed, being present and able to focus on physical/mental tasks and enhanced sleep, including sleep latency, duration, and quality (Harrison et al., 2025).

Mindfulness can also induce 'flow state' for performers. Flow state can be described as a mindset when an individual perceives balance between the challenges associated with a situation and their capabilities to meet those demands (Csikszentmihalyi, 2008). Dancers have reported that they feel they have performed best while in flow state, increasing feelings of positive emotions and enhanced well-being. Flow qualities include centring of attention, perceptions of control over actions and environment, lower self-consciousness, losing track of time, merging of action and awareness, and greater intrinsic satisfaction. Davidson et al. (2003) have delineated several characteristics of peak-performance moments in athletes. Relaxation, confidence, high energy, present-centred focus, extraordinary awareness, feeling in control, and detachment from distractions are among the major factors that have been identified.

A six-week mindfulness and acceptance-based intervention was tested in this cohort by Harrison et al. (2025); dancers reported that the intervention was valuable, however found it challenging to dedicate time in their busy schedule. Integrating mindfulness and acceptance-based interventions into the company schedule would be beneficial.

The PLA uses Progressive Muscle Relaxation (PMR) to attenuate stress both in the body and mind. Dancers can also use this activity, either guided or self-guided, before going to sleep. It allows them to disconnect and 'de-role' from their performance, promoting mindfulness and present moment awareness (The Arts Wellbeing Collective, 2025). The PMR technique is a powerful method to reduce oxygen metabolism, respiration, blood pressure, muscle tension, and negative thoughts (Toussaint et al., 2021). Research has shown that there is a positive correlation between the use of PMR and sports performance (Parnabas et al., 2014).

As touring is a key time when dancers struggle to maintain their well-being, a 20-minute weekly PMR session is scheduled into the dancers' timetable. Sessions at TAB headquarters are one-on-one or in small groups and are usually outside the timetabled schedule. Educational content in relation to mindfulness and PMR is distributed to dancers via infographics.

Recovery or 'rest days' have been introduced into the company's schedule following the 2023 TAB Enterprise Bargaining Agreement (2024), as a strategy to reduce dancer fatigue. Recovery techniques such as PMR sessions or education sessions on well-being can be scheduled during these 'rest days'.

Insights from TAB: A professional ballet dancer's perspective

Life as a professional dancer goes far beyond what is contracted for. The idiom 'performing is not a job, but a lifestyle' is true for many of us. Mentally it is hard to switch off from something you are so engaged and passionate about, and we are physically so attuned to our bodies; waking up sore in the morning can cause serious anxiety about making it through a long day of class, rehearsals, and performance.

Mental and physical recovery is a learned skill in a professional ballet company and a personal choice. Recovery is not explicitly built into our day, and seeing the importance of switching off mentally and allowing enough physical recovery time is a difficult choice to make. This is specifically difficult when you are inspired and motivated by repertoire, hungry to progress through the ranks, or feel the internal pressure to perform at all costs. The Australian Ballet's Health Team is world-leading. Company artists have incredible access to physiotherapists, strength and conditioning and rehabilitation coaches, a gym, Pilates and recovery facilities with full support through injury rehabilitation as well as psychological and nutritional support. Dancers have been educated about the science of sleep, valuing well-being and offered artistic support with intimacy coordinators and cultural advisors including how to 'de-role' after emotionally challenging roles. But with all that is offered, it can be a full-time job to engage with all the advice. Day-to-day scheduling, touring and traditional ballet mentalities can present some challenges to implement the recommended health and recovery policies. Supported by a healthy company culture, stemming from the artistic director, and educated by a team of health professionals, you can find what resonates with you from what is offered, so you are mentally and physically able to have a long and fulfilling career.

Contractually, company artists are required to follow up on advice from the TAB medical team and maintain our physical fitness as supported by ready access to rehabilitation ballet staff, medical staff and facilities. Time is not specifically allocated within our schedule to implement our programmes for injury prevention and physical and mental recovery strategies after gruelling rehearsals. Despite this, there is a very healthy culture at TAB. Gym and Pilates spaces buzz an hour before work starts, during lunches and breaks, and the ice-bath is usually overflowing with dancers at the end of the day. What you can manage does fluctuate substantially during the year depending on repertoire and touring seasons. Though a slower return to work may be more beneficial in the long run, the 'Return-to-work policy' can be very hard to follow when a technical week for a challenging full-length ballet is only four weeks away. Internal and external pressures make it difficult to be completely objective about how you are physically coping and how strictly you follow the protocol.

Dancers also have post-flight recovery strategies in place for touring, which include reduced dance workload for the first two days, but that is sometimes not possible when long technical rehearsal days or dress rehearsals are scheduled the day after interstate travel. It can be difficult to immediately establish physical routines and nutritional preparation when schedules are tight, and tensions can become high. International touring schedules can be even more challenging with very demanding turn-arounds post flight, questionable gym access and no kitchen facilities. Although recommended to stick to light intensity exercise, especially in a pool for gentle mobilisation, the temptation to sight-see and spend every break walking around a new city is hard to resist.

Progression of our strength-building exercises after holidays at the start and middle of the year during rehearsal periods, tends to be in our homes. Maintenance of that level is the aim during performance seasons, but it can start to get very challenging when fatigue sets in and access to facilities changes dramatically. Equipment access is greatly reduced when interstate and/or in the theatre, so greater motivation is needed to travel to a gym in a break between rehearsal and performance. Mental fatigue can mean that you do not have the energy to add to or even change a routine, leading to a 'just hold on and pick up the pieces later' mentality in long seasons. It is important to establish healthy routines around physical and mental recovery in the rehearsal periods, so that they can be followed mindlessly when exhausted. Our longest seasons are spent away from our usual support systems – home, family, friends and pets – which can lead to a work-heavy/life balance.

Sports and scientific research around strength training, recovery, and fatigue does not resonate easily with every artistic mind. Trust and communication are so important between the dancers and the health team. It can be hard to relate the maintenance of a 100 kg leg press to the beauty and refinement of a ballet solo and to trust that rest or tapering can be more beneficial than an extra rehearsal. The traditional ballet mindset of working past breaking point and not showing mental weakness also makes the idea of acknowledging physical and mental struggle challenging. Education is challenging 'old-school' thoughts of strength meaning bulk, injury as weakness overcome by mental determination and that emotions should be left outside the studio. Being given greater autonomy and responsibility in rehearsal so that the focus shifts to what is needed by the dancer, rather than what pleases the person at the front of the room helps. A company culture that values personal development and mental and physical health can help shift the focus to what is important: a healthy and inspired dancer capable of maintaining a high level of performance through long performance seasons.

Conclusion and recommendations for practice

For professional ballet dancers to continue to perform at the highest level, recovery and well-being must be prioritised. This includes understanding physiological processes such as mental and physical fatigue, fostering environments in which discussing well-being is safe and utilising evidence-based methods for recovery. This chapter highlights the physical and mental challenges faced by professional ballet dancers and the importance of load management, as well as the role of tailored exercise programmes to build capacity and attenuate physical fatigue. Educating dancers on the early signs of physical fatigue and how to mitigate fatigue can help prevent injury. The impact of mental fatigue in professional ballet needs to be considered, and strategies that have been observed to reduce the accumulation of mental fatigue can be introduced, initially through education and then implementation. Managing stressors, optimising sleep and nutrition, and finding opportunities to get exposure to nature can all help to recover from mental fatigue.

Integrated, holistic support from various members of a multidisciplinary health team can assist in the management of fatigue and can help provide dancers with a more sustainable work environment. Scheduling within a professional company is challenging, and some of the practical strategies utilised within the company have been described, such as a graduated return to full workload, scheduled progressive muscle relaxation sessions and education sessions on recovery strategies, and could be adopted by other arts companies. Finally, it is important to recognise that while professional ballet dancers are incredibly resilient, they require support on their journey to balanced health and well-being in a demanding profession.

Note

1 Flat-based dancers wear soft ballet shoes, while pointe-based dancers wear pointe shoes.

References

Bahr, R. (2016). Why screening tests to predict injury do not work—and probably never will…: A critical review. *British Journal of Sports Medicine*, *50*, 776–780.
Bailey, R. R. (2017). Goal setting and action planning for health behavior change. *American Journal of Lifestyle Medicine*, *13*(6), 615–618.
Beckmann, J., Kellmann, M., & Jakowski, S. (2023). Recovery is more than just healing: Advocating a broader perspective on recovery in physical and mental health. In M. Kellmann, S. Jakowski, & J. Beckmann (Eds.), *The importance of recovery for physical and mental health: Negotiating the effects of underrecovery* (pp. 266–270). Routledge.
Birnkraut, T., Kellmann, M., & Jakowski, S. (2025). Effect of daily mindfulness fluctuations on sleep and recovery-stress states in elite level judoka: An observational study. *Frontiers in Sports and Active Living*, *7*, 1583058. https://doi.org/10.3389/fspor.2025.1583058
Blevins, P., Erskine, S., Hopper, L., & Moyle, G. M. (2019). Finding your balance: An investigation of recovery–stress balance in vocational dance training. *Journal of Dance Education*, *20*(1), 12–22.
Borghini, G., Astolfi, L., Vecchiato, G., Mattia, D., & Babiloni, F. (2014). Measuring neurophysiological signals in aircraft pilots and car drivers for the assessment of mental workload, fatigue and drowsiness. *Neuroscience & Biobehavioral Reviews*, *44*, 58–75.
Botonis, P. G., Toubekis, A. G., Hill, D. W., & Mundel, T. (2025). Impact of long-haul airline travel on athletic performance and recovery: A critical review of the literature. *Experimental Physiology*, *110*(11), 1584–1602.
Burnell, L., Ong, C. W., Pitt, T., Butt, J., & Eubank, M. (2023). Exploring the perceived benefits of engaging with Spotlight personality profiling in performance domains. *Sport & Exercise Psychology* Review, *18*(1), 76–95.
Charest, J., & Grandner, M. A. (2020). Sleep and athletic performance: Impacts on physical performance, mental performance, injury risk and recovery, and mental health. *Sleep Medicine Clinics*, *15*(1), 41–57.
Csikszentmihalyi, M. (2008). *Flow: The psychology of optimal experience*. Harper Perennial.
Dantas, A. G., Alonso, D. A., Sánchez-Miguel, P. A., & del Río Sánchez, C. (2018). Factors dancers associate with their body dissatisfaction. *Body Image*, *25*, 40–47.
Davidson, R. J., Kabat-Zinn, J., Schumacher, J., Rosenkranz, M., Muller, D., Santorelli, S. F., Urbanowski, F., Harrington, A., Bonus, K., & Sheridan, J. F. (2003). Alterations in brain and immune function produced by mindfulness meditation. *Psychosomatic Medicine*, *65*(4), 564–570.
De Wet, J. S., Africa, E., & Venter, R. (2022). Recovery-stress states of professional ballet dancers during different phases of a ballet season. *Journal of Dance Medicine & Science*, *26*(1), 8–15.
Du, J. (2024). Health and wellbeing assessment in sport. In V. Girginov & Y. Inoue (Eds.), *Routledge resources online - Sport studies* (pp. 1–11). Routledge. https://doi.org/10.4324/9780367766924-RESS89-1

Dwarika, M. S., & Haraldsen, H. M. (2023). Mental health in dance: A scoping review. *Frontiers in Psychology, 14*, 1090645. https://doi.org/10.3389/fpsyg.2023.1090645

Fair Play AMS. (2025). *Athlete management system.* Retrieved June 10, 2025 from https://fairplayams.com/

Farmer, C., & Brouner, J. (2021). Perceptions of strength training in dance. *Journal of Dance Medicine & Science, 25*(3), 160–168.

Gardiner, C., Weakley, J., Burke, L. M., Roach, G. D., Sargent, C., Maniar, N., Townshend, A., & Halson, S. L. (2023). The effect of caffeine on subsequent sleep: A systematic review and meta-analysis. *Sleep Medicine Reviews, 69*, 101764. https://doi.org/10.1016/j.smrv.2023.101764

Harrison, C., Ruddock, S., Mayes, S., Cook, J., O'Halloran, P., Ferrar, K., Li, X., & Ruddock, M. (2025). A 6-week mindfulness-acceptance-commitment intervention to improve professional ballet dancers' psychological states around performance. *Journal of Dance Medicine & Science, 29*(2), 67–76.

Jakowski, S., Kiel, A., Kullik, L., & Erlacher, D. (2023). Sleep to heal and restore: The role of sleep in the recovery and regeneration process. In J. Beckmann, M. Kellmann, & S. Jakowski (Eds.), *The importance of recovery for physical and mental health: Negotiating the effects of underrecovery* (pp. 141–153). Routledge.

Jamtvedt, G., Herbert, R. D., Flottorp, S., Odgaard-Jensen, J., Håvelsrud, K., Barratt, A., Mathieu, E., Burls, A., & Oxman, A. D. (2010). A pragmatic randomised trial of stretching before and after physical activity to prevent injury and soreness. *British Journal of Sports Medicine, 44*(14), 1002–1009.

Kaufman, K. A., Glass, C. R., & Arnkoff, D. B. (2009). Evaluation of mindful sport performance enhancement (MSPE): A new approach to promote flow in athletes. *Journal of Clinical Sport Psychology, 3*(4), 334–356.

Kellmann, M., Pelka, M., & Beckmann, J. (2024). Psychological relaxation techniques to enhance recovery in sports. In M. Kellmann & J. Beckmann (Eds.), *Fostering recovery and well-being in a healthy lifestyle: Psychological, somatic, and organizational prevention approaches* (pp. 117–130). Routledge.

Kużdżał, A., Trybulski, R., Muracki, J., Klich, S., Clemente, F. M., & Kawczyński, A. (2025). Dry needling in sports and sport recovery: A systematic review with an evidence gap map. *Sports Medicine, 55*(4), 811–844.

Leach, M. J. (2005). Rapport: A key to treatment success. *Complementary Therapies in Clinical Practice, 11*(4), 262–265.

Loch, F., Jakowski, S., Hof zum Berge, A., & Kellmann, M. (2022). Mental fatigue and the concept of mental recovery in sport. In M. Kellmann & J. Beckmann (Eds.), *Recovery and well-being in sport and exercise* (pp. 187–200). Routledge.

Long, K. L., Milidonis, M. K., Wildermuth, V. L., Kruse, A. N., & Parham, U. T. (2021). The impact of dance-specific neuromuscular conditioning and injury prevention training on motor control, stability, balance, function and injury in professional ballet dancers: A mixed-methods quasi-experimental study. *International Journal of Sports Physical Therapy, 16*(2), 404–417.

Maloney, B. M., Mattiussi, A. M., Cleather, D. J., Price, P., & Shaw, J. W. (2024). Jumping demands during classical ballet class. *Scandinavian Journal of Medicine & Science in Sports, 34*(1), e14502. https://doi.org/10.1111/sms.14502

Marcora, S. M., Staiano, W., & Manning, V. (2009). Mental fatigue impairs physical performance in humans. *Journal of Applied Physiology, 106*(3), 857–864.

McCormack, M., Bird, H., De Medici, A., Haddad, F., & Simmonds, J. (2019). The physical attributes most required in professional ballet: A delphi study. *Sports Medicine International Open*, *3*(01), E1–E5. https://doi.org/10.1055/a-0798-3570

Mindflick. (2025). *Spotlight*. Software from Mindflick. Hathersage, United Kingdom.

Mountjoy, M., Ackerman, K. E., Bailey, D. M., Burke, L. M., Constantini, N., Hackney, A. C., Heikura, I. A., Melin, A., Pensgaard, A. M., Stellingwerff, T., Sundgot-Borgen, J. K., Torstveit, M. K., Jacobsen, A. U., Verhagen, E., Budgett, R., Engebretsen, L., & Erdener, U. (2023). 2023 International Olympic Committee's (IOC) consensus statement on Relative Energy Deficiency in Sport (REDs). *British Journal of Sports Medicine*, *57*(17), 1073–1097.

Moyle, G. M. (2016). Mindfulness and dancers. In A. L. Baltzell (Ed.), *Mindfulness and performance* (pp. 367–388). Cambridge University Press.

Nogueira, L. F. R., Pellegrino, P., Cipolla-Neto, J., Moreno, C. R. C., & Marqueze, E. C. (2021). Timing and composition of last meal before bedtime affect sleep parameters of night workers. *Clocks & Sleep*, *3*(4), 536–546.

Parnabas, V. A., Mahamood, Y., Parnabas, J., & Abdullah, N. M. (2014). The relationship between relaxation techniques and sport performance. *Universal Journal of Psychology*, *2*(3), 108–112.

Schantz, P. G., & Åstrand, P. (1984). Physiological characteristics of classical ballet. *Medicine & Science in Sports & Exercise*, *16*(5), 472–476.

Schoenfeld, B. J., Grgic, J., Van Every, D. W., & Plotkin, D. L. (2021). Loading recommendations for muscle strength, hypertrophy, and local endurance: A re-examination of the repetition continuum. *Sports*, *9*(2), 32. https://doi.org/10.3390/sports9020032

Shaw, J. W., Mattiussi, A. M., Brown, D. D., Williams, S., Kelly, S., Springham, M., Pedlar, C. R., & Tallent, J. (2021). Dance exposure, individual characteristics, and injury risk over five seasons in a professional ballet company. *Medicine and Science in Sports and Exercise*, *53*(11), 2290–2297.

Sun, H., Soh, K. G., Mohammadi, A., Toumi, Z., Zhang, L., Ding, C., Gao, X., & Tian, J. (2024). Counteracting mental fatigue for athletes: A systematic review of the interventions. *BMC Psychology*, *12*(1), 67. https://doi.org/10.1186/s40359-023-01476-w

TAB Enterprise Bargaining Agreement. (2024). *Annual Report | 2023–24*. Retrieved July 07, 2025 from https://www.meaa.org/download/meaa-annual-report-2023-24/

The Arts Wellbeing Collective. (2025). *Your pocket guide to de-role*. Retrieved June 10, 2025 from https://www.artswellbeingcollective.com.au/resources/your-pocket-guide-to-post-show-de-role/

The Australian Ballet. (2018). *Strength beats stretch*. Retrieved March 04, 2025 from https://australianballet.com.au/blog/strength-beats-stretch?srsltid=AfmBOoqL8JJPoZEMjVHXDKIOEMJKQutcMk5iBhRmtne3NjQnLeArC7xh

The Australian Ballet. (2020). *Injury risk management program*. Retrieved March 04, 2025 from https://assets.australianballet.com.au/documents/Other-Documents/TAB-injury-risk-reduction-program-2020.pdf

The Australian Ballet. (2024). *Body image and disordered eating guidelines: A framework for action and prevention of eating disorders*. Retrieved March 04, 2025 from https://assets.australianballet.com.au/documents/Health/Body-Image-and-Disordered-Eating-Guidelines-A-framework-for-action-and-prevention-of-eating-disorders.pdf

The Australian Ballet. (2025a). *Ballet frequently asked questions*. Retrieved June 03, 2025 from https://australianballet.com.au/ballet-101/ballet-faq#:~:text=How%20many%20times%20does%20The,Perth%2C%20and%20regularly%20tours%20overseas

The Australian Ballet. (2025b). *Injury risk management program*. Retrieved March 04, 2025 from https://assets.australianballet.com.au/documents/Health/Injury-Management-and-Risk-Reduction-Program-2025.pdf

Tornero-Aguilera, J. F., Jimenez-Morcillo, J., Rubio-Zarapuz, A., & Clemente-Suárez, V. J. (2022). Central and peripheral fatigue in physical exercise explained: A narrative review. *International Journal of Environmental Research and Public Health*, *19*(7), 3909. https://doi.org/10.3390/ijerph19073909

Toussaint, L., Nguyen, Q. A., Roettger, C., Dixon, K., Offenbächer, M., Kohls, N., Hirsch, J., & Sirois, F. (2021). Effectiveness of progressive muscle relaxation, deep breathing, and guided imagery in promoting psychological and physiological states of relaxation. *Evidence-based Complementary and Alternative Medicine*, *eCAM*, 5924040. https://doi.org/10.1155/2021/5924040

Wang, W., Schweickle, M. J., Arnold, E. R., & Vella, S. A. (2025). Psychological interventions to improve elite athlete mental wellbeing: A systematic review and meta-analysis. *Sports Medicine*, *55*(4), 877–897.

Warden, S. J., Davis, I. S., & Fredericson, M. (2014). Management and prevention of bone stress injuries in long-distance runners. *The Journal of Orthopaedic and Sports Physical Therapy*, *44*(10), 749–765.

Wirdnam, M., Ferrar, K., Mayes, S., MacMahon, C., Cook, J., & Rio, E. (2024). "A sprained ankle is the biggest sign of mental fatigue": A qualitative study of the perceptions and experiences of mental fatigue in professional ballet. *Physical Therapy in Sport, 65*, 154–161.

World Health Organisation. (2025). *Mental health*. Retrieved on the June 03, 2025 from https://www.who.int/health-topics/mental-health#tab=tab_1

12

CREATING MAGIC ON AND OFF THE STAGE

Cirque du Soleil contextual recovery and well-being approaches

Veronique Richard, Chad Fraser, and Bernard Petiot

Introduction

Cirque du Soleil (CDS) is renowned for its innovative approach to live circus performances, delivered in a variety of models and formats (see Lavers & Leroux, 2018, for details). Over the past 40 years, CDS has evolved from its iconic *Big Top* touring shows to permanent *theatre* spectacles and fast-paced *arena* productions designed to reach smaller markets. Despite this evolution, the essence of the CDS experience remains consistent – captivating audiences with awe-inspiring performances (Weisberger, 2018).

> Without beautiful choreography, intriguing costumes, wonderful make up, phenomenal music, superb theatrical lighting, hi-tech projection and stunning scenography, acrobatics cannot speak. However, without acrobatics, the story cannot be told the Cirque du Soleil way. This narrative is possible because the company allows us to experiment, to be innovative, and thus acrobatics create a tale of poetry in motion that turn heads and capture the hearts of our audiences
>
> *Boris Verkhovsky – key pioneers of Cirque du Soleil human performance*

When attending a CDS show, most audience members sit back and relax to enjoy the spectacular performance, likely contributing to their own recovery

Richard, V., Fraser, C., & Petiot, B. (2026). Creating magic on and off the stage: Cirque du Soleil contextual recovery and well-being approaches. In E. Altenmüller, M. Kellmann, J. Beckmann, & G. M. Moyle (Eds.), *Recovery and well-being in the performing arts* (pp. 205–222). Routledge.

DOI: 10.4324/9781003566885-15

and well-being (Renton et al., 2012; Shim et al., 2021; Siu et al., 2016). But what happens when the curtain falls, and the applause fades? How do these performers recover and sustain their health and well-being amid the demands of their craft?

Research on professional circus artists' health and well-being is scarce and mixed. For example, Donohue et al. (2020) found that CDS professionals reported fewer social, performance-related challenges and greater support than student-artists as well as lower depression than normative samples. In contrast, van Rens and Heritage (2021) found that circus artists had higher levels of depression, anxiety, and stress but also greater resilience compared to normative samples. These contrasting findings highlight the complexity of addressing health and well-being in professional circus contexts.

To support the health and well-being of circus performers, implementing effective recovery strategies is essential (Decker et al., 2019; Filho et al., 2016; Shrier & Hallé, 2011). Hence, this chapter offers a framework for designing flexible recovery plans tailored to the unique constraints of CDS performers. Acting as the ultimate backstage access pass, it provides a vivid glimpse into the diverse ecosystem of CDS, highlighting the rich variety of performers and the complex tasks and environments they navigate.

An ecological dynamic perspective

Altenmüller et al. (this volume, Chapter 1) introduce the performing arts as inherently complex, calling for a systemic and interaction-focused approach to learning and performance. We argue that the same approach is essential for understanding recovery – especially in environments like CDS where physical, psychological, and social demands are high. Recovery is more than just physical rest; it's a dynamic process that helps restore balance across body, mind, and social relationships (Kellmann et al., 2018).

To explore how recovery and well-being unfold in the CDS context, we draw on ecological dynamics – a framework that looks at how individuals interact with their environments over time. Hence, rather than viewing recovery as something that happens in isolation, we argue that it is emerging from the ongoing relationship between performers and their environment, such as training spaces, the schedule, the team, the pressures of performance, etc.

This approach brings together ideas from several fields:

- Ecological psychology conceptualises how people make sense of their environments and respond in real time (Rietveld & Kiverstein, 2014).
- Nonlinear dynamics highlights how small changes – like a shift in team communication or a short recovery pause – can have big impacts (Phillips et al., 2010).

- Complexity science views performers not as machines, but as adaptable systems shaped by physical, mental, and social factors all at once (Davids et al., 2013; Seifert & Davids, 2017).

In practical terms, this means recognising that recovery in CDS is not one-size-fits-all. It is a moving target shaped by how performers interact with their roles, their bodies, their teammates, and the demands of the show. By understanding these interactions, we can better support sustainable performance and long-term well-being.

A constraint-led approach to recovery

Within the ecological dynamics framework, the constraint-led approach (CLA) offers a relevant lens to analyse and optimise recovery and well-being. Constraints are defined as "boundary conditions, limitations, or design features that apply restrictions to the degrees of freedom of a system, thereby indicating the trajectories that the system may exhibit" (Chow et al., 2006, p. 262; referring to Newell, 1986). Newell's (1986) conceptualisation categorises constraints into three domains: individual/organismic, environmental, and task constraints (see Balagué et al., 2019 for complete review).

Organismic constraints are related to personal characteristics, such as an artist's body composition, personality, cultural background, or psychological state at a specific moment. Environmental constraints are external to the individual. At CDS, these may include the show format, travel schedules, and socio-cultural norms and expectations. Task constraints, on the other hand, are defined by the specific requirements of the task at hand. CDS presents a wide variety of tasks, ranging from high-risk acrobatics to emotionally grounded physical acting.

While the CLA has been extensively explored in skill acquisition (Clark et al., 2018; Orth et al., 2019; Renshaw et al., 2010; Seifert et al., 2017) and preliminarily discussed in rehabilitation (Wikstrom et al., 2013) and injury risk reduction in sport (Pol et al., 2019), its application to recovery and well-being in performing artists remains underexplored. Yet, recovery, as a process of restoring biopsychosocial balance after periods of physical and/or mental stress (Kellmann et al., 2018), necessitates an understanding of the constraints that may hinder or facilitate this process.

The Constraint-Led Wheel of Recovery and Well-being Framework

The CLA's emphasis on the interplay of constraints aligns seamlessly with the multifaceted demands of recovery in CDS contexts. The unique constraints of CDS – such as the interplay of individual capabilities, task demands, and

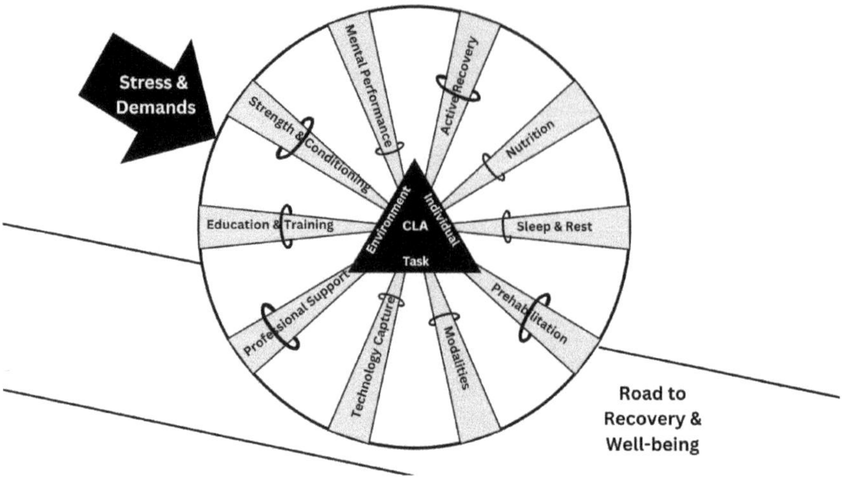

FIGURE 12.1 The Constraint-Led Wheel of Recovery and Well-being Framework.

environmental conditions – offer a rich and complex landscape to apply this approach. By identifying and leveraging these constraints, the CLA provides a structured yet flexible framework for optimising recovery strategies, ensuring that performers' biopsychosocial balance is effectively restored. When combined with specific recovery strategies employed in CDS settings, it forms the *Constraint-Led Wheel of Recovery and Well-being Framework* (Figure 12.1). This evidence-informed framework supports the development of individualised and adaptive recovery plans for performers. Figure 14.1 illustrates the ten addressed components of overall recovery strategies available on a CDS show. In no particular order, they consist of:

- **Active recovery:** Engaging in low-intensity aerobic activities such as swimming, walking, or recreational cycling to promote blood flow without overstraining the body. This may also include dynamic stretching and mobility exercises to prevent stiffness.
- **Strength and conditioning:** Incorporating functional training and core stability exercises designed to mimic the movements performed in an artist's act. This helps develop strength, endurance, power, and agility in relevant muscle groups.
- **Nutrition:** Ensuring proper hydration to support overall bodily functions and maintaining a balanced diet rich in essential nutrients to fuel performance and aid muscle repair.
- **Sleep and rest:** Prioritising appropriate quantity of quality sleep per night to facilitate natural recovery. Regularly scheduled rest days are also essential to prevent overtraining and support long-term performance.
- **Prehabilitation:** Addressing concerns promptly with appropriate interventions designed to strengthen and/or prepare vulnerable areas (i.e., soft

tissue or joint ranges) and reduce injury risk incorporating targeted exercises (e.g., rotator cuff) or mobility (e.g., PNF stretching)

- **Mental performance:** Developing appropriate mental skills and strategies to enhance performance, deal with stressors, and maintain overall well-being.
- **Recovery modalities:** Employing various treatment methods, including manual therapy (e.g., massage and joint mobilisation) to alleviate muscle tension and improve circulation. Additional techniques may involve Instrument Assisted Soft Tissue Mobilisation (i.e., muscle scraping), cupping, foam rolling, and ball therapy. Temperature-based approaches, such as thermotherapy (e.g., heat pads, hot tubs), cryotherapy (e.g., icing, cold plunges), and contrast therapy (alternating hot/cold), can help reduce muscle soreness and inflammation.
- **Technology capture:** Leveraging technology such as video analysis, biomechanics testing, GPS tracking, and biometric data to monitor performance, optimise training loads, and tailor recovery strategies to individual needs.
- **Education and training:** Engaging in workshops and learning opportunities focused on injury prevention, recovery techniques, and overall well-being.
- **Professional support:** Seeking guidance from sports medicine professionals who understand the specific demands of circus artists and can provide specialised care and advice.

Under conditions of high stress and demands (illustrated by the top-left arrow in Figure 12.1), recovery strategies should not be applied ad hoc. Instead, they must be carefully tailored to the unique individual, environmental, and task constraints central to each performer's context (illustrated by the triangle in the middle of the wheel in Figure 14.1). Hence, each spoke of the recovery wheel functions as a sliding scale, adjustable based on the specific context of the performer (illustrated by the ellipse surrounding each spoke in Figure 14.1). We argue that this constraint-led approach sets performers on a road to recovery and well-being, increasing the likelihood of achieving sustainable high-level performance.

The following sections examine the environmental, task, and individual constraints that shape recovery strategies at CDS, highlighting how the CLA can inform a nuanced and systemic understanding of recovery and well-being in this unique context.

Environmental constraints: From theatre to big top to arena

While environmental constraints may be more consistent across artists compared to individual and task constraints, understanding the three major environments in which artists perform, along with their respective constraints, is essential for identifying recovery opportunities. Table 12.1 provides an overview of the environmental constraints that could influence recovery processes.

TABLE 12.1 Cirque du Soleil environmental conditions x show format.

	Resident shows	*Big top shows*	*Arena shows*
Number of shows in operations as of December 2025	6 (Drawn to Life, KA, Mad Apple, MJ One, Mystere, O)	5 (Alegria, Echo, Kooza, Kurios, Luzia)	2 (Corteo, OVO)
Total number of shows performed in 2023	3,280	1,759	643
Average number of shows/year	469	293	213
Typical number of days off/ week	2	2	3
Typical show schedule	5 double shows days consecutives	Wed: 1 show Thu: 1 show Fri: 1 or 2 shows Sat: 2 or 3 shows Sun: 2 shows	Thu: 1 show Fri: 1 show Sat: 2 or 3 shows Sun: 1 or 2 shows
Number of artists	567	292	157
Artist breakdown/show	Drawn to Life: 76 KA: 84 Mad Apple: 65 MJ One: 85 Mystere: 73 O: 95	Alegria: 49 Echo: 54 Kooza: 53 Kurios: 51 Luzia: 50	Corteo: 60 OvO: 52
Average number of artists	81	49	52
Inter-city travel mode	n/a	Bus, commercial or charter flight	Bus, commercial or chartered flight
Average time in a city	n/a	4–12 weeks	5 days
Average days off between performance city	n/a	10	3
Average days of training prior to first performance after breaks	n/a	3	1
Lodging	Personal residence	Corporate apartment in each city	Hotel rooms in every city
Family accompanying artist	Live with their family at home	Able to travel with family	Family is not supported
Food	Not supported	On-site full kitchen with 4 full-time CDS chefs	On-site catering from external company

Theatre environment

The theatre format at CDS emerged as a milestone in the organisation's history, starting with *Mystère* in 1993 at Treasure Island in Las Vegas. It marked the company's transition to permanent productions, offering a stable and high-calibre entertainment experience. Theatre productions allow for a custom-designed performance space tailored to the storyline, accommodating 70 to over 90 artists, with acrobatic performers constituting 50–60% of the cast. Shows run five nights a week with two performances per evening, totalling more than 470 shows annually. The schedule offers artists consistency, with two weekly days off and periodic two-week vacations. The predictable environment enables performers to integrate into a stable lifestyle, contrasting the nomadic nature of touring formats. Artists dedicate seven to more than nine hours daily to performances, rehearsals, and training, supported by two or three Performance Medicine Therapists and a robust coaching team made up of full-time coach(es) as well as designated artist-coaches for larger group acts.

Big top environment

Big top touring shows represent CDS's foundational format, perfected over the years since the company's inception in 1984. These productions feature around 49 performers, with acrobats making up the majority. Each show runs for 100 minutes of performance with a 30-minute intermission, and is presented between six and ten times weekly, typically over five working days. Tour stops range from 4 to 14 weeks depending upon the size of the market city, interspersed with one to two-week breaks between touring cities. A performer's daily schedule includes up to twelve hours on-site, encompassing show prep, showtime, act-specific rehearsals, physical conditioning, and injury risk reduction care from on-site medical therapists. Performers are provided accommodations, split between apartments and hotels, with daily commutes ranging from 15 to 45 minutes. Annual performance counts range from 310 to 360, making this format highly intensive yet structured for long-term touring.

Arena environment

The arena format allows CDS to expand its reach into smaller markets by reducing travel size requirements. This fast-paced touring model features one-week stops in different cities, with five to seven performances weekly. Arena shows maintain a similar structure to big top productions, with a 100-minute performance and a cast of 45 to 60 artists. However, the logistical demands are higher, with weekly city transfers by bus or flight, often late at night. Performers encounter varying conditions at each location, from new dressing rooms and commuting arrangements to environmental challenges such as cold arenas or isolated venues situated far from amenities to maintain proximity to the performance space. The tight turnaround limits settling-in time, with artists constantly adapting. Despite the challenges, the format offers CDS a unique opportunity to bring its creative productions to diverse audiences, presenting 200 to 250 shows annually.

Environment-led recovery processes and strategies

To the best of our knowledge, no research has specifically examined the impact of these three distinct environmental contexts on performers' recovery and well-being. However, a study conducted at the National Circus School – from which CDS frequently recruits artists – revealed that student-artists' perceived fatigue fluctuated in response to variations in training demands throughout the school year (Decker et al., 2019). Specifically, student-artists reported higher fatigue levels during periods of increased training load and stress, whereas perceived fatigue was lower following extended break periods. Building on this evidence, the consistency and quantity of time off available in each of the three CDS environments might be an important environmental constraint to consider to adjust the recovery plan of performers.

For instance, because resident shows provide consistent yet limited time off, they offer a greater sense of normalcy and routine, more closely resembling a 'normal weekend' similar to many non-performance careers. Since artists in resident shows typically live in permanent lodging of their own, their environment affords greater potential to implement recovery strategies consistently. They benefit from the stability of established routines, such as regularly consuming the same recovery drinks or food, visiting the same massage therapist, or attending the same facility for thermo-, cryo-, and/or contrast therapy (i.e., alternating hot and cold treatments). This environmental familiarity may help reduce their perception of stress, positively contributing to recovery and well-being.

Conversely, arena or big top artists, who perform in various locations worldwide, usually stay in hotels or corporate apartments and may have as little as one day off or as many as three. However, many use this time to explore and engage in local attractions or activities, as their time in each location is brief. This can lead to artists sacrificing time typically dedicated to recovery in favour of personal and social enjoyment. While social activities support important aspects of well-being on tour (Newman et al., 2022), it can also leave artists feeling physically, socially, and/or mentally fatigued upon returning to work. Additionally, constantly changing beds may disrupt sleep quality, being in a foreign country may limit access to familiar foods that aid recovery, and distance from family can impact their sense of community – all of which can affect their biopsychological balance.

Consequently, artists performing in arena and big top environments may need to adjust the weighting of each spoke on the wheel to reflect their current conditions (Figure 14.1). The environment may not always afford the same opportunities for recovery, sometimes requiring artists to be creative in replenishing their physiological and psychological resources.

Task constraints

Regardless of show format, CDS performances share common task constraints. On each show, the selection of acts is guided by the storyline, with act content and music carefully harmonised to enhance the required energy, tempo, and mood. Act-specific costumes are designed to balance aesthetics with performance functionality and safety. Shows typically feature ten to twelve acts, with up to four acts created specifically for a particular production. Act durations generally range from six to eight minutes but can extend to twelve minutes for more complex or content-dense performances, whether involving solo artists, small ensembles, or larger groups of ten to twelve performers. Regardless of the structure of the act, the replicability and sustainability of performance over time are key to each artist's task. To ensure flexibility, at least one act is kept in rotation (i.e., backup act) to fill gaps if another act is unavailable or requires recovery. Larger group acts often have surplus performers, allowing for rotation and providing a contingency for injuries or other absences.

Furthermore, the composition of the global cast highlights the diversity of human performances on stage. The cast is divided into two primary categories: acrobatic and artistic performers. Comprising up to two-thirds of the cast, acrobatic performers' tasks are characterised by high physical demands, significant risk, dependence on partners, teamwork, and reliance on equipment (e.g., tumbling, aerials, juggling, equilibrium, contortions, etc.). In contrast, artistic performers making up the remaining third of the cast include musicians, singers, dancers, and physical actors, with notable contributions from pantomime and clown artists. While they tend to face fewer physical risks, their contributions are no less taxing.

The performances of artistic cast members depend heavily on emotional expression, stage presence, and sustained interaction with both fellow performers and live audiences. These requirements create an emotional load which involves the ongoing modulation of affect, energy, and empathy in real time. Unlike physical exertion, emotional labour may not be as visibly taxing, but it can be deeply fatiguing, especially over long tours and repetitive performances (Holman et al., 2008). Performing with emotional authenticity while managing audience feedback, maintaining group synchrony, and adapting to the subtle cues of live performance imposes a cognitive-emotional toll that can lead to mental and physical exhaustion. For some artists, the repeated summoning of intense emotional states – whether joy, melancholy, tension, or humour – can blur the boundaries between performance and self, adding further complexity to their recovery needs (Liu et al., 2023).

Beyond their primary act responsibilities, performers participate in cue tracks – short performances such as dancing or character expressions that add artistry to the show. These cues, which vary across performances and often involve rotation among performers, introduce unique movement demands. While these demands may align with or differ from those of the performer's main act, they still contribute significantly to the overall workload (Faltus & Richard, 2022).

Finally, the risk exposure of performers also varies based on the nature of the act, equipment, and environment. Acts may occur on stage level (e.g., juggling), mid-air (e.g., banquine), or high above the ground (e.g., trapeze), with some acts combining these elements. Risk mitigation measures – such as mats, spotters, safety lines, airbags, or nets – are employed where possible. However, certain acts, such as tissue or straps (i.e., aerials) performed over the stage, may increase safety risks, increasing psychological stress in addition to physical and technical demands.

Task-led recovery and well-being processes and strategies

Task constraints must be carefully considered when planning the recovery of circus performers as they have the potential to impact every spoke of the wheel. For instance, research reveals that acrobatic performers are slightly more prone to physical injury than their artistic counterparts (Shrier et al., 2009). This suggests that physical stress is more pronounced for artists engaged in acrobatic tasks, highlighting the need for targeted recovery interventions to optimise physical restoration and mitigate injury risk (Greenspan et al., 2022).

At CDS, when an artist transitions from injured phase to functional recovery and prevention, it is essential to assess whether the issue is an isolated incident or part of a recurring trend (Bolling et al., 2019). If necessary, adjustments can be made to their existing physical routine to minimise the risk of re-injury. At this stage, emphasis shifts to the *Strength and Conditioning* and *Prehabilitation* spokes of the wheel, integrating area-specific exercises into their preparation and priming routine. These exercises are tailored to the nature of their previous injury and the demands of their performance. This comprehensive approach ensures that both the affected and surrounding structures are re-patterned and sufficiently prepared for the rigours of performance.

The purpose of *Prehabilitation* movements is to elicit a specific tissue response. For instance, a trapeze artist recovering from shoulder impingement might incorporate controlled eccentric movements in a rotator cuff stabilisation programme as part of their priming and accessory work. Simultaneously, a structured upper-extremity loading programme – including compound movements like shoulder presses and pull-ups – would be tailored to their discipline, with varying strength and plyometric components.

The *Technology* spoke of the wheel also plays a valuable role in establishing task-led recovery strategies. While GPS tracking is extensively utilised in sports to analyse movement patterns and evaluate external load, internal load, fatigue, and athletic performance (Ferraz et al., 2023), its application in the circus environment is challenging. However, Barker and colleagues (2020) demonstrated the potential of accelerometer-based monitoring, which tracks forces exerted on performers both during injury recovery and under normal training conditions. Their study utilised a wearable shirt equipped with an accelerometer and sensors that collect heart rate and breathing data. By using commercial accelerometers, coaches can assess the mechanical demands of various acts and adjust training intensities accordingly. This approach may be particularly beneficial for structuring artists' workload substitution tapping into the *Rest and Sleep* spoke of the wheel.

Once these elements are in place, other spokes of the wheel would be addressed as needed to support all facets of recovery, not just the physical components. Collaboration among the performer, medical provider, strength and conditioning coach, mental performance consultant, and artistic coach further enhances recovery. Together, they can design innovative and engaging exercises that reflect the physical, cognitive, affective, and social demands of a given skill, ensuring a more holistic approach to recovery and well-being plan (Bolling et al., 2019; Faltus & Richard, 2022). For instance, Filho et al. (2016) propose a performance pressure model that tailors mental training to the specific demands of each discipline. Contortionists, for instance, may benefit from relaxation techniques and biofeedback training to maintain a healthy stress-recovery balance and manage pain, while jugglers might find mindfulness-based acceptance training particularly effective in alleviating performance anxiety and mitigating the fear of failure.

This integrated approach highlights the need for recovery strategies tailored to both the physical and psychological demands of each discipline. By considering the biopsychological load of each artist's task, each spoke of the wheel can be carefully adjusted to ensure appropriate resource replenishment. Beyond enhancing recovery, these practices may also support overall well-being by exposing artists to manageable levels of physical and mental stress.

Performers' constraints: Embracing diversity

While it is impossible to account for all the individual constraints affecting recovery and well-being at CDS, several key categories warrant attention. Each specific constraint is immediately followed by relevant recovery processes and strategies.

Physical characteristics

One of the many marvels of CDS performers is the remarkable diversity of physical attributes displayed on stage. From the muscular, well-defined upper body of a strap artist to the slight, lean physique of a contortionist, or the powerful lower body and core of a Russian Cradle porter – each performer must meticulously adapt their *Active Recovery*, *Strength and Conditioning*, and *Nutrition* spokes of the wheel to meet the demands of their craft. Their dedication to these recovery components enables them to execute high-risk, awe-inspiring feats with precision and consistency at the highest level.

Psychological characteristics

Psychological characteristics can also play a crucial role in influencing the recovery and well-being of circus artists. For instance, empirical evidence underscores that CDS artists with low self-efficacy are twice as likely to sustain injuries compared to those with high self-efficacy, while factors such as social stress or a lack of personal accomplishment can also heighten injury risk (Shrier & Hallé, 2011). Similarly, evidence shows that the interaction of personality, perception of risk, and emotion regulation skills influences safety outcomes in circus arts. Namely, floor acrobats report higher accident rates than aerial acrobats or object manipulators, while aerial acrobats exhibit stronger emotion regulation skills and score higher in traits like conscientiousness and agreeableness (van Rens & Filho, 2021). Moreover, psychological skills such as confidence, focus, energy management, and emotional regulation have been identified as integral to success in circus performance, differing from traditional sports by emphasising emotional expression and audience connection (Burtt & Lavers, 2017; Ross & Shapiro, 2017).

To develop appropriate mental skills, Certified Mental Performance Consultants (CMPCs) provide *Education and Training* through the CDS Mental Performance and Well-being Service. On demand, they visit shows for periods ranging from a few days to two weeks, delivering show-specific workshops and meeting with artists seeking to develop mental skills. Given the global nature of CDS productions, online one-on-one sessions are also available, allowing artists to work with a CMPC to enhance their mental performance and well-being.

Background

At CDS, artists primarily come from two backgrounds: elite athletes transitioning from disciplines such as gymnastics, trampoline, diving, and action sports, or professional circus artists. While those from the professional circus community are typically accustomed to the multifaceted demands of this unique environment, transitioning athletes may face identity shifts as they adapt to the artistic and creative aspects of circus performance. Moving from the structured and goal-oriented world of sports to the dynamic and improvisational nature of circus arts can be challenging. Successfully navigating this transition is essential for performers to thrive both mentally and physically in their new roles (Filho et al., 2016; Ménard & Hallé, 2014; Ross & Shapiro, 2017; van Rens & Filho, 2020).

These backgrounds can also influence recovery processes. For example, former high-performance athletes often possess extensive knowledge of recovery techniques and are accustomed to having access to advanced resources and support systems, which may not always be available on CDS shows. A study on elite gymnasts transitioning to professional circus found that physical recovery was a significant challenge during the adaptation phase, often resulting in pain and exhaustion (van Rens & Filho, 2020). However, some participants highlighted the exceptional support provided by CDS, noting that "the physio department was incredible" (van Rens & Filho, 2020, p. 139).

The primary goal of the 'physio department' – formally known as the Performance Medicine (PMed) department within CDS – is to provide comprehensive support for artists while upholding the quality of show production. The *Professional Support* spoke of the wheel extends beyond the physical, encompassing emotional well-being by fostering a safe and supportive environment (Bolling et al., 2019; Donohue et al., 2020; Faltus & Richard, 2022). PMed therapists serve as the artists' first – and sometimes only – link to medical support, highlighting the importance of establishing a strong bond built on trust and rapport. As they observe performances each night and oversee most training sessions beyond the audience's view, they develop a keen ability to detect even the subtlest variations in an artist's biomechanical movements and overall psychological state. This expertise allows PMed to intervene preemptively, sometimes identifying concerns before the artists themselves are aware of them.

As opposed to artists coming from a sporting background, artists from circus families may have little to no exposure to recovery strategies and may assume they will manage 'just fine' without them. This mindset often overlooks the significantly higher task demands of CDS shows compared to those of other companies. This is where trust and rapport with the show therapists become vital, as the PMed staff plays a key role in introducing the *Education and Training* spoke of the wheel to artists new to this unique operational environment. One of the key distinctions from smaller circus models is guiding artists to understand the broader perspective of cumulative performance volume and individual workload. Whether through one-on-one sessions or small group discussions, assessing each artist's starting point and upskilling them in various recovery strategies through workshops and dialogue is essential. Encouraging artists to adopt these strategies proactively rather than reactively is crucial for optimising their success and enhancing their performance longevity.

Culture

In addition to physical, psychological, and background diversities, multiple cultures coexist within every CDS show. On average, performers from 18 different countries are represented in each production. To collaborate effectively, performers must navigate language barriers and cultivate cross-cultural awareness, enabling them to communicate clearly and build trust with their fellow artists (Ménard & Hallé, 2014). Sharing training and performance spaces with international fellows also fosters ongoing exchanges on recovery and well-being practices, allowing artists to continually refine their individual routines. For example, on one show, a Russian contortionist leads stretching sessions; on another, an Australian dancer teaches ballet; while on a third, a Hungarian performer directs short films with a group of 'creative junky' artists. Whether for relaxing over taxed systems or to stress under stimulated ones (see Kellmann, 2002, for details), one of the unique aspects of CDS is its openness to leverage the individualities of artists on each show. Recovery and well-being choices are always respected, and adaptation is a natural part of the shared environment. To summarise how artists adapt their own *Constraint-Led Wheel of Recovery and Well-being*, four artists coming from different cultures and backgrounds share their recovery philosophies (Table 12.2).

Conclusion and recommendations for practice

Cirque du Soleil performers navigate a unique and demanding ecosystem, requiring a structured yet flexible approach to recovery and well-being. This chapter applied an ecological dynamics perspective, introducing a constraint-led framework that considers the interplay of environmental, task, and individual constraints in shaping recovery strategies.

The *Constraint-Led Wheel of Recovery and Well-being Framework* provides an adaptable model where recovery is viewed as an ongoing, integrated process rather than an isolated intervention. Given the physical and emotional demands of CDS performances, fostering a pro-active recovery culture is essential. As artists continuously adapt to changing environments, workloads, and performance expectations, equipping them with tailored strategies enhances their ability to maintain or restore biopsychological balance. While we are offering a framework in this chapter based on existing evidence, much more research is needed to refine recovery approaches in the circus arts, ensuring performers receive the same level of scientific and medical support as elite athletes.

TABLE 12.2 Artists' recovery philosophies.

Origin	*Discipline*	*Recovery philosophies*
America	Figure skating	*"Recovery is something I stay mindful of throughout the day, especially when it comes to properly fuelling my body. Even if I incorporate every active recovery method I know, I can still feel the difference if I'm not giving my body the nutrition it craves. As a professional figure skater, my post-training recovery always includes mind-body practices like yoga, allowing me to slow down, connect with my body, and identify areas that need attention. I also prioritise Pilates to support joint health and mobility. Breathing through movement not only aids my physical recovery but also helps me reset mentally."*
Belgium	Teeterboard flyer	*"Recovery, for me, is just as important as training and performing—it's a constant balance between physical and mental restoration to ensure I can perform at my best. I strive for a 50:50 ratio, integrating recovery throughout my day with simple yet effective habits: fuelling my body with balanced meals, using breathing techniques to manage stress, incorporating short foam rolling and stretching sessions, soaking up as much sunlight as possible, and prioritising my favourite – sleep! I aim for nine hours a night because, ultimately, optimal recovery isn't about complexity; it's about consistency"*
Russia	Power track tumbler	*"Recovery is a big thing. It's important for my health and for doing a good show every night. It's not always easy to recover every day, as often there is not enough time, but I try my best to sleep enough and make sure I eat well too. I also get some massage on my body sometimes"*
India	Mallakhamb	*"Recovery is all about letting my body heal after my performance or intense physical activity. It also helps me mentally recharge for the next day, so I can start my day stronger and train again. It's a process that helps me feel more positive, allowing me to continue my performance journey. As part of my daily practice, I make sure to stay hydrated, stretch and focus on mobility after performances or strength training, eat healthy, and, most importantly, get enough sleep."*

Now that the backstage tour is complete and we have uncovered practical strategies used by CDS artists to support recovery and optimise performance and well-being, the question becomes: how can these insights be applied to artists of all levels and backgrounds?

A first step is for artists and those who support them to assess the key elements shaping the artist's experience – namely, their environment, the nature of their tasks, and their individual characteristics. This evaluation can inform the development of an initial recovery and well-being plan, which should be treated as dynamic – tested, refined, and adapted in response to individual needs and evolving contexts. Over time, artists can build awareness of what works best for them in different situations, gradually developing a personalised and flexible recovery toolbox. As illustrated in Figure 14.1, activating their *Wheel* allows artists to navigate this ongoing journey, supporting sustainable well-being and high performance.

Ultimately, optimising recovery creates conditions that enable circus artists to thrive artistically, physically, and psychologically, allowing them to continue captivating audiences worldwide with their poetry in motion.

References

Balagué, N., Pol, R., Torrents, C., Ric, A., & Hristovski, R. (2019). On the relatedness and nestedness of constraints. *Sports Medicine - Open*, *5*, 6. https://doi.org/10.1186/s40798-019-0178-z

Barker, L., Burnstein, B., & Mercer, J. (2020). Acceleration profile of an acrobatic act during training and shows using wearable technology. *Sports Biomechanics*, *19*(2), 201–211.

Bolling, C., Mellette, J., Pasman, H. R., van Mechelen, W., & Verhagen, E. (2019). From the safety net to the injury prevention web: Applying systems thinking to unravel injury prevention challenges and opportunities in Cirque du Soleil. *BMJ Open Sport & Exercise Medicine*, *5*, e000492. https://doi.org/10.1136/bmjsem-2018-000492

Burtt, J., & Lavers, K. (2017). Re-imagining the development of circus artists for the twenty-first century. *Theatre, Dance and Performance Training*, *8*(2), 143–155.

Chow, J. Y., Davids, K., Button, C., Shuttleworth, R., Renshaw, I., & Araujo, D. (2006). Nonlinear pedagogy: A constraints-led framework for understanding emergence of game play and movement skills. *Nonlinear Dynamics, Psychology, and Life Sciences*, *10*, 71–103.

Clark, M. E., McEwan, K., & Christie, C. J. (2018). The effectiveness of constraints-led training on skill development in interceptive sports: A systematic review. *International Journal of Sports Science & Coaching*, *14*(2), 229–240.

Davids, K., Araújo, D., Vilar, L., Renshaw, I., & Pinder, R. (2013). An ecological dynamics approach to skill acquisition: Implications for development of talent in sport. *Talent Development & Excellence*, *5*, 21–34.

Decker, A., Aubertin, P., & Kriellaars, D. (2019). Sleep and fatigue of elite circus student-artists during one year of training. *Science & Medicine*, *34*(3), 125–131.

Donohue, B., Gavrilova, Y., Galante, M., Burnstein, B., Aubertin, P., Gavrilova, E., Funk, A., Light, A., & Benning, S. D. (2020). Empirical development of a screening method for mental, social, and physical wellness in amateur and professional circus artists. *Psychology of Aesthetics, Creativity, and the Arts*, *14*(3), 313–324.

Faltus, J., & Richard, V. (2022). Considerations for the medical management of the circus performance artist and acrobat. *International Journal of Sports Physical Therapy*, *17*(2), 307–316.

Ferraz, A., Duarte-Mendes, P., Sarmento, H., Valente-Dos-Santos, J., & Travassos, B. (2023). Tracking devices and physical performance analysis in team sports:

A comprehensive framework for research—trends and future directions. *Frontiers in Sports and Active Living*, *5*, 1284086. https://doi.org/10.3389/fspor.2023.1284086
Filho, E., Aubertin, P., & Petiot, B. (2016). The making of expert performers at Cirque du Soleil and the National Circus School: A performance enhancement outlook. *Journal of Sport Psychology in Action*, *7*(2), 68–79.
Greenspan, S., Munro, D., Nicholas, J., Stubbe, J., Stuckey, M. I., & van Rijn, R. M. (2022). Circus-specific extension of the International Olympic Committee 2020 consensus statement: Methods for recording and reporting of epidemiological data on injury and illness in sport. *BMJ Open Sport & Exercise Medicine*, *8*(3), e001394. https://doi.org/10.1136/bmjsem-2022-001394
Holman, D., Martinez-Iñigo, D., & Totterdell, P. (2008). Emotional labor, well-being, and performance. In S. Cartwright & C. L. Cooper (Eds.), *The Oxford handbook of organizational well-being* (pp. 331–355). Oxford University Press.
Kellmann, M. (2002). Underrecovery and overtraining: Different concepts – Similar impact? In M. Kellmann (Ed.), *Enhancing recovery: Preventing underperformance in athletes* (pp. 3–24). Human Kinetics.
Kellmann, M., Bertollo, M., Bosquet, L., Brink, M., Coutts, A. J., Duffield, R., Erlacher, D., Halson, S. L., Hecksteden, A., Heidari, J., Kallus, K. W., Meeusen, R., Mujika, I., Robazza, C., Skorski, S., Venter, R., & Beckmann, J. (2018). Recovery and performance in sport: Consensus statement. *International Journal of Sports Physiology and Performance*, *13*(2), 240–245.
Lavers, K., & Leroux, L. P. (2018). The multiple narratives of Cirque du Soleil. In B. Sellers-Young, & J. R. McCutcheon (Eds.), *Narrative in performance* (pp. 111–132). Macmillan.
Liu, X., Liao, Y., Tan, J., Duan, J., & Gao, R. (2023). Emotional labor mediates the associations between self-consciousness and flow in dancers. *Scientific Reports*, *13*, 17382. https://doi.org/10.1038/s41598-023-44730-2
Ménard, J. F., & Hallé, M. (2014). Circus also needs performance psychology: Facts and realities of consulting at Cirque du Soleil. In L. Tashman & J. G. Cremades (Eds.), *Becoming a sport, exercise, and performance psychology professional: A global perspective* (pp. 127–134). Psychology Press.
Newell, K. M. (1986). Constraints on the development of coordination. In M. G. Wade & T. A. Whiting (Eds.), *Motor development in children: Aspects of coordination and control* (pp. 341–360). Martinus Nijhoff.
Newman, C., George, R. P., Beitz, T., Bergson, Z., & Zemon, V. (2022). Mental health issues among international touring professionals in the music industry. *Journal of Psychiatric Research*, *145*, 243–249.
Orth, D., Van Der Kamp, J., & Button, C. (2019). Learning to be adaptive as a distributed process across the coach–athlete system: Situating the coach in the constraints-led approach. *Physical Education and Sport Pedagogy*, *24*, 146–161.
Phillips, E., Davids, K., Renshaw, I., & Portus, M. (2010). Expert performance in sport and the dynamics of talent development. *Sports Medicine*, *40*, 271–283.
Pol, R., Hristovski, R., Medina, D., & Balague, N. (2019). From microscopic to macroscopic sports injuries. Applying the complex dynamic systems approach to sports medicine: A narrative review. *British Journal of Sports Medicine*, *53*(19), 1214–1220.
Renshaw, I., Chow, J. Y., Davids, K., & Hammond, J. (2010). A constraints-led perspective to understanding skill acquisition and game play: A basis for integration of motor learning theory and physical education praxis? *Physical Education and Sport Pedagogy*, *15*, 117–137.

Renton, A., Phillips, G., Daykin, N., Yu, G., Taylor, K., & Petticrew, M. (2012). Think of your art-eries: Arts participation, behavioural cardiovascular risk factors and mental well-being in deprived communities in London. *Public Health, 126*, 57–64.

Rietveld, E., & Kiverstein, J. (2014). A rich landscape of affordances. *Ecological Psychology, 26*, 325–352.

Ross, A., & Shapiro, J. (2017). Under the big top: An exploratory analysis of psychological factors influencing circus performers. *Performance Enhancement & Health, 5*(3), 115–121.

Seifert, L., Araújo, D., Komar, J., & Davids, K. (2017). Understanding constraints on sport performance from the complexity sciences paradigm: An ecological dynamics framework. *Human Movement Science, 56*, 178–180.

Seifert, L., & Davids, K. (2017). Ecological dynamics: A theoretical framework for understanding sport performance, physical education and physical activity. In A. Peñalver, C. Sánchez, & A. G. Pereira (Eds.), *Complex systems digital campus 2015: Proceedings of the first complex systems digital campus World E-conference 2015* (pp. 29–40). Springer.

Shim, Y., Jebb, A. T., Tay, L., & Pawelski, J. O. (2021). Arts and humanities interventions for flourishing in healthy adults: A mixed studies systematic review. *Review of General Psychology, 25*(3), 258–282.

Shrier, I., & Hallé, M. (2011). Psychological predictors of injuries in circus artists: An exploratory study. *British Journal of Sports Medicine, 45*(5), 433–436.

Shrier, I., Meeuwisse, W. H., Matheson, G. O., Wingfield, K., Steele, R. J., Prince, F., Hanley, J., & Montanaro, M. (2009). Injury patterns and injury rates in the circus arts: An analysis of 5 years of data from Cirque du Soleil. *American Journal of Sports Medicine, 37*(6), 1143–1149.

Siu, N. Y.-M., Kwan, H.-Y., Zhang, T. J.-F., & Ho, C. K.-Y. (2016). Arts consumption, customer satisfaction and personal well-being: A study of performing arts in Hong Kong. *Journal of International Consumer Marketing, 28*(2), 77–91.

van Rens, F. E. C. A., & Filho, E. (2020). Realizing, adapting, and thriving in career transitions from gymnastics to contemporary circus arts. *Journal of Clinical Sport Psychology, 14*(2), 127–148.

van Rens, F. E. C. A., & Filho, E. (2021). Not just clowning around: Investigating psychological mechanisms underlying accidents in a heterogeneous group of contemporary circus artists. *Psychology of Aesthetics, Creativity, and the Arts, 15*(2), 377–385.

van Rens, F. E. C. A., & Heritage, B. (2021). Mental health of circus artists: Psychological resilience, circus factors, and demographics predict depression, anxiety, stress, and flourishing. *Psychology of Sport and Exercise, 53*, 101850. https://doi.org/10.1016/j.psychsport.2020.101850

Weisberger, M. (2018). *Here's your brain on Cirque du Soleil: Performers spark awe, scans show. Live Science.* Retrieved June 15, 2025 from https://www.livescience.com/64047-neuroscience-awe-cirque-du-soleil.html?utm_source=chatgpt.com

Wikstrom, E. A., Hubbard-Turner, T., & McKeon, P. O. (2013). Understanding and treating lateral ankle sprains and their consequences. *Sports Medicine, 43*(6), 385–393.

PART IV

Performing arts as a resource for recovery in our society

13

MUSIC AND ARTS INTERVENTIONS FOR WELL-BEING AND HEALTHY BRAIN AGEING

Nella Moisseinen and Teppo Särkämö

Introduction

In the late 1980s, a group of researchers invited nearly 500 community-dwelling older adults to participate in a study, where they would report their daily leisure activities while receiving neuropsychological assessments approximately once a year. The plan was to find out whether the choice of ordinary leisure activities, such as reading, swimming, or playing a musical instrument, would influence their mood or risk of developing dementia. Activity reports and neuropsychological assessments were gathered up to two decades, until the long-awaited results came out. Now a classic research article, Verghese and colleagues (2003) reported that more frequent participation in leisure activities was associated with reduced depression across various types of physically and/or cognitively engaging activities. With respect to dementia risk, however, the results turned out to be more limited: out of the 15 most common leisure activities, only reading, dancing, and playing a musical instrument or board games were associated with a reduced risk for developing dementia. Moreover, Verghese et al. (2003) found that frequent participation in cognitive leisure activities reduced the participants' dementia risk by 63% compared to participating once a week or less.

While ageing is often associated with a negative image, it is important to distinguish between normal ageing, which occurs and continues throughout one's life, and degenerative diseases and conditions, such as Alzheimer's

Moisseinen, N., & Särkämö, T. (2026). Music and arts interventions for well-being and healthy brain ageing. In E. Altenmüller, M. Kellmann, J. Beckmann, & G. M. Moyle (Eds.), *Recovery and well-being in the performing arts* (pp. 225–240). Routledge.

DOI: 10.4324/9781003566885-17

disease and other dementia-causing diseases, which are often associated with (but not restricted to) advanced age. Our genetic predisposition for dementia, for instance, is something which we cannot influence; our lifestyle choices, on the other hand, can have remarkable effects on how the natural biological mechanisms of ageing unfold (Rodriguez et al., 2025). The fact is that the ageing trajectory of any individual can materialise in countless different forms – and fail at fulfilling our negative expectations.

Ageing in the ever-changing brain

In everyday language, we use the word *ageing* for many types of age-associated decline, be it in hearing, sight, memory, or something else, perhaps thinking of young adulthood as the supremacy of sensory or cognitive capacity. Many of the 'ageing effects' we see in daily life are thought to stem from gradual degradation of *grey matter* (Bethlehem et al., 2022; Salat et al., 2004; Vinke et al., 2018), that is, the cell bodies and dendrites (receiving connections) of neurons as well as other valuable building blocks of the brain, and *white matter*, the myelinated axons through which the neurons communicate to one another (Charlton et al., 2006; Nicolas et al., 2020; Ritchie et al., 2015). Together, grey and white matter form numerous small and large-scale networks across the brain, which enable the brain's remarkable ability to learn and perform the countless variations of daily tasks, from sensing and remembering to moving and imagining. Ageing, on the other hand, leads to disruptions in vital maintenance processes, including cellular metabolism and repair (Mattson & Arumugam, 2018). As the cells of the brain deteriorate, so does the composition of its valuable networks – a key process associated with cognitive decline (Koini et al., 2018; Manard et al., 2016; Nicolas et al., 2020; Ritchie et al., 2015).

It should be noted, however, that cell death and structural decline are a normal and necessary part of brain plasticity. Several measures of brain structure, such as total volume of the cerebrum, reach their peak already before adolescence, and the thickness of the cortex begins to decline already around the age of two (Bethlehem et al., 2022). Normal structural decline occurs in many forms throughout life (Bethlehem et al., 2022; Mattson & Arumugam, 2018), partially to allow the brain to focus on our unique needs. This means that the brain aims to *specialise*, i.e., fine-tune itself in response to real-life experiences. With proper training and choice of daily activities, it is possible then to induce favourable changes in brain structure – also in parallel with the accelerating declines with advancing age (Boyke et al., 2008; Colcombe et al., 2006; Kühn et al., 2017; Lövdén et al., 2010).

Musical activities support brain structure with advancing age

Music is a beautiful example of brain specialisation. For example, professional opera singers train vocal control persistently, and their brains show increased grey matter volume in the somatosensory regions representing the larynx (Kleber et al., 2016; for more examples on musical specialisation, see Cheng et al., 2023; Halwani et al., 2011; Perron et al., 2021; Rus-Oswald et al., 2022). However, music goes beyond regional specialisation effects. Even when not rehearsing a particular musical skill, such as the classical vocal technique, music requires complex auditory processing and domain-general cognitive processing, such as attention and working memory, while inducing emotional responses, memories, and sometimes the urge to move to its beat. Consequently, it trains an exceptionally large variety of brain networks simultaneously (Sihvonen et al., 2017; Sutcliffe et al., 2020).

Various musical activities have been associated with structural enhancements in the ageing brain (Bidelman & Alain, 2015; Böttcher et al., 2022; Chaddock-Heyman et al., 2021; Gaser & Schlaug, 2003; Jünemann et al., 2022; Moisseinen et al., 2024; Worschech et al., 2023). For instance, a cross-sectional study (Moisseinen et al., 2024) with healthy adults found that, across adulthood (aged 21–88 years), longer choir singing experience is associated with enhanced structural connectivity (estimated with quantitative anisotropy) in white matter pathways supporting auditory and language function (e.g., arcuate and inferior fronto-occipital fasciculi), somatomotor control (e.g., corticospinal tract), and emotional and cognitive function (e.g., cingulum and corpus callosum) at the whole-brain level.

Since ageing-associated declines do not occur evenly across the whole brain, however, it is also important to consider more localised specialisation effects that become particularly relevant after midlife. For instance, correlational evidence on choir singing (Moisseinen et al., 2024) as well as intervention studies on dance (Burzynska et al., 2017) and piano playing (Jünemann et al., 2022) suggest that musical activities can help maintain the structural integrity of the *fornix*, a core memory-supporting pathway serving as the main output tract of the hippocampus.

While such effects are unlikely to be unique to music (Klimecki et al., 2023), their localisation in the fornix, a structure highly vulnerable to ageing (Korbmacher et al., 2023; Zhu et al., 2025), illustrates the benefits of musical practice not only in young and healthy brains but also with respect to simultaneously ongoing decline. Indeed, these results seem to offer one potential mechanism for how music can act as a protective factor for dementia (Rodriguez et al., 2025). Jünemann et al. (2022), for instance, also reported evidence for parallel improvements in a memory task (delayed recall in the Rey Auditory Verbal Learning Test) after piano training – albeit more supporting evidence from behavioural as well as functional brain data is still needed.

Connecting musical memories and emotions in the ageing brain

We know from everyday life that music tends to intertwine with our memories and emotions (Ren & Brown, 2024). A classical finding, shown also in many viral online videos, suggests that our personal connection with our musical memories and emotions is long preserved, also in the advanced stage of Alzheimer's disease (for a suggestion on underlying brain mechanisms, see Jacobsen et al., 2015). Functional brain imaging data from young (Taruffi et al., 2017; Wilkins et al., 2014) and older adults (Hennessy et al., 2025) suggests that musical pieces that are personally preferred, nostalgic, or sad, thus possibly inducing more self-reflective thought (Taruffi et al., 2017), activate the brains' default mode network (DMN), a network of brain regions which communicate in a coordinated fashion to support our 'internal narrative' involving episodic memory and sense of self, for instance (for more suggested functions of DMN in cognition, see Menon, 2023; Smallwood et al., 2021). Specifically, musical memories and pleasure seem to activate the medial prefrontal cortex (mPFC; Belfi et al., 2018; Belfi & Loui, 2020; Hennessy et al., 2025; Janata, 2009; Quinci et al., 2022), a key region in DMN associated with various integrative, self-referential processes (Levorsen et al., 2025; for a brief review, see also Menon, 2023).

The functional connectivity of DMN, i.e., the ability of its constituents to communicate in a coordinated fashion, is susceptible to dysfunction in normal and pathological ageing, including Alzheimer's disease; this is thought to mediate, to some degree, the associated memory decline (Ferreira & Busatto, 2013; Menon, 2023) or losing one's sense of self (Menon, 2023). The questions of whether music can enhance the functional connectivity of this network and whether such enhancements would support healthy ageing seem appealing. Indeed, tentative evidence from cross-sectional (Liebscher et al., 2024) and follow-up studies (Faber et al., 2024; Quinci et al., 2022) suggests that musical activities can support the functional connectivity of, for instance, mPFC (during rest and music listening, respectively) in the ageing brain. While assessing the utility of such effects requires further investigation (for discussion and suggestions for future works, see Faber et al., 2024; Liebscher et al., 2024; Quinci et al., 2022), these results do suggest that music can be used to enhance functional connectivity in the ageing brain. A similar mechanism has been suggested to promote, for instance, the sense of self when persons with dementia listen to their favourite music (Baird & Thompson, 2018); also, this account emphasises the role of mPFC and the personal emotional value of music in this context.

Finally, musical emotions can contribute to well-being through the transient yet rapid influence of music on brain chemistry. Specifically, music listening can evoke rich emotional responses in the brain through the dopaminergic reward system, stress hormone cortisol, and social hormone oxytocin (Fancourt et al., 2014; Greenberg et al., 2021; Koelsch, 2014). These may contribute to the pain-alleviating (analgesic) effects of music (Lunde et al., 2019), for instance, consequently supporting the well-being and quality of life (QOL) in various patient groups.

Music interventions for the recovering and degenerating brain

After acute brain damage, caused by stroke for example, neural stimulation provided by the environment plays an important role in recovery, leading to many types of neuroplasticity changes, such as increased synaptic plasticity and neurogenesis (Nithianantharajah & Hannan, 2006). In this context, the broad extent of the cortical and subcortical neural networks activated by music can be a form of environmental enrichment, which can stimulate the recovery of brain areas surrounding the lesion and in the contralesional (unaffected) hemisphere (Sihvonen et al., 2017). This idea is supported by recent fMRI studies showing that music processing evokes a complex pattern of functional connectivity across both close and distant brain regions (Karmonik et al., 2016; Wu et al., 2019). Also the positive effects of music on affective state via the dopaminergic reward system, on physiological arousal via the autonomic nervous system, and on stress reduction via the hypothalamic-pituitary-adrenal axis make music a powerful tool to enhance recovery (Sihvonen et al., 2017). In neurological rehabilitation, the therapeutic use of music can be either receptive, focusing on music listening, or expressive, focusing on active music production in the form of singing or instrument playing.

Regarding the receptive use of music, daily music listening during the first months after stroke has been shown to enhance cognitive recovery, especially in the domains of memory and attention, improve mood, and increase motor activity in the home setting (Baylan et al., 2020; Fan et al., 2024; Forsblom et al., 2010; Särkämö et al., 2008; Wang et al., 2025), coupled with increase in grey matter volume in spared prefrontal and limbic regions associated with cognitive and emotional functions (Särkämö, Ripollés et al., 2014). Music listening can also be targeted for the rehabilitation of specific post-stroke deficits. In patients with aphasia, listening to sung music with lyrics can also enhance the recovery of speech production as well as increase grey matter volume, structural (white matter) connectivity, and functional connectivity in the language network of the brain (Sihvonen, Pitkäniemi et al., 2021; Sihvonen, Soinila et al., 2021, 2022; Sihvonen et al., 2020). In patients with unilateral spatial neglect, music listening can temporarily enhance the orientation of attention to the neglected (left) side of space (Chen et al., 2013; Kaufmann et al., 2022). In patients with hemiparesis, training movements with the help of rhythmic music can enhance gait, overall motor function, and balance (Ghai & Ghai, 2019; Thaut et al., 1997; Wang et al., 2022).

Expressive music interventions can be effectively used to facilitate the recovery of cognitive, motor, and language deficits. Singing-based interventions, such as Melodic Intonation Therapy and choir singing, in turn can improve the recovery of communication and speech production and enhance psychosocial well-being (Popescu et al., 2022; Siponkoski et al., 2022; van der Meulen et al., 2014) as well as induce structural and functional neuroplasticity changes in the bilateral language network (Marchina et al., 2023; Sihvonen et al., 2024) in aphasic stroke patients. Music interventions utilising instrument playing, such as music-supported training, have been shown to improve the recovery of upper limb movements and enhance connectivity between auditory and motor cortical brain regions in hemiparetic stroke patients (Grau-Sánchez et al., 2020; Ripolles et al., 2026; Schneider et al., 2010) as well as improve executive function and enhance the structure and connectivity of the right prefrontal cortex in patients with traumatic brain injury (Sihvonen, Siponkoski et al., 2022; Siponkoski et al., 2020). Finally, different forms of dance and movement therapy show promise for improving mobility, balance, and motor coordination after stroke (Patterson et al., 2018; Young et al., 2021), but larger clinical trials are still needed to determine their clinical efficacy.

In addition to aiding recovery, musical activities also hold great potential in supporting better cognitive and socioemotional functioning and reducing the risk of ageing-related neurocognitive decline (Verghese et al., 2003; Walsh et al., 2021) as well as in maintaining these functions across different stages of neurodegeneration. Within the dementia continuum, especially expressive music interventions, which involve singing, instrument playing, and/or dancing, have been shown to enhance cognitive functioning (e.g., memory, attention) in mild cognitive impairment (Doi et al., 2017; Dorris et al., 2021; Quan et al., 2025) as well as in the early (mild) stage of dementia (Lyu et al., 2018; Särkämö, Tervaniemi et al., 2014; Särkämö et al., 2016). In more advanced (moderate-severe) stages of dementia, both receptive and expressive music interventions can effectively reduce neuropsychiatric symptoms, such as depression, and caregiver distress as well as improve QOL (Baker et al., 2022; Lin et al., 2023; Lyu et al., 2018; Särkämö, Tervaniemi et al., 2014; van der Steen et al., 2025). In Parkinson's disease, rhythm-based music interventions, including dancing, can also alleviate motor symptoms, such as gait, balance and mobility impairments, and improve cognitive functioning (Kalyani et al., 2019; Lee & Ko, 2023).

All in all, current evidence suggests that music is a versatile and effective tool for enhancing motor, cognitive, verbal, and emotional recovery and inducing structural and functional brain reorganisation after a neurological illness as well as in countering the effects of neurodegeneration on cognitive and socioemotional functioning.

Regular engagement with music and arts promotes subjective well-being

While music is currently the best covered art form in neurocognitive research literature, the well-being effects of various art forms encourage exploring their potential for supporting healthy ageing and brain recovery. Regular and sustained engagement with music as well as other art forms can enhance mood, reduce depression, and promote well-being in healthy ageing (Coulton et al., 2015; Tymoszuk et al., 2020) and across various clinical target groups (for reviews, see Fancourt & Finn, 2019; Koh et al., 2024; Trupp et al., 2025). A longitudinal cohort study (Tymoszuk et al., 2020) with over 3,000 respondents (aged 50 and above at baseline), for example, reported that going to the theatre, concerts, galleries, and exhibitions was associated with greater well-being when continued up to a decade (Beauchet et al., 2020; Meeks et al., 2018). Further, it has been suggested that group-based arts activities, such as group singing (Coulton et al., 2015; Galinha et al., 2023; Skingley et al., 2016), can amplify the emotional benefits of arts (Livesey et al., 2012; Moss et al., 2018; for systematic reviews involving clinical populations, see Daykin et al., 2018; Williams et al., 2018), potentially due to the added value from social engagement (Lonsdale & Day, 2021; Maury & Rickard, 2022; Stewart & Lonsdale, 2016). Suggested specific mechanisms, such as experiences of higher autonomy (Tymoszuk et al., 2020), autobiographical significance associated with relational aesthetics (Rose & Lonsdale, 2016), or finding generic enjoyment in colours and textures in visual arts (Reynolds, 2010), also illustrate the potential for participants to find personal meaning and motivation in arts interventions.

Conclusions and recommendations for practice

In this chapter, we have reviewed research literature on how music and arts can be used to support healthy ageing and enhance recovery in ageing-related neurological disorders. While the brain is constantly changing and many of the major ageing effects in the brain begin rather early in life, our lifestyle choices, including engagement with music and arts, can have wide-ranging positive effects on brain structure and function as well as on cognitive and socioemotional well-being. With increasing evidence for their efficacy, music and arts are now advocated by many healthcare organisations, including WHO (Fancourt & Finn, 2019) and Global Council on Brain Health (2020), and they are increasingly included also in the national treatment and rehabilitation guidelines for neurological disorders (e.g., stroke, dementia) in many countries, although more systematic research and large-scale clinical trials are still needed, especially for arts interventions other than music. Also, more multimodal research exploring the links between the neural and the behavioural (cognitive, verbal, motor, and emotional) effects of music and arts interventions is needed to broaden our understanding of their complex underlying mechanisms.

References

Baird, A., & Thompson, W. F. (2018). The impact of music on the self in dementia. *Journal of Alzheimer's Disease*, *61*(3), 827–841.

Baker, F. A., Lee, Y. C., Sousa, T. V., Stretton-Smith, P. A., Tamplin, J., Sveinsdottir, V., Geretsegger, M., Wake, J. D., Assmus, J., & Gold, C. (2022). Clinical effectiveness of music interventions for dementia and depression in elderly care (MIDDEL): Australian cohort of an international pragmatic cluster-randomised controlled trial. *Lancet Healthy Longevity*, *3*(3), e153–e165.

Baylan, S., Haig, C., MacDonald, M., Stiles, C., Easto, J., Thomson, M., Cullen, B., Quinn, T. J., Stott, D., Mercer, S. W., Broomfield, N. M., Murray, H., & Evans, J. J. (2020). Measuring the effects of listening for leisure on outcome after stroke (MELLO): A pilot randomized controlled trial of mindful music listening. *International Journal of Stroke*, *15*(2), 149–158.

Beauchet, O., Bastien, T., Mittelman, M., Hayashi, Y., & Hau Yan Ho, A. (2020). Participatory art-based activity, community-dwelling older adults and changes in health condition: Results from a pre–post intervention, single-arm, prospective and longitudinal study. *Maturitas*, *134*, 8–14.

Belfi, A. M., Karlan, B., & Tranel, D. (2018). Damage to the medial prefrontal cortex impairs music-evoked autobiographical memories. *Psychomusicology: Music, Mind, and Brain*, *28*(4), 201–208.

Belfi, A. M., & Loui, P. (2020). Musical anhedonia and rewards of music listening: Current advances and a proposed model. *Annals of the New York Academy of Sciences*, *1464*(1), 99–114.

Bethlehem, R. A. I., Seidlitz, J., White, S. R., Vogel, J. W., Anderson, K. M., Adamson, C., Adler, S., Alexopoulos, G. S., Anagnostou, E., Areces-Gonzalez, A., Astle, D. E., Auyeung, B., Ayub, M., Bae, J., Ball, G., Baron-Cohen, S., Beare, R., Bedford, S. A., Benegal, V., ... Alexander-Bloch, A. F. (2022). Brain charts for the human lifespan. *Nature*, *604*(7906), 525–533.

Bidelman, G. M., & Alain, C. (2015). Musical training orchestrates coordinated neuroplasticity in auditory brainstem and cortex to counteract age-related declines in categorical vowel perception. *Journal of Neuroscience*, *35*(3), 1240–1249.

Böttcher, A., Zarucha, A., Köbe, T., Gaubert, M., Höppner, A., Altenstein, S., Bartels, C., Buerger, K., Dechent, P., Dobisch, L., Ewers, M., Fliessbach, K., Freiesleben, S. D., Frommann, I., Haynes, J. D., Janowitz, D., Kilimann, I., Kleineidam, L., Laske, C., ... Wirth, M. (2022). Musical activity during life is associated with multi-domain cognitive and brain benefits in older adults. *Frontiers in Psychology*, *13*, 945709. https://doi.org/10.3389/fpsyg.2022.945709

Boyke, J., Driemeyer, J., Gaser, C., Büchel, C., & May, A. (2008). Training-induced brain structure changes in the elderly. *Journal of Neuroscience*, *28*(28), 7031–7035.

Burzynska, A. Z., Jiao, Y., Knecht, A. M., Fanning, J., Awick, E. A., Chen, T., Gothe, N., Voss, M. W., McAuley, E., & Kramer, A. F. (2017). White matter integrity declined over 6-months, but dance intervention improved integrity of the fornix of older adults. *Frontiers in Aging Neuroscience*, *9*, 59. https://doi.org/10.3389/fnagi.2017.00059

Chaddock-Heyman, L., Loui, P., Weng, T. B., Weisshappel, R., Mcauley, E., & Kramer, A. F. (2021). Musical training and brain volume in older adults. *Brain Sciences*, *11*(1), 50. https://doi.org/10.3390/brainsci11010050

Charlton, R. A., Barrick, T. R., McIntyre, D. J., Shen, Y., O'Sullivan, M., Howe, F. A., Clark, C. A., Morris, R. G., & Markus, H. S. (2006). White matter damage on diffusion tensor imaging correlates with age-related cognitive decline. *Neurology*, *66*(2), 217–222.

Chen, M. C., Tsai, P. L., Huang, Y. T., & Lin, K. C. (2013). Pleasant music improves visual attention in patients with unilateral neglect after stroke. *Brain Injury*, *27*(1), 75–82.

Cheng, L., Chiu, Y., Lin, Y., Li, W., Hong, T., Yang, C., Shih, C., Yeh, T., Tseng, W. I., Yu, H., Hsieh, J., & Chen, L. (2023). Long-term musical training induces white matter plasticity in emotion and language networks. *Human Brain Mapping*, *44*(1), 5–17.

Colcombe, S. J., Erickson, K. I., Scalf, P. E., Kim, J. S., Prakash, R., McAuley, E., Elavsky, S., Marquez, D. X., Hu, L., & Kramer, A. F. (2006). Aerobic exercise training increases brain volume in aging humans. *Journals of Gerontology Series A: Biological Sciences and Medical Sciences*, *61*(11), 1166–1170.

Coulton, S., Clift, S., Skingley, A., & Rodriguez, J. (2015). Effectiveness and cost-effectiveness of community singing on mental health-related quality of life of older people: Randomised controlled trial. *British Journal of Psychiatry*, *207*(3), 250–255.

Daykin, N., Mansfield, L., Meads, C., Julier, G., Tomlinson, A., Payne, A., Grigsby Duffy, L., Lane, J., D'Innocenzo, G., Burnett, A., Kay, T., Dolan, P., Testoni, S., & Victor, C. (2018). What works for wellbeing? A systematic review of wellbeing outcomes for music and singing in adults. *Perspectives in Public Health*, *138*(1), 39–46.

Doi, T., Verghese, J., Makizako, H., Tsutsumimoto, K., Hotta, R., Nakakubo, S., Suzuki, T., & Shimada, H. (2017). Effects of cognitive leisure activity on cognition in mild cognitive impairment: Results of a randomized controlled trial. *Journal of the American Medical Directors Association*, *18*(8), 686–691.

Dorris, J. L., Neely, S., Terhorst, L., VonVille, H. M., & Rodakowski, J. (2021). Effects of music participation for mild cognitive impairment and dementia: A systematic review and meta-analysis. *Journal of American Geriatric Society*, *69*(9), 2659–2667.

Faber, S., Belden, A., Loui, P., & McIntosh, A. R. (2024). Network connectivity differences in music listening among older adults following a music-based intervention. *Aging Brain*, *6*, 100128. https://doi.org/10.1016/j.nbas.2024.100128

Fan, L. P., Quijano-Ruiz, A., Wang, C., Zhao, H. W., Wang, D. N., Wu, H. M., Liu, L., Zhan, Y. H., & Zhou, X. B. (2024). Effects of personalized music listening on post-stroke cognitive impairment: A randomized controlled trial. *Complementary Therapies in Clinical Practice*, *57*, 101885. https://doi.org/10.1016/j.ctcp.2024.101885

Fancourt, D., & Finn, S. (2019). *What is the evidence on the role of the arts in improving health and well-being? A scoping review*. WHO Regional Office for Europe. Retrieved June 18, 2025 from https://iris.who.int/handle/10665/329834

Fancourt, D., Ockelford, A., & Belai, A. (2014). The psychoneuroimmunological effects of music: A systematic review and a new model. *Brain, Behavior, and Immunity*, *36*, 15–26.

Ferreira, L. K., & Busatto, G. F. (2013). Resting-state functional connectivity in normal brain aging. *Neuroscience & Biobehavioral Reviews*, *37*(3), 384–400.

Forsblom, A., Särkämö, T., Laitinen, S., & Tervaniemi, M. (2010). The effect of music and audio book listening on people recovering from stroke: The patient's point of view. *Music and Medicine*, *2*(4), 229–234.

Galinha, I. C., Fernandes, H. M., Lima, M. L., & Palmeira, A. L. (2023). Intervention and mediation effects of a community-based singing group on older adults' perceived physical and mental health: The Sing4Health randomized controlled trial. *Psychology & Health*, *38*(1), 73–93.

Gaser, C., & Schlaug, G. (2003). Brain structures differ between musicians and non-musicians. *Journal of Neuroscience*, *23*(27), 9240–9245.

Ghai, S., & Ghai, I. (2019). Effects of (music-based) rhythmic auditory cueing training on gait and posture post-stroke: A systematic review & dose-response meta-analysis. *Scientific Reports*, *9*(1), 2183. https://doi.org/10.1038/s41598-019-38723-3

Global Council on Brain Health. (2020). *Music on our minds: The rich potential of music to promote brain health and mental well-being*. Retrieved June 18, 2025 from https://doi.org/10.26419/pia.00103.001

Grau-Sánchez, J., Münte, T. F., Altenmüller, E., Duarte, E., & Rodríguez-Fornells, A. (2020). Potential benefits of music playing in stroke upper limb motor rehabilitation. *Neuroscience & Biobehavioral Reviews*, *112*, 585–599.

Greenberg, D. M., Decety, J., & Gordon, I. (2021). The social neuroscience of music: Understanding the social brain through human song. *American Psychologist*, *76*(7), 1172–1185.

Halwani, G., Loui, P., Rueber, T., & Schlaug, G. (2011). Effects of practice and experience on the arcuate fasciculus: Comparing singers, instrumentalists, and non-musicians. *Frontiers in Psychology*, *2*, 156. https://doi.org/10.3389/fpsyg.2011.00156

Hennessy, S., Janata, P., Ginsberg, T., Kaplan, J., & Habibi, A. (2025). Music-evoked nostalgia activates default mode and reward networks across the lifespan. *Human Brain Mapping*, *46*(4), e70181. https://doi.org/10.1002/hbm.70181

Jacobsen, J.-H., Stelzer, J., Fritz, T. H., Chételat, G., La Joie, R., & Turner, R. (2015). Why musical memory can be preserved in advanced Alzheimer's disease. *Brain*, *138*(8), 2438–2450.

Janata, P. (2009). The neural architecture of music-evoked autobiographical memories. *Cerebral Cortex*, *19*(11), 2579–2594.

Jünemann, K., Marie, D., Worschech, F., Scholz, D. S., Grouiller, F., Kliegel, M., Van De Ville, D., James, C. E., Krüger, T. H. C., Altenmüller, E., & Sinke, C. (2022). Six months of piano training in healthy elderly stabilizes white matter microstructure in the fornix, compared to an active control group. *Frontiers in Aging Neuroscience*, *14*, 817889. https://doi.org/10.3389/fnagi.2022.817889

Kalyani, H. H. N., Sullivan, K., Moyle, G. M., Brauer, S., Jeffrey, E. R., Roeder, L., Berndt, S., & Kerr, G. (2019). Effects of dance on gait, cognition, and dual-tasking in Parkinson's disease: A systematic review and meta-analysis. *Journal of Parkinson's Disease*, *9*(2), 335–349.

Karmonik, C., Brandt, A., Anderson, J., Brooks, F., Lytle, J., Silverman, E., & Frazier, J. T. (2016). Music listening modulates functional connectivity and information flow in the human brain. *Brain Connectivity*, *6*(8), 632–641.

Kaufmann, B. C., Cazzoli, D., Bartolomeo, P., Frey, J., Pflugshaupt, T., Knobel, S., Nef, T., Müri, R. M., & Nyffeler, T. (2022). Auditory spatial cueing reduces neglect after right-hemispheric stroke: A proof of concept study. *Cortex*, *148*, 152–167.

Kleber, B., Veit, R., Moll, C. V., Gaser, C., Birbaumer, N., & Lotze, M. (2016). Voxel-based morphometry in opera singers: Increased gray-matter volume in right somatosensory and auditory cortices. *NeuroImage*, *133*, 477–483.

Klimecki, O. M., Liebscher, M., Gaubert, M., Hayek, D., Zarucha, A., Dyrba, M., Bartels, C., Buerger, K., Butryn, M., Dechent, P., Dobisch, L., Ewers, M., Fliessbach, K., Freiesleben, S. D., Glanz, W., Hetzer, S., Janowitz, D., Kilimann, I., Kleineidam, L., … Wirth, M. (2023). Long-term environmental enrichment is associated with better fornix microstructure in older adults. *Frontiers in Aging Neuroscience*, *15*, 1170879. https://doi.org/10.3389/fnagi.2023.1170879

Koelsch, S. (2014). Brain correlates of music-evoked emotions. *Nature Reviews Neuroscience*, *15*(3), 170–180.

Koh, W. Q., Wora, N., Liong, N. W. L., Ludlow, K., Pachana, N. A., & Liddle, J. (2024). Non–exercise-based interventions to support healthy aging in older adults: A systematic review and meta-analysis of randomized controlled trials. *Gerontologist*, *65*(2), gnae156. https://doi.org/10.1093/geront/gnae156

Koini, M., Duering, M., Gesierich, B. G., Rombouts, S. A. R. B., Ropele, S., Wagner, F., Enzinger, C., & Schmidt, R. (2018). Grey-matter network disintegration as predictor of cognitive and motor function with aging. *Brain Structure and Function*, *223*(5), 2475–2487.

Korbmacher, M., de Lange, A. M., van der Meer, D., Beck, D., Eikefjord, E., Lundervold, A., Andreassen, O. A., Westlye, L. T., & Maximov, I. I. (2023). Brain-wide associations between white matter and age highlight the role of fornix microstructure in brain ageing. *Human Brain Mapping*, *44*(10), 4101–4119.

Kühn, S., Lorenz, R. C., Weichenberger, M., Becker, M., Haesner, M., O'Sullivan, J., Steinert, A., Steinhagen-Thiessen, E., Brandhorst, S., Bremer, T., & Gallinat, J. (2017). Taking control! Structural and behavioural plasticity in response to game-based inhibition training in older adults. *NeuroImage*, *156*, 199–206.

Lee, H., & Ko, B. (2023). Effects of music-based interventions on motor and non-motor symptoms in patients with Parkinson's disease: A systematic review and meta-analysis. *International Journal of Environmental Research and Public Health*, *20*(2), 1046. https://doi.org/10.3390/ijerph20021046

Levorsen, M., Aoki, R., Sedikides, C., & Izuma, K. (2025). Decomposing cognitive processes in the mPFC during self-thinking. *Journal of Neuroscience*, *45*(22), e2378242025. https://doi.org/10.1523/JNEUROSCI.2378-24.2025

Liebscher, M., Dell'Orco, A., Doll-Lee, J., Buerger, K., Dechent, P., Ewers, M., Fliessbach, K., Glanz, W., Hetzer, S., Janowitz, D., Kilimann, I., Laske, C., Lüsebrink, F., Munk, M., Perneczky, R., Peters, O., Preis, L., Priller, J., Rauchmann, B., … Wirth, M. (2024). Lifetime musical activity and resting-state functional connectivity in cognitive networks. *PLoS ONE*, *19*(5), e0299939. https://doi.org/10.1371/journal.pone.0299939

Lin, T. H., Liao, Y. C., Tam, K. W., Chan, L., & Hsu, T. H. (2023). Effects of music therapy on cognition, quality of life, and neuropsychiatric symptoms of patients with dementia: A systematic review and meta-analysis of randomized controlled trials. *Psychiatry Research*, *329*, 115498. https://doi.org/10.1016/j.psychres.2023.115498

Livesey, L., Morrison, I., Clift, S., & Camic, P. (2012). Benefits of choral singing for social and mental wellbeing: Qualitative findings from a cross-national survey of choir members. *Journal of Public Mental Health*, *11*(1), 10–26.

Lonsdale, A. J., & Day, E. R. (2021). Are the psychological benefits of choral singing unique to choirs? A comparison of six activity groups. *Psychology of Music*, *49*(5), 1179–1198.

Lövdén, M., Bodammer, N. C., Kühn, S., Kaufmann, J., Schütze, H., Tempelmann, C., Heinze, H.-J., Düzel, E., Schmiedek, F., & Lindenberger, U. (2010). Experience-dependent plasticity of white-matter microstructure extends into old age. *Neuropsychologia*, *48*(13), 3878–3883.

Lunde, S. J., Vuust, P., Garza-Villarreal, E. A., & Vase, L. (2019). Music-induced analgesia: How does music relieve pain? *Pain*, *160*(5), 989–993.

Lyu, J., Zhang, J., Mu, H., Li, W., Champ, M., Xiong, Q., Gao, T., Xie, L., Jin, W., Yang, W., Cui, M., Gao, M., & Li, M. (2018). The effects of music therapy on cognition, psychiatric symptoms, and activities of daily living in patients with Alzheimer's disease. *Journal of Alzheimer's Disease*, *64*(4), 1347–1358.

Manard, M., Bahri, M. A., Salmon, E., & Collette, F. (2016). Relationship between grey matter integrity and executive abilities in aging. *Brain Research*, *1642*, 562–580.

Marchina, S., Norton, A., & Schlaug, G. (2023). Effects of melodic intonation therapy in patients with chronic nonfluent aphasia. *Annals of the New York Academy of Sciences*, *1519*(1), 173–185.

Mattson, M. P., & Arumugam, T. V. (2018). Hallmarks of brain aging: Adaptive and pathological modification by metabolic states. *Cell Metabolism*, *27*(6), 1176–1199.

Maury, S., & Rickard, N. (2022). The benefits of participation in a choir and an exercise group on older adults' wellbeing in a naturalistic setting. *Musicae Scientiae*, *26*(1), 144–171.

Meeks, S., Vandenbroucke, R. J., & Shryock, S. K. (2018). Psychological benefits of attending the theatre associated with positive affect and well-being for subscribers over age 60. *Aging & Mental Health*, *24*(2), 333–340.

Menon, V. (2023). 20 years of the default mode network: A review and synthesis. *Neuron*, *111*(16), 2469–2487.

Moisseinen, N., Ahveninen, L., Martínez-Molina, N., Sairanen, V., Melkas, S., Kleber, B., Sihvonen, A. J., & Särkämö, T. (2024). Choir singing is associated with enhanced structural connectivity across the adult lifespan. *Human Brain Mapping*, *45*(7), e26705. https://doi.org/10.1002/hbm.26705

Moss, H., Lynch, J., & O'Donoghue, J. (2018). Exploring the perceived health benefits of singing in a choir: An international cross-sectional mixed-methods study. *Perspectives in Public Health*, *138*(3), 160–168.

Nicolas, R., Hiba, B., Dilharreguy, B., Barse, E., Baillet, M., Edde, M., Pelletier, A., Periot, O., Helmer, C., Allard, M., Dartigues, J.-F., Amieva, H., Pérès, K., Fernandez, P., & Catheline, G. (2020). Changes over time of diffusion MRI in the white matter of aging brain, a good predictor of verbal recall. *Frontiers in Aging Neuroscience*, *12*, 218. https://doi.org/10.3389/fnagi.2020.00218

Nithianantharajah, J., & Hannan, A. J. (2006). Enriched environments, experience-dependent plasticity and disorders of the nervous system. *Nature Reviews Neuroscience*, *7*(9), 697–709.

Patterson, K. K., Wong, J. S., Nguyen, T. U., & Brooks, D. (2018). A dance program to improve gait and balance in individuals with chronic stroke: A feasibility study. *Topics in Stroke Rehabilitation*, *25*(6), 410–416.

Perron, M., Theaud, G., Descoteaux, M., & Tremblay, P. (2021). The frontotemporal organization of the arcuate fasciculus and its relationship with speech perception in young and older amateur singers and non-singers. *Human Brain Mapping*, *42*(10), 3058–3076.

Popescu, T., Stahl, B., Wiernik, B. M., Haiduk, F., Zemanek, M., Helm, H., Matzinger, T., Beisteiner, R., & Fitch, W. T. (2022). Melodic intonation therapy for aphasia: A multi-level meta-analysis of randomized controlled trials and individual participant data. *Annals of the New York Academy of Sciences*, *1516*(1), 76–84.

Quan, Y., Lo, C. Y., Wolff, L., Wang, J., Olsen, K. N., & Thompson, W. F. (2025). Cognitive benefits of music in aerobic exercise: Evidence from a Bayesian network meta-analysis in adults with mild cognitive impairment. *Archives of Gerontology and Geriatrics*, *134*, 105848. https://doi.org/10.1016/j.archger.2025.105848

Quinci, M. A., Belden, A., Goutama, V., Gong, D., Hanser, S., Donovan, N. J., Geddes, M., & Loui, P. (2022). Longitudinal changes in auditory and reward systems following receptive music-based intervention in older adults. *Scientific Reports*, *12*(1), 11517. https://doi.org/10.1038/s41598-022-15687-5

Ren, Y., & Brown, T. I. (2024). Beyond the ears: A review exploring the interconnected brain behind the hierarchical memory of music. *Psychonomic Bulletin & Review*, *31*(2), 507–530.

Reynolds, F. (2010). 'Colour and communion': Exploring the influences of visual art-making as a leisure activity on older women's subjective well-being. *Journal of Aging Studies*, *24*(2), 135–143.

Ripolles, P., Rojo, N., Grau-Sanchez, J., Amengual, J., Camara, E., Marco-Pallares, J., Juncadella, M., Vaquero, L., Rubio, F., Duarte, E., Garrido, C., Altenmüller, E., Münte, T. F., & Rodríguez-Fornells, A. (2016). Music supported therapy promotes motor plasticity in individuals with chronic stroke. *Brain Imaging and Behavior*, *10*(4), 1289e1307. https://doi.org/10.1007/s11682-015-9498-x

Ritchie, S. J., Bastin, M. E., Tucker-Drob, E. M., Maniega, S. M., Engelhardt, L. E., Cox, S. R., Royle, N. A., Gow, A. J., Corley, J., Pattie, A., Taylor, A. M., Valdés Hernández, M. del C., Starr, J. M., Wardlaw, J. M., & Deary, I. J. (2015). Coupled changes in brain white matter microstructure and fluid intelligence in later life. *Journal of Neuroscience*, *35*(22), 8672–8682.

Rodriguez, F. S., Hofbauer, L. M., Reppermund, S., Samtani, S., & Röhr, S. (2025). Updating risk and protective factors for dementia in older adults. *Nature Reviews Psychology*, *4*, 322–335.

Rose, E., & Lonsdale, S. (2016). Painting place: Re-imagining landscapes for older people's subjective wellbeing. *Health & Place*, *40*, 58–65.

Rus-Oswald, O. G., Benner, J., Reinhardt, J., Bürki, C., Christiner, M., Hofmann, E., Schneider, P., Stippich, C., Kressig, R. W., & Blatow, M. (2022). Musicianship-related structural and functional cortical features are preserved in elderly musicians. *Frontiers in Aging Neuroscience*, *14*, 807971. https://doi.org/10.3389/fnagi.2022.807971

Salat, D. H., Buckner, R. L., Snyder, A. Z., Greve, D. N., Desikan, R. S. R., Busa, E., Morris, J. C., Dale, A. M., & Fischl, B. (2004). Thinning of the cerebral cortex in aging. *Cerebral Cortex*, *14*(7), 721–730.

Särkämö, T., Laitinen, S., Numminen, A., Kurki, M., Johnson, J. K., & Rantanen, P. (2016). Clinical and demographic factors associated with the cognitive and emotional efficacy of regular musical activities in dementia. *Journal of Alzheimer's Disease*, *49*(3), 767–781.

Särkämö, T., Ripollés, P., Vepsäläinen, H., Autti, T., Silvennoinen, H. M., Salli, E., Laitinen, S., Forsblom, A., Soinila, S., & Rodríguez-Fornells, A. (2014). Structural changes induced by daily music listening in the recovering brain after middle cerebral artery stroke: A voxel-based morphometry study. *Frontiers in Human Neuroscience*, *8*, 245. https://doi.org/10.3389/fnhum.2014.00245

Särkämö, T., Tervaniemi, M., Laitinen, S., Forsblom, A., Soinila, S., Mikkonen, M., Autti, T., Silvennoinen, H. M., Erkkilä, J., Laine, M., Peretz, I., & Hietanen, M. (2008). Music listening enhances cognitive recovery and mood after middle cerebral artery stroke. *Brain*, *131*(3), 866–876.

Särkämö, T., Tervaniemi, M., Laitinen, S., Numminen, A., Kurki, M., Johnson, J. K., & Rantanen, P. (2014). Cognitive, emotional, and social benefits of regular musical activities in early dementia: Randomized controlled study. *Gerontologist*, *54*(4), 634–650.

Schneider, S., Münte, T., Rodriguez-Fornells, A., Sailer, M., & Altenmüller, E. (2010). Music-supported training is more efficient than functional motor training for recovery of fine motor skills in stroke patients. *Music Perception*, *27*(4), 271–280.

Sihvonen, A. J., Leo, V., Ripollés, P., Lehtovaara, T., Ylönen, A., Rajanaro, P., Laitinen, S., Forsblom, A., Saunavaara, J., Autti, T., Laine, M., Rodríguez-Fornells, A., Tervaniemi, M., Soinila, S., & Särkämö, T. (2020). Vocal music enhances memory and language recovery after stroke: Pooled results from two RCTs. *Annals of Clinical and Translational Neurology*, *7*(11), 2272–2287.

Sihvonen, A. J., Pitkäniemi, A., Leo, V., Soinila, S., & Särkämö, T. (2021). Resting-state language network neuroplasticity in post-stroke music listening: A randomized controlled trial. *European Journal of Neuroscience*, *54*(11), 7886–7898.

Sihvonen, A. J., Pitkäniemi, A., Siponkoski, S.-T., Kuusela, L., Martínez-Molina, N., Laitinen, S., Särkämö, E. R., Pekkola, J., Melkas, S., Schlaug, G., Sairanen, V., & Särkämö, T. (2024). Structural neuroplasticity effects of singing in chronic aphasia. *eNeuro*, *11*(5), ENEURO.0408-23.2024. https://doi.org/10.1523/eneuro.0408-23.2024

Sihvonen, A. J., Särkämö, T., Leo, V., Tervaniemi, M., Altenmüller, E., & Soinila, S. (2017). Music-based interventions in neurological rehabilitation. *Lancet Neurology*, *16*(8), 648–660.

Sihvonen, A. J., Siponkoski, S.-T., Martínez-Molina, N., Laitinen, S., Holma, M., Ahlfors, M., Kuusela, L., Pekkola, J., Koskinen, S., & Särkämö, T. (2022). Neurological music therapy rebuilds structural connectome after traumatic brain injury: Secondary analysis from a randomized controlled trial. *Journal of Clinical Medicine*, *11*(8), 2184. https://doi.org/10.3390/jcm11082184

Sihvonen, A. J., Soinila, S., & Särkämö, T. (2022). Post-stroke enriched auditory environment induces structural connectome plasticity: Secondary analysis from a randomized controlled trial. *Brain Imaging and Behavior*, *16*(4), 1813–1822.

Siponkoski, S.-T., Martínez-Molina, N., Kuusela, L., Laitinen, S., Holma, M., Ahlfors, M., Jordan-Kilkki, P., Ala-Kauhaluoma, K., Melkas, S., Pekkola, J., Rodriguez-Fornells, A., Laine, M., Ylinen, A., Rantanen, P., Koskinen, S., Lipsanen, J., & Särkämö, T. (2020). Music therapy enhances executive functions and prefrontal structural neuroplasticity after traumatic brain injury: Evidence from a randomized controlled trial. *Journal of Neurotrauma*, *37*(4), 618–634.

Siponkoski, S.-T., Pitkäniemi, A., Laitinen, S., Särkämö, E.-R., Pentikäinen, E., Eloranta, H., Tuomiranta, L., Melkas, S., Schlaug, G., Sihvonen, A. J., & Särkämö, T. (2022). Efficacy of a multicomponent singing intervention on communication and psychosocial functioning in chronic aphasia: A randomized controlled crossover trial. *Brain Communications*, *5*(1), fcac337. https://doi.org/10.1093/braincomms/fcac337

Skingley, A., Martin, A., & Clift, S. (2016). The contribution of community singing groups to the well-being of older people. *Journal of Applied Gerontology*, *35*(12), 1302–1324.

Smallwood, J., Bernhardt, B. C., Leech, R., Bzdok, D., Jefferies, E., & Margulies, D. S. (2021). The default mode network in cognition: A topographical perspective. *Nature Reviews Neuroscience*, *22*(8), 503–513.

Stewart, N. A. J., & Lonsdale, A. J. (2016). It's better together: The psychological benefits of singing in a choir. *Psychology of Music*, *44*(6), 1240–1254.

Sutcliffe, R., Du, K., & Ruffman, T. (2020). Music making and neuropsychological aging: A review. *Neuroscience & Biobehavioral Reviews*, *113*, 479–491.

Taruffi, L., Pehrs, C., Skouras, S., & Koelsch, S. (2017). Effects of sad and happy music on mind-wandering and the default mode network. *Scientific Reports*, *7*(1), 14396. https://doi.org/10.1038/s41598-017-14849-0

Thaut, M. H., McIntosh, G. C., & Rice, R. R. (1997). Rhythmic facilitation of gait training in hemiparetic stroke rehabilitation. *Journal of the Neurological Sciences*, *151*(2), 207–212.

Trupp, M. D., Howlin, C., Fekete, A., Kutsche, J., Fingerhut, J., & Pelowski, M. (2025). The impact of viewing art on well-being — A systematic review of the evidence base and suggested mechanisms. *The Journal of Positive Psychology*, *20*(6), 978–1002.

Tymoszuk, U., Perkins, R., Spiro, N., Williamon, A., & Fancourt, D. (2020). Longitudinal associations between short-term, repeated, and sustained arts engagement and well-being outcomes in older adults. *Journals of Gerontology: Series B*, *75*(7), 1609–1619.

van der Meulen, I., van de Sandt-Koenderman, W. M., Heijenbrok-Kal, M. H., Visch-Brink, E. G., & Ribbers, G. M. (2014). The efficacy and timing of melodic intonation therapy in subacute aphasia. *Neurorehabilitation & Neural Repair*, *28*(6), 536–544.

van der Steen, J. T., van der Wouden, J. C., Methley, A. M., Smaling, H. J. A., Vink, A. C., & Bruinsma, M. S. (2025). Music-based therapeutic interventions for people with dementia. *Cochrane Database of Systematic Reviews*, *3*(3), CD003477. https://doi.org/10.1002/14651858.cd003477.pub5

Verghese, J., Lipton, R. B., Katz, M. J., Hall, C. B., Derby, C. A., Kuslansky, G., Ambrose, A. F., Sliwinski, M., & Buschke, H. (2003). Leisure activities and the risk of dementia in the elderly. *New England Journal of Medicine*, *348*(25), 2508–2516.

Vinke, E. J., de Groot, M., Venkatraghavan, V., Klein, S., Niessen, W. J., Ikram, M. A., & Vernooij, M. W. (2018). Trajectories of imaging markers in brain aging: The Rotterdam Study. *Neurobiology of Aging*, *71*, 32–40.

Walsh, S., Causer, R., & Brayne, C. (2021). Does playing a musical instrument reduce the incidence of cognitive impairment and dementia? A systematic review and meta-analysis. *Aging & Mental Health*, *25*(4), 593–601.

Wang, L., Peng, J. L., Xiang, W., Huang, Y. J., & Chen, A. L. (2022). Effects of rhythmic auditory stimulation on motor function and balance ability in stroke: A systematic review and meta-analysis of clinical randomized controlled studies. *Frontiers in Neuroscience*, *16*, 1043575. https://doi.org/10.3389/fnins.2022.1043575

Wang, Z., Xue, Y., Sun, G., Yun, J., Li, Y., Chen, Q., Wang, R., Wang, J., & Ren, C. (2025). Effects of music-supported therapy for depression and cognitive disorders in people living with stroke and its impact on quality of life: A systematic evaluation and meta-analysis. *Cerebrovascular Disorders*, *54*(6), 959–984.

Wilkins, R. W., Hodges, D. A., Laurienti, P. J., Steen, M., & Burdette, J. H. (2014). Network science and the effects of music preference on functional brain connectivity: From Beethoven to Eminem. *Scientific Reports*, *4*(1), 6130. https://doi.org/10.1038/srep06130

Williams, E., Dingle, G. A., & Clift, S. (2018). A systematic review of mental health and wellbeing outcomes of group singing for adults with a mental health condition. *European Journal of Public Health*, *28*(6), 1035–1042.

Worschech, F., James, C. E., Jünemann, K., Sinke, C., Krüger, T. H. C., Scholz, D. S., Kliegel, M., Marie, D., & Altenmüller, E. (2023). Fine motor control improves in older adults after 1 year of piano lessons: Analysis of individual development and its coupling with cognition and brain structure. *European Journal of Neuroscience*, *57*(12), 2040–2061.

Wu, K., Anderson, J., Townsend, J., Frazier, T., Brandt, A., & Karmonik, C. (2019). Characterization of functional brain connectivity towards optimization of music selection for therapy: A fMRI study. *International Journal of Neuroscience*, *129*(9), 882–889.

Young, H. J., Mehta, T., Herman, C., Baidwan, N. K., Lai, B., & Rimmer, J. H. (2021). The effects of a movement-to-music (M2M) intervention on physical and psychosocial outcomes in people poststroke: A randomized controlled trial. *Archives of Rehabilitation Research and Clinical Translation*, *3*(4), 100160. https://doi.org/10.1016/j.arrct.2021.100160

Zhu, A. H., Nir, T. M., Javid, S., Villalón-Reina, J. E., Rodrigue, A. L., Strike, L. T., de Zubicaray, G. I., McMahon, K. L., Wright, M. J., Medland, S. E., Blangero, J., Glahn, D. C., Kochunov, P., Williamson, D. E., Håberg, A. K., Thompson, P. M., & Jahanshad, N. (2025). Lifespan reference curves for harmonizing multi-site regional brain white matter metrics from diffusion MRI. *Scientific Data*, *12*(1), 748. https://doi.org/10.1038/s41597-025-05028-2

14

RECOVERY APPROACHES IN MUSIC-BASED INTERVENTIONS AND MUSIC THERAPY

Thomas Stegemann and Michael J. Silverman

Introduction

Within an adult mental health context, recovery can be defined in a number of ways and as both a process and outcome (Leonhardt et al., 2017; Warner, 2009). For example, "recovery can be conceptualized as a process of change where people improve their health and well-being, live a self-directed, purposeful, and meaningful life, and strive to reach their full potential" (Silverman, 2022, p. 97). Kellmann and Kallus (2001) described recovery as a more specific approach that goes beyond regeneration or 'being cured' or 'being normal again' (Beckmann et al., 2023). This perspective addresses recovery as a process of change as well as a resource that enables individuals to recover from stress and develop resilience to health-threatening stress. Kallus (2016, p. 42) defined recovery as "an inter- and intraindividual multilevel (e.g., psychological, physiological, social) process in time for the re-establishment of personal resources and their full functional capacity". As music can function as a coping strategy or be used as a treatment medium as in music therapy, music can be an integral component of recovery. Therefore, the purpose of this chapter is to describe music therapy in recovery contexts, differentiate music listening from music therapy, and describe music therapy in clinical and non-clinical settings. First, as a foundational model for understanding recovery mechanisms mediated by sound, we propose a neurobiological framework explaining the stress-reducing and relaxing effects of music.

Stegemann, T., & Silverman, M. J. (2026). Recovery approaches in music-based interventions and music therapy. In E. Altenmüller, M. Kellmann, J. Beckmann, & G. M. Moyle (Eds.), *Recovery and well-being in the performing arts* (pp. 241–254). Routledge.

DOI: 10.4324/9781003566885-18

Neurobiological model of the stress-reducing and relaxing effects of music

In the following, we will briefly describe a model (Figure 14.1) that seeks to integrate neurobiological concepts and research findings to elucidate the mechanisms wherein music mediates stress reduction and relaxation: *Music-Related Neurobiological Relaxation Model* (Stegemann, 2013, 2021). This model is based on the assumption that the ascending pathways of the central auditory system (i.e., the connections from the inner ear to the neocortex) can be differentiated into a *classical* and a *non-classical* auditory system (Möller, 2013). The non-classical pathway differs from the classical pathway in that it does not project into the primary auditory cortex, but communicates with other areas of the brain via the dorsal part of the medial geniculate body. These include the components of the limbic system that are of particular interest in our context, such as the hypothalamus and the amygdala. The auditory system is connected to the motor system via reflex arcs and influences arousal (wakefulness) as well as the autonomic and endocrine systems (Möller, 2013).

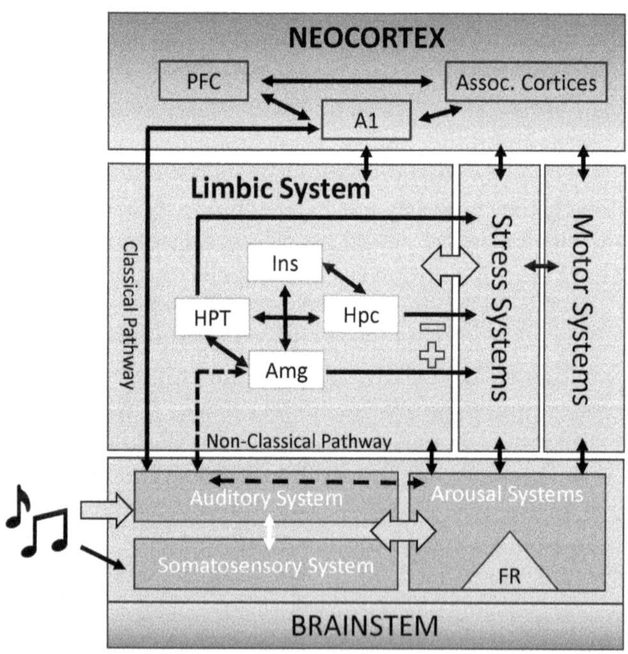

FIGURE 14.1 *Music-related Neurobiological Relaxation Model* translated from Stegemann (2013).

Note: A1 – primary auditory cortex; Amg – amygdala; FR – reticular formation; Hpc – hippocampus; HPT – hypothalamus; Ins – Insula; and PFC – prefrontal cortex.

As described above, the *classical pathway* of the central auditory pathway leads to the primary auditory cortex, while the *non-classical pathway* connects the auditory system directly to the amygdala. When someone listens to music, the sound waves are received through the auditory system (and possibly also via the somatosensory system as vibrations) and processed in parallel via the two pathways of the central auditory pathway. It is assumed that general musical parameters – including volume, dynamics, rhythm – have a direct effect on arousal, stress, and limbic regulatory systems via the non-classical pathway. Without the influence of higher cognitive areas (i.e., bottom-up), music can have an activating or relaxing/stress-reducing effect on the organism. At the same time, top-down mechanisms that integrate individual preferences or previous experiences – thus modulating the psychological and physical reactions to the music stimulus – take effect via the classical pathway involving the neocortex. In summary, the *Music-Related Neurobiological Relaxation Model* allows the integration of current music-psychological and neurobiological findings with regard to a music-mediated relaxation response with the interplay of bottom-up and top-down processes.

This perspective on recovery processes supported by the effects of music listening or music making (see below) is also congruent with recent research on the neurobiology of stress resilience: as Kalisch et al. (2024) explained in a review article, "functions of the hippocampus, the prefrontal cortex, and the reward system support resilience and are in turn supported by factors promoting neuroplasticity, immunoregulation, gut microbiome composition, and integrity of the gut barrier and the blood-brain barrier" (p. 1205). More than two decades of neuroimaging research have revealed that music – similar to other primary reinforcers – is able to engage the brain's reward system (Mas-Herrero et al., 2021). In addition, there is growing evidence for the impact of music-based interventions and music therapy on enhancing neuroplastic and neurodevelopmental processes in the brain including neurological disorders (Sihvonen et al., 2017), autism (Sharda et al., 2018), and neonatal care (Haslbeck et al., 2023). According to Sihvonen et al. (2017), "the psychological effects and neurobiological mechanisms underlying the effects of music interventions are likely to share common neural systems for reward, arousal regulation, learning, and activity-driven plasticity" (p. 648). In summary, music-based interventions and music therapy likely facilitate and support recovery processes by engaging a wide range of brain circuits in concert with factors that enhance neuroplasticity, regulate the immune and digestive systems, and stabilise the blood-brain barrier. Music's positive effects on health and recovery processes are achieved through interventions that are relatively inexpensive, have minimal side effects, and are highly accepted by service users (Stegemann et al., 2019).

Defining music therapy

Music therapy is a healthcare profession wherein a qualified professional uses music interventions to meet the needs of a service user within the relationships that develop between the music, service user, and music therapist (European Music Therapy Confederation, n.d.). To practice music therapy, music therapists undergo "rigorous" (Sena Moore, 2015, p. 82) academic training consisting of music theory and history, various musical instruments and voice, psychology, therapeutic theories and orientations, and anatomy. Music therapists also complete supervised clinical training during their academic coursework in addition to internships. To meet the clinical needs of service users, music therapists have strong music skills[1] and are able to improvise and compose music.

Although music therapists can work with a number of clinical and non-clinical populations, music therapists often practice in a variety of inpatient and outpatient settings wherein recovery constitutes the ultimate objective. Clinically based settings may include addiction, mental health, and physical rehabilitation. Music therapists tailor, design, and implement interventions based on the motivations and clinical goals of the service user, the service user's music preferences and experiences, an assessment of the service user's abilities and strengths, as well as their philosophical orientation to treatment. Music therapists can work in individual or group settings and deliver services via in-person or remote formats (Clements-Cortés et al., 2025; Knight & Blank, 2025; Wang et al., 2023).

Music therapy is typically used as an intervention to address a service user's non-music clinical objectives (e.g., stress reduction, coping strategies, community reintegration, social supports). However, music therapy also has the potential to be used in non-clinical groups for prevention. For example, Gold et al. (2017) studied the effects of group music therapy as a preventive intervention for young people at risk of developing mental health conditions. Although there was no between-group difference in the group music therapy and self-directed music listening conditions, both groups showed improvements in mental health outcomes. Music therapists can work with musicians (Bruscia, 2012) and treat professional musicians' performance anxiety (Zhukov, 2019).

Differentiating music therapy from music medicine and music-based interventions

Although listening to music can be helpful for many people, a key component of music therapy is that it is provided by a qualified practitioner who uses the relationships between the service user, music, and music therapist to address clinical objectives (Bruscia, 2014). For example, a music therapist might conduct a lyric analysis session to identify adaptive coping strategies with a group of patients hospitalised on a mental health unit. The group

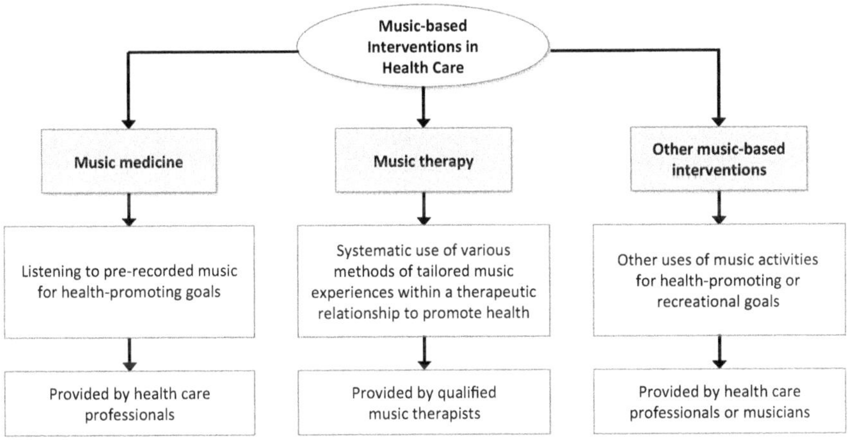

FIGURE 14.2 Differentiating music medicine, music therapy, and other music-based interventions adopted from Stegemann et al. (2019).

would first listen to the song and then process the lyrics and identify ways to cope. Therefore, music listening can be a component of music therapy when a music therapist is present. Listening to music alone can be self-regulating, but also has the potential to result in maladaptive impacts on people's health (Silverman et al., 2020). Music listening without a music therapist may be especially detrimental to people experiencing depression as they may not have the insight to know how the music impacts them (Stewart et al., 2019). For example, self-directed music listening has the potential for unhealthy music use such as rumination and avoidance (Saarikallio et al., 2015). In cases wherein music may activate a service user's trauma, specifically qualified music therapists are trained to help people process and contain these emotions to keep them safe. As non-music therapists can use music for people's health promotion, Figure 14.2 differentiates music therapy from music medicine and other music-based interventions.

Recovery

Recovery is increasingly guiding service provision and policy in contemporary adult mental healthcare. In applying the recovery approach to clinical practice, people with mental health conditions have hope, the power to make decisions, and lives of self-directed meaning and purpose (Corrigan et al., 1999; Hancock et al., 2015). Recovery-oriented practitioners have moved away from the historically paternalistic and medically dominated philosophy (Sowers et al., 2004) and believe that people with mental health conditions have the potential to recover, have a fulfilling vocation, and live productive and satisfying lives (Bellack, 2006).

Music therapy and recovery

Because music therapy is a flexible psychosocial intervention, music therapists can address clinical objectives related to mental health recovery. To date, music therapy scholars have highlighted the alignment between music therapy and recovery (Fletcher et al., 2019; Grocke et al., 2008; McCaffrey & Edwards, 2016; McCaffrey et al., 2011, 2018; Silverman, 2022; Solli et al., 2013). For example, McCaffrey et al. (2020) investigated how service users perceived the role of group songwriting in recovery-oriented mental health services. An analysis of the composed song lyrics reflected mental health service users' growth, empowerment and freedom using music engagement, and empathy for other people. The authors analysed interviews after songwriting and found four themes: (1) group songwriting breaks down barriers in ways that help to promote equality; (2) group songwriting offered new perspectives; (3) group songwriting can expose perceived vulnerabilities; and (4) group songwriting may be approached with knowledge of music's capacity to promote well-being (McCaffrey et al., 2020).

Music therapy and addiction

Music therapists often work in various types of addiction settings (i.e., detoxification, intensive inpatient programmes, and longer-term outpatient programmes) and treat people with substance use conditions (SUC). To date, the results of systematic reviews and meta-analyses of music therapy for adults with SUC have been positive and indicate that music therapy can have positive impacts on recovery-related constructs including craving, change readiness, and motivation (Carter & Panisch, 2021; Ghetti et al., 2022; Hohmann et al., 2017; Megranahan & Lynskey, 2018). In addiction settings, music therapists often use song discussion, lyric analysis, songwriting, improvisation, and recreational music therapy to address aspects of recovery that can include motivation for change, social connectedness, community resources, and coping strategies (Silverman, 2009).

Songwriting is a commonly used music therapy intervention involving the creation of music, lyrics, or music and lyrics that has widespread therapeutic application across Europe, Australia, and the Americas (Baker & Wigram, 2005; Baker et al., 2008). In a clinical example of single-session group songwriting with adults on a detoxification unit, a clinician-researcher used a twelve-bar blues progression to facilitate the lyrical composition of two verses that focus on recovery will-power (verse 1) and recovery way-power (verse 2). The theoretical framework for this songwriting intervention is based on *Snyder's Hope Theory* (Snyder, 1994, 2002), and the protocol can be found in Silverman (2023, 2024a).[2] An example of composed lyrics is as follows:

Verse 1: Recovery will power	*Verse 2: Recovery way power*
Sick of the sneaking	Gotta be honest
Tired of the lies	And know that it's true
You'd think I'd know better	Hold my boundaries
It's time to get wise	And be humble too
Head's stuck in the sand	Faith in the higher power
From not following through	Will help me be true
I got them detox...	Fighting them detox...
I got them detox blues.	Fighting them detox blues.

Music and health

Because of music's accessibility, widespread popularity, and strong connection to personal identity (MacDonald et al., 2017), individuals often engage with music as a self-directed tool for emotional regulation in everyday life. For example, people may deliberately select music to calm themselves when anxious, to energise themselves when fatigued, or to reflect on personal experiences, all without the involvement of a qualified music therapist. Listening to preferred music can have positive impacts on people in high-stress occupations including air traffic controllers (Lesiuk, 2008) and professional computer information systems developers (Lesiuk, 2010).

For people interested in music listening for health promotion without a qualified music therapist, their preferred music genres will typically have the greatest positive impact. To date, there is a lack of literature noting that there is a superior type or genre of music to be used for health promotion. For example, listening to Mozart may not result in augmented intelligence (Helding, 2014). Moreover, listening to heavy metal does not result in suicidal ideation (Brown, 2025). When considering music choices for health promotion, the function of the music for the individual person – not the genre – is the consequential and therapeutic aspect. The impact of music is a result of the listener's relationship with music and their music preferences (Jiang et al., 2016; North & Hargreaves, 2012). Although the media may promote or imply that certain music genres – typically rock and hip hop and their related derivatives including heavy metal and rap – result in adverse behaviours such as violence or substance use (Anglada-Tort, 2019), specific music genres are not necessarily harmful (Lozon & Bensimon, 2014). In fact, although rap is often criticised as promoting violence, rap can provide social connection and a uniting alternative commentary not found in mainstream media that can name oppression and discrimination (Allen & Randolf, 2020; Epps & Dixon, 2017; Mozie, 2022) as well as express and change people's negative affective states (Powell et al., 2022).

Unfortunately, certain types of music are vilified and considered problematic without the proper evidence (Silverman, 2024b).

Prevention, promotion, management, and treatment through the arts

The field of arts and health is a broad and expanding interdisciplinary domain, encompassing a diverse range of professions working with varied clientele and objectives (see Figure 14.2 to differentiate music medicine, music therapy, and other music-based interventions). Recovery-oriented interventions may be well-suited as an overarching or unifying philosophy for these various initiatives, even if the term 'recovery' itself is not consistently used or uniformly applied across contexts. A Health Evidence Network synthesis report by the WHO (Fancourt & Finn, 2019), based on the analysis of over 3,000 studies, emphasised the importance of the arts in health policy, identifying "a major role for the arts in the prevention of ill health, promotion of health, and management and treatment of illness across the lifespan" (p. ii). Specifically, positive effects were observed in the following areas:

Within *prevention and promotion*, findings showed how the arts can:

- affect the social determinants of health;
- support child development;
- encourage health-promoting behaviours;
- help to prevent ill health;
- support caregiving.

Within *management and treatment*, findings showed how the arts can:

- help people experiencing mental illness;
- support care for people with acute conditions;
- help to support people with neurodevelopmental and neurological disorders;
- assist with the management of noncommunicable diseases; and
- support end-of-life care (Fancourt & Finn, 2019, pp. vii/viii).

Situated at the intersection of music therapy and other music-based interventions, we will briefly present a research project illustrating the relevance of the recovery approach in the health sector. As part of an international and multisite research project, we developed the Professional Excellence in Meaningful Music in Healthcare (ProMiMiC) as an intervention for the radiation oncology department at a University Hospital in Austria to investigate interprofessional collaboration between music therapists and musicians in a hospital setting (Bezold et al., 2023; van der Wal-Huisman et al., 2023). Music therapy, particularly as a complementary therapy, can support recovery processes in oncology. A Cochrane review by Bradt et al. (2021, p. 3) concluded that music therapy and music medicine interventions may have a beneficial effect on anxiety, depression, hope, pain, fatigue, heart rate and blood pressure in adults with cancer. Music therapy but not music medicine interventions may improve adult patients' quality of life and levels of fatigue.

Although oncological care primarily focuses on addressing a patient's somatic needs, the ProMiMiC project aimed to provide a person-centred, holistic approach through specially tailored live bedside music. Based on the patient's musical preferences and immediate needs, an ensemble of music therapists and musicians performed pieces from their repertoire or created spontaneous improvisations, translating prompts such as landscapes, past vacations, or moods into music. Results from a thematic qualitative content analysis revealed four overarching themes: emotional release, positive distraction, alterations in contact, and shared humanity (van der Wal-Huisman et al., 2023). In addition, the ProMiMiC project and its pilot investigation found that patients and hospital staff – including nurses and doctors 'witnessing' the live music on the ward – can benefit from these interventions, especially in terms of motivation and work satisfaction (Smilde et al., 2019). These findings highlight the impact of music therapy and music-based interventions on recovery processes, including their effects at both systemic and organisational levels.

Conclusion and recommendations for practice

With technological advances, music has become increasingly accessible. However, music use and listening can be a privilege as not everyone has access to devices, internet, and other resources necessary for music use. Professional musicians and performing artists might consult with music therapists regarding how to use music for self-care to augment their health and well-being. Professional musicians could also partner with music therapists to deliver music-based interventions in healthcare settings. This may result in additional revenue sources for professional musicians as well as the ability to reach clinical populations who can benefit from live music as a health-promoting resource. However, future work is needed to better differentiate unhealthy and healthy music use (Riedl & Stegemann, 2018; Saarikallio et al., 2015) to ensure people use music in a manner that promotes recovery and health. As music therapy is a relatively diminutive profession, additional research from all paradigms is warranted to increase access to services.

Notes

1 Musical skills are a required prerequisite for admission to music therapy training programmes, and their further development forms an important part of the curricula in several European countries. This includes a wide range of musical instruments (including voice and body), with particular emphasis on improvisation, which plays a central role in many training programmes (Stegemann et al., 2016).

2 The second author extends his gratitude and appreciation to the service users who shared their narratives and ideas to compose these lyrics.

References

Allen, T. N., & Randolph, A. (2020). Listening for the interior in hip-hop and R&B music. *Sociology of Race and Ethnicity*, *6*(1), 46–60.

Anglada-Tort, M. (2019). Measuring stereotypes in music: A commentary on Susino and Schubert (2019). *Empirical Musicology Review*, *14*(1–2), 16–21.

Baker, F., & Wigram, T. (2005). *Songwriting: Methods, techniques and clinical applications for music therapy clinicians, educators and students*. Jessica Kingsley Publishers.

Baker, F., Wigram, T., Stott, D., & McFerran, K. (2008). Therapeutic songwriting in music therapy: Part I: Who are the therapists, who are the clients, and why is songwriting used? *Nordic Journal of Music Therapy*, *17*(2), 105–123.

Beckmann, J., Kellmann, M., & Jakowski, S. (2023). Recovery is more than just healing: Advocating a broader perspective on recovery in physical and mental health. In M. Kellmann, S. Jakowski, & J. Beckmann (Eds.), *The importance of recovery for physical and mental health: Negotiating the effects of underrecovery* (pp. 266–270). Routledge.

Bellack, A. S. (2006). Scientific and consumer models of recovery in schizophrenia: Concordance, contrasts, and implications. *Schizophrenia Bulletin*, *32*, 432–442.

Bezold, L., Bork, M., & Stegemann, T. (2023). Musiktherapie [Music therapy]. In A. Petri-Preis & J. Voit (Eds.), *Handbuch Musikvermittlung – Studium, Lehre, Berufspraxis* (pp. 325–327). Transcript Verlag.

Bradt, J., Dileo, C., Myers-Coffman, K., & Biondo, J. (2021). Music interventions for improving psychological and physical outcomes in people with cancer. *Cochrane Database of Systematic Reviews*, *10*(10), CD006911. https://doi.org/10.1002/14651858.CD006911.pub4

Brown, A. R. (2025). Songs in the key of depression, suicide and death. In J. Heimerdinger, H. Riedl, & T. Stegemann (Eds.), *Musik und Suizidalität. Interdisziplinäre Perspektiven* (pp. 79–103). mdwPress.

Bruscia, K. E. (Ed.). (2012). *Case examples of music therapy for musicians*. Barcelona Publishers.

Bruscia, K. E. (2014). *Defining music therapy* (3rd ed.). Barcelona Publishers.

Carter, T. E., & Panisch, L. S. (2021). A systematic review of music therapy for psychosocial outcomes of substance use clients. *International Journal of Mental Health and Addiction*, *19*, 1551–1568.

Clements-Cortés, A., Fuller, A., Kelly, L., Pranjić, M., Selvarajah, I., Brotons, M. M., & Bridi, N. (2025). Music therapists' global perspectives on telehealth music therapy: A qualitative interview inquiry. *Music Therapy Perspectives*, *43*(1), miae030. https://doi.org/10.1093/mtp/miae030

Corrigan, P. W., Giffort, D., Rashid, F., Leary, M., & Okeke, I. (1999). Recovery as a psychological construct. *Community Mental Health Journal*, *35*, 231–239.

Epps, A. C., & Dixon, T. L. (2017). A comparative content analysis of anti- and prosocial rap lyrical themes found on traditional and new media outlets. *Journal of Broadcasting & Electronic Media*, *61*(2), 467–498.

European Music Therapy Confederation. (n.d.). *What is music therapy?* Retrieved August 04, 2025 from https://emtc-eu.com/faq/

Fancourt, D., & Finn, S. (2019). *What is the evidence on the role of the arts in improving health and well-being? A scoping review* (Health Evidence Network synthesis report, No. 67). WHO Regional Office for Europe. https://www.ncbi.nlm.nih.gov/books/NBK553773/

Fletcher, A., Hackett, S., & Carr, S. M. (2019). The 4P participatory arts recovery model: Peers, product, personhood and positive interaction. *Journal of Applied Arts & Health*, *10*(1), 41–56.

Ghetti, C., Chen, X. J., Brenner, A. K., Hakvoort, L. G., Lien, L., Fachner, J., & Gold, C. (2022). Music therapy for people with substance use disorders. *Cochrane Database of Systematic Reviews*, (5), CD012576. https://doi.org/10.1002/14651858.CD012576.pub3

Gold, C., Saarikallio, S., Crooke, A. H. D., & McFerran, K. S. (2017). Group music therapy as a preventive intervention for young people at risk: Cluster-randomized trial. *Journal of Music Therapy*, *54*(2), 133–160.

Grocke, D., Bloch, S., & Castle, D. (2008). Is there a role for music therapy in the care of the severely mentally ill? *Australasian Psychiatry*, *16*, 442–445.

Hancock, N., Scanlan, J. N., Honey, A., Bundy, A. C., & O'Shea, K. (2015). Recovery Assessment Scale – Domains and Stages (RAS-DS): Its feasibility and outcome measurement capacity. *Australian & New Zealand Journal of Psychiatry*, *49*, 624–633.

Haslbeck, F. B., Adams, M., Schmidli, L., Bassler, D., Bucher, H. U., & Natalucci, G. (2023). Creative music therapy for long-term neurodevelopment in extremely preterm infants: Results of a feasibility trial. *Acta Paediatrica*, *112*(12), 2524–2531.

Helding, L. (2014). The Mozart effect turns twenty. *Journal of Singing*, *70*(4), 473–479.

Hohmann, L., Bradt, J., Stegemann, T., & Kolesch, S. (2017). Effects of music therapy and music-based interventions in the treatment of substance use disorders: A systematic review. *PLoS ONE*, *12*(11), e0187363. https://doi.org/10.1371/journal.pone.0187363

Jiang, J., Rickson, D., & Jiang, C. (2016). The mechanism of music for reducing psychological distress: Music preference as the mediator. *The Arts in Psychotherapy*, *48*, 62–68.

Kalisch, R., Russo, S. J., & Müller, M. B. (2024). Neurobiology and systems biology of stress resilience. *Physiological Reviews*, *104*(3), 1205–1263.

Kallus, K. W. (2016). Stress and recovery: An overview. In K. W. Kallus & M. Kellmann (Eds.), *The Recovery-Stress Questionnaires: User manual* (pp. 27–48). Pearson.

Kellmann, M., & Kallus, K. W. (2001). *The Recovery-Stress Questionnaire for Athletes: User manual*. Human Kinetics.

Knight, A., & Blank, C. A. (2025). An analysis of caregiver perceptions of early childhood music therapy telehealth groups. *Approaches: An Interdisciplinary Journal of Music Therapy*, 17(3), 486–505. https://doi.org/10.56883/aijmt.2025.589

Leonhardt, B. L., Huling, K., Hamm, J. A., Roe, D., Hasson-Ohayon, I., McLeod, H. J., & Lysaker, P. H. (2017). Recovery and serious mental illness: A review of current clinical and research paradigms and future directions. *Expert Review of Neurotherapeutics*, *17*(11), 1117–1130.

Lesiuk, T. (2008). The effect of preferred music listening on stress levels of air traffic controllers. *The Arts in Psychotherapy*, *35*(1), 1–10.

Lesiuk, T. (2010). The effect of preferred music on mood and performance in a high-cognitive demand occupation. *Journal of Music Therapy*, *47*(2), 137–154.

Lozon, J., & Bensimon, M. (2014). Music misuse: A review of the personal and collective roles of "problem music". *Aggression and Violent Behavior*, *19*(3), 207–218.

MacDonald, R., Hargreaves, D. J., & Miell, D. (Eds.). (2017). *Handbook of musical identities*. Oxford University Press.

Mas-Herrero, E., Maini, L., Sescousse, G., & Zatorre, R. J. (2021). Common and distinct neural correlates of music and food-induced pleasure: A coordinate-based meta-analysis of neuroimaging studies. *Neuroscience and Biobehavioral Reviews*, *123*, 61–71.

McCaffrey, T., Carr, C., Solli, H. P., & Hense, C. (2018). Music therapy and recovery in mental health: Seeking a way forward. *Voices: A World Forum for Music Therapy*, *18*(1), 1–16. https://doi.org/10.15845/voices.v18i1.918

McCaffrey, T., & Edwards, J. (2016). "Music therapy helped me get back *doing*": Perspectives of music therapy participants in mental health services. *Journal of Music Therapy*, *53*, 121–148.

McCaffrey, T., Edwards, J., & Fannon, D. (2011). Is there a role for music therapy in the recovery approach in mental health? *Arts in Psychotherapy*, *38*, 185–189.

McCaffrey, T., Higgins, P., Monahan, C., Moloney, S., Nelligan, S., Clancy, A., & Cheung, P. S. (2020). Exploring the role and impact of group songwriting with multiple stakeholders in recovery-oriented mental health services. *Nordic Journal of Music Therapy*, *30*(1), 41–60.

Megranahan, K., & Lynskey, M. T. (2018). Do creative arts therapies reduce substance misuse? A systematic review. *The Arts in Psychotherapy*, *57*, 50–58.

Möller, A. R. (2013). *Hearing* (3rd ed.). Plural Publishing.

Mozie, D. (2022). "They killin' us for no reason": Black lives matter, police brutality, and hip-hop music: A quantitative content analysis. *Journalism & Mass Communication Quarterly*, *99*(3), 826–847.

North, A. C., & Hargreaves, D. J. (2012). Pop music subcultures and wellbeing. In R. McDonald, G. Kreutz, & L. Mitchell (Eds.), *Music, health, and wellbeing* (pp. 502–512). Oxford University Press.

Powell, M., Olsen, K. N., & Thompson, W. F. (2022). Does music help regulate depressive symptoms for fans of violently themed music? *Psychology of Music*, *50*(4), 1296–1311.

Riedl, H., & Stegemann, T. (2018). Die Übersetzung der Healthy-Unhealthy Uses of Music Scale (HUMS) vom Englischen ins Deutsche [Translation of the Healthy-Unhealthy Uses of Music Scale (HUMS) from English into German]. *Musiktherapeutische Umschau*, *39*(3), 229–240.

Saarikallio, S., Gold, C., & McFerran, K. (2015). Development and validation of the Healthy-Unhealthy music Scale. *Child and Adolescent Mental Health*, *20*(4), 210–217.

Sena Moore, K. (2015). Music therapy advocacy for professional recognition: A historical perspective and future directions. *Music Therapy Perspectives*, *33*(1), 76–85.

Sharda, M., Tuerk, C., Chowdhury, R., Jamey, K., Foster, N., Custo-Blanch, M., Tan, M., Nadig, A., & Hyde, K. (2018). Music improves social communication and auditory-motor connectivity in children with autism. *Translational Psychiatry*, *8*(1), 231. https://doi.org/10.1038/s41398-018-0287-3

Sihvonen, A. J., Särkämö, T., Leo, V., Tervaniemi, M., Altenmüller, E., & Soinila, S. (2017). Music-based interventions in neurological rehabilitation. *The Lancet Neurology*, *16*(8), 648–660.

Silverman, M. J. (2009). A descriptive analysis of music therapists working with consumers in substance abuse rehabilitation. *The Arts in Psychotherapy*, *36*, 123–130.

Silverman, M. J. (2022). *Music therapy in mental health for illness management and recovery* (2nd ed.). Oxford University Press.
Silverman, M. J. (2023). A cluster-randomized comparison of music therapy interventions as measured by craving and commitment in adults on a detoxification unit. *Substance Use and Misuse*, *58*(14), 1847–1854.
Silverman, M. J. (2024a). A proposed critical theory of music vilification to explain "problem music." *The Arts in Psychotherapy*, *91*, 102223. https://doi.org/10.1016/j.aip.2024.102223
Silverman, M. J. (2024b). Comparing music therapy interventions in adults with substance use disorder on a detoxification unit as measured by the group relationship: A three-group cluster-randomized study. *International Journal of Systemic Therapy*, *35*(3), 245–265.
Silverman, M. J., Gooding, L. F., & Yinger, O. S. (2020). It's…complicated: A theoretical model of music-induced harm. *Journal of Music Therapy*, *57*(3), 251–281.
Smilde, R., Heineman, E., de Wit, K., Dons, K., & Alheit, P. (2019). *If music be the food of love, play on: Meaningful music in healthcare*. Eburon.
Snyder, C. R. (1994). *The psychology of hope: You can get there from here*. Simon and Schuster.
Snyder, C. R. (2002). Hope theory: Rainbows in the mind. *Psychological Inquiry*, *13*(4), 249–275.
Solli, H. P., Rolvsjord, R., & Borg, M. (2013). Toward understanding music therapy as a recovery-oriented practice within mental health care: A meta-synthesis of service users' experiences. *Journal of Music Therapy*, *50*, 244–273.
Sowers, W., Huskshorn, K., & Ashcraft, L. (2004). *Transforming systems of care: Translation of recovery to mental health treatment settings* [Paper presentation]. National Consensus Conference on Mental Health Recovery and Systems Transformation, Rockville, United States.
Stegemann, T. (2013). *Stress, Entspannung und Musik – Untersuchungen zu rezeptiver Musiktherapie im Kindes- und Jugendalter* [Stress, relaxation, and music – Studies on receptive music therapy in childhood and adolescence; doctoral dissertation]. Hochschule für Musik und Theater Hamburg. Retrieved August 22, 2025 from https://ediss.sub.uni-hamburg.de/handle/ediss/5168
Stegemann, T. (2021). Neurobiologische Grundlagen [Neurobiological principles]. In H. H. Decker-Voigt & E. Weymann (Eds.), *Lexikon Musiktherapie* (3rd ed., pp. 437–445). Hogrefe.
Stegemann, T., Geretsegger, M., Phan Quoc, E., Riedl, H., & Smetana, M. (2019). Music therapy and other music-based interventions in pediatric health care: An overview. *Medicines*, *6*(1), 25. https://doi.org/10.3390/medicines6010025
Stegemann, T., Schmidt, H. U., Fitzthum, E., & Timmermann, T. (Eds.). (2016). *Music therapy training programmes in Europe: Theme and variations*. Reichert.
Stewart, J., Garrido, S., Hense, C., & McFerran, K. (2019). Music use for mood regulation: Self-awareness and conscious listening choices in young people with tendencies to depression. *Frontiers in Psychology*, *10*, 1199. https://doi.org/10.3389/fpsyg.2019.01199
van der Wal-Huisman, H., van den Berg, N. M., Paans, W., Bezold, L., Stegemann, T., de Graeff, P., & Van Leeuwen, B. L. (2023). Live bedside music for hospitalized older adults: A qualitative descriptive interview study. *International Journal of Older People Nursing*, *18*, e12574. https://doi.org/10.1111/opn.12574

Wang, S. G., Cevasco-Trotter, A. M., Silverman, M. J., & Yuan, S. H. (2023). A narrative review of music therapy for neuropsychiatric symptoms in Alzheimer's disease and rationale for protocolized music teletherapy. *Frontiers in Medicine*, *10*, 1248245. https://doi.org/10.3389/fmed.2023.1248245

Warner, R. (2009). Recovery from schizophrenia and the recovery model. *Current Opinion in Psychiatry*, *22*, 374–380.

Zhukov, K. (2019). Current approaches for management of music performance anxiety: An introductory overview. *Medical Problems of Performing Artists*, *34*(1), 53–60.

15

DANCE – A LIFELINE FOR HOLISTIC RECOVERY AND CREATIVE AGEING

Erica R. Jeffrey, Clare Guss-West, and David Leventhal

Introduction: Dancing, adapting, and transforming

Beyond its intrinsic value as an art form and cultural means of expression, dance provides a transformative context for narrative communication, social connection, and individual adaptation. Dance, in its myriad forms, has for millennia offered pathways for individuals to explore their evolving identities, nurture their creativity, and experience embodied communication. Today, harnessing dance as a vehicle for health provides reflective opportunities to deepen parallel understandings of recovery. Kellmann and Kallus (2001, 2025) propose a broader understanding of recovery that extends beyond notions of regeneration, cure, or a return to "normal" functioning (Beckmann et al., 2023, p. 6). This perspective positions recovery as a vital resource, supporting not only restoration from stress but also the development of resilience against health-threatening stress. Kallus defines recovery as "an inter- and intraindividual, multilevel (e.g., psychological, physiological, social) process in time for the re-establishment of personal resources and their full functional capacity" (Kallus, 2016, p. 42). This chapter extends the discussion to consider recovery in the context of *dance for health* and those living with degenerative conditions.

Dance for health invites participants to experience meaningful physical, emotional, and psychological change, fostering a sense of wholeness through dance, rather than dance being the cause of injury (Blevins et al., 2020; De Wet et al., 2022). In this context dance emerges as a unique vehicle

Jeffrey, E. R., Guss-West, C., & Leventhal, D. (2026). Dance – A lifeline for holistic recovery and creative ageing. In E. Altenmüller, M. Kellmann, J. Beckmann, & G. M. Moyle (Eds.), *Recovery and well-being in the performing arts* (pp. 255–266). Routledge.

DOI: 10.4324/9781003566885-19

for transformation, as a form of creative physical rehabilitation, a multidimensional holistic journey of recovery, discovery, creativity, and resilience. Honouring the significant ways in which dance has played a role in community and cultural well-being throughout history, this chapter focuses on the interaction of *dance for health* with concepts of recovery through the shared experiences of *dance for health* leaders across three continents.

The role and function of dance continues to expand beyond the artistic stage and studio to encompass the support of well-being, health, and personal growth. This growing field, known as *dance for health* underscores the potential of dance to meaningfully impact lives, particularly for individuals managing degenerative conditions such as Parkinson's disease (PD), Multiple Sclerosis (MS), and the ageing process itself (Bruyneel, 2019; Chappell et al., 2021). For these populations, dance transcends the boundaries of physical activity to offer artistry and creativity that enrich life beyond functional recovery. Expanding rehabilitation pathways, dance incorporates elements of music, using improvisation, to stimulate creativity and connection – unlocking new dimensions of aliveness and presence.

To understand the transformative potential of dance and its role in recovery, it is crucial to start from a holistic understanding of recovery, the unique components of dance that support this process, and the perspectives of both participants and teaching artists (Booth, 2003; Fortin et al., 2023). Through narrative storytelling and ethnographic interviews, this chapter explores how dance fosters a nuanced understanding of recovery and agency. Building on Kellmann and Kallus's (2001, 2025) expanded perspectives of recovery, *dance for health* offers a key context for investigating the multilevel inter and intraindividual processes at work (Kallus, 2016), especially when framed by the experiences of those living with degenerative conditions from which there is no cure.

Medical philosopher Friedman (2021) views recovery as a journey towards a new state of well-being rather than a return to a former state. This approach highlights patient participation in achieving wholeness. Friedman's view extends beyond biomedical recovery to include personal and social dimensions, requiring adaptation in work and social life. The biomedical, personal, and social aspects of recovery are interconnected but can progress independently such that one may recover physically yet struggle socially and personally, or never fully recover physically yet still attain a sense of personal well-being and wholeness. Recovery is thus a dynamic process of continuous adaptation rather than a fixed destination (Huber et al., 2011).

Context: *Dance for health* in practice

Recently, the integration of dance into health and wellness initiatives has grown exponentially. Programmes such as Dance for PD (McRae et al., 2018; Westheimer, 2008) and other community-based initiatives highlight how dance can support individuals living with chronic and degenerative conditions. Research has shown that dance improves balance, other motor skills, and cognitive function in individuals with PD while fostering social connections and emotional well-being (Bearss & DeSouza, 2021; Haputhanthirige et al., 2023; Kalyani et al., 2019, 2020). For older adult populations, dance offers similar benefits and promotes positive health, encouraging individuals to remain active, and socially connected, while combating the decline provoked by isolation (Clifford et al., 2023; Podolski et al., 2023; Waugh et al., 2024). These dance initiatives cater to diverse populations, and aim to address the physical, emotional and psychological challenges of living with a degenerative condition. By focusing on creativity, connection, and artistic expression, dance provides participants with tools to navigate their conditions with resilience and optimism (Bruyneel, 2019).

The authors of this chapter are recognised *dance for health* leaders, facilitators, and artists, with established creative *dance for health* programmes. They share an artistic focus, drawing on formal dance training and professional performance, to deliver a multigenre approach of dance, musical theatre, opera, Eastern movement, and somatic practice that addresses the artistic objectives and contextual needs of participants and programmes. They contribute to the training and development of next-generation teaching artists and initiate parallel, ongoing research in the field.

The qualitative study presented in this chapter combines a process of collaborative autoethnography and grounded analysis drawing on the lived experience of three *dance for health* leaders across three continents: Australia, Europe, and North America. Collaborative autoethnography is a qualitative research method involving reflective dialogue and collective meaning-making, where personal stories are situated within broader societal, cultural, or institutional frameworks and collective insights can provide a deeper understanding (Hernandez et al., 2017; Lapadat, 2017; Malorni et al., 2023).

Through focus group discussions, the authors investigated their experiences as artists, their observations of participants, questions of practice, and considerations for further investigation, alongside analysis of existing research with their respective programmes.

Reframing recovery through dance

The implication of established definitions of recovery is that of a returning journey to a state of prior health or functionality. In the context of permanent loss of motor capacity or of degenerative health conditions such as certain cancers, MS and PD, or the condition of ageing itself, this returning journey narrative perpetuates unrealistic, unattainable goals, and reinforces a sense of failure to recover. The biomedical focus on the measurement of loss of function and faculties exacerbates this sense of failure to recover. Disease is understood as an objective physiological process on a fixed timeline, whereas the patient experiences illness subjectively, distinct from its medical classification (Carel, 2007). In the context of progressive or irreversible health conditions, recovery might be reframed as adaptation to new circumstances, to new physical, mental, and social health challenges and as the ability to successfully self-manage (Huber et al., 2011).

> Through a medical lens everything is about measuring the loss and managing the symptoms ... in a dance for health context ... We're only looking at what's possible now, today ... that's a great relief because it allows a sort of freedom to be better than a measure.
>
> *(Guss-West, personal communication, February 13, 2025)*

This perspective changes the focus of the journey of recovery from one of a restoration of a previous state to an emphasis on new possibilities and potential for new learning, skill development, and creative self-determination. Moving away from the *restoration narrative* a degenerative condition promotes a *quest narrative* (Frank, 1995), much like Campbell's Hero's Journey (1990) of reinvention. Leventhal shared that, "it's not 'getting back'. It's making a new sense and creating a new reality for oneself. That, to me, is the recovery that I see happening when people engage in dance" (personal communication, December 11, 2024).

Guss-West described recovery as the spiral path of Buddhist philosophy. "There's kind of no such thing as recovery to baseline for anybody ... It's the baseline shifted on that spiral", that leads onwards to a new perspective, promoting organic personal growth, agency, and adaptation to living with a degenerative health condition (personal communication, December 11, 2024). For many community participants, dance opens up multiple possibilities and an opportunity to explore scenarios extending beyond initial fixed perceptions and experiences, with a focus on personalised creative solutions. The creative process embraces the potential of the unexpected and proposes an ongoing journey of adaptation and self-discovery. Recovery in the face of such health challenges and loss of faculties demands a heightened presence and openness to the new, rather than a focus on past losses and paths traversed. Jeffrey highlighted the role of new identity formation: "a key element through dance is the opportunity for exploration, creative journeys that bring out the individual person, as opposed to the medical system where sometimes you become just another number" (personal communication, February 13, 2025).

Participants in Dance for PD programmes, for example, often report feeling "more like themselves" during and after sessions (Leventhal, personal communication, February 13, 2025). Participants frequently describe discovering a sense of freedom and flourishing in dance that transcends the limitations imposed by their conditions. From this perspective, recovery becomes a deeply personal journey of adaptation and new growth, shaped by the unique interplay of physical, emotional, social and artistic elements within the dance experience (Andreasson et al., 2024). This adaptability spans multiple domains, responding to personal bodily changes rather than external factors. It follows a cycle of disruption and response, highlighting the creative process of adaptation rather than its challenges and connects to finding health within illness (Carel, 2007).

Paradox in action – Perspectives of quality of life

A point of ongoing academic dialogue within *dance for health* is the frequent discrepancy between participants' positive, self-reported experiences of transformation and possibility, and new identity gathered in qualitative research (Andreasson et al., 2024; Houston, 2019; see Figure 15.1) and the seeming mismatch in correlation with quantitative data. Huber et al. (2011) address this potential gap in terms of self-reported health and recovery: "if people are able to develop successful strategies for coping, [age related] impaired functioning does not strongly change the perceived quality of life, a phenomenon known as the Disability Paradox" (2011, p. 2). The Disability Paradox refers to the experiences of many people living with disabilities who report a high quality of life despite facing significant physical limitations, health challenges, or societal barriers. This paradox challenges common assumptions

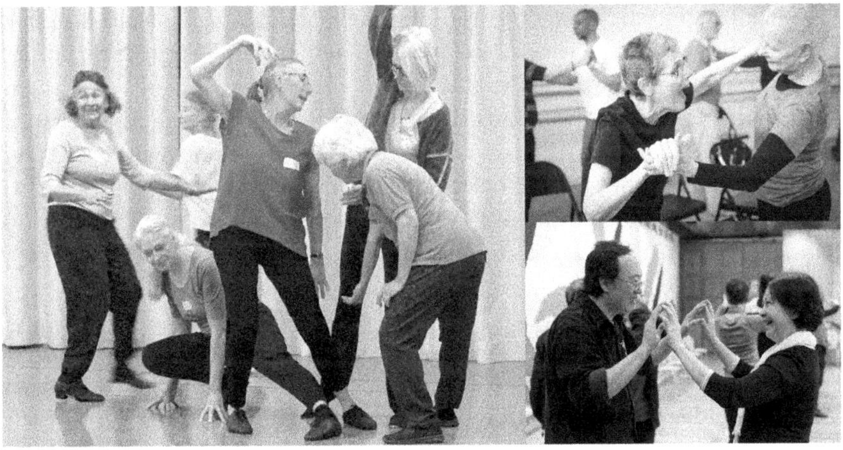

FIGURE 15.1 "Trilogy – Recovery through dance across three continents", a collage of dance for health classes in North America, Europe, and Australia, led by facilitators Erica Rose Jeffrey, Clare Guss-West, and David Leventhal.

Photo credits: Ellis Gaskell, Daniel Boud, and Nathalie Jufer.

that living with a disability inevitably leads to unhappiness or a lower quality of life (Albrecht & Devlieger, 1999; Fellinghauer et al., 2012). Carel (2007) observes that illness creates a divide between the biological and lived body, necessitating significant adaptation in social and physical interactions. This process highlights the interplay between adversity and creativity, reinforcing the notion that adaptability emerges as a positive response to illness.

Although researched in the field of medical philosophy, this phenomenon has not been widely accepted in medical practice, where in some cases up to 82% of doctors believe that people living with significant disabilities have a lower quality of life (Iezzoni et al., 2021). Recently there is a growing body of empirical research in the related area of the well-being paradox, according to which a more severe clinical condition is associated with a reported higher well-being and quality of life (Andonian et al., 2021).

Dance as a catalyst for health

The spaces where dance occurs are described by community participants as unique environments fostering exploration and reframing potential. Participants can find a new sense of belonging that contrasts with daily experiences of isolation (Carapellotti et al., 2023). Leventhal emphasised the transformative potential of dance spaces: "We tend to undervalue how significant it is for people with chronic conditions to walk into a space that is dedicated to dancing and acknowledge that they have a place there, that they're welcome" (personal communication, February 13, 2025).

Dance invites participants to reframe their abilities and identities, offering opportunities to experience joy, beauty, and agency within their bodies. The collective energy of a dance group can instigate a kind of entrainment effect that lifts the group's mindset, encouraging a shared adaptive perspective (Cross et al., 2019). As Guss-West noted, "you're seeing a kind of 'group effect' … bringing those who are less courageous or positive upwards into an 'I can do, I can manage, I can overcome' mindset" (personal communication, February 13, 2025).

Embodied, social, and emotional dimensions

The benefits of dance as a physical activity have been extensively researched within the older adult population (Clifford et al., 2023). Results show practical benefits such as improved walking speeds and balance as a result of creative dance programmes that naturally support day-to-day activities (Schärli & Guss-West, 2025).

Encouraging safe physical challenges is essential to supporting well-being outcomes (Clifford et al., 2023). In various mixed-methods studies of a creative dance programme, participants highlighted, "that their movement repertoire had increased and that, within the dance sessions, they dare to do things they would not normally do" (Schärli & Guss-West, 2025, p. 6). "You act differently. You stand differently. You walk differently. You really move differently when you dance" (Mataj, 2023, p. 20).[1]

The authors of this chapter agreed on the importance of providing challenges and spaces which foster risk-taking and develop courage (Rehfeld et al., 2018). Leventhal reflected that, "participants are encouraged to push boundaries safely, leading to physical, cognitive and psychological growth and enhanced neuroplasticity" (personal communication, December 11, 2024). Guss-West highlighted the benefits of challenges proposed through improvisation (Fong Yan et al., 2024). Opportunities for improvisation increase participants' spontaneity, "allowing yourself to be in a space, to not control the response or try to plan it that's a huge psychological development and a shift in mindset" (Guss-West, personal communication, February 13, 2025).

The participants in Schärli and Guss-West's (2025) study echoed these sentiments: "I've actually become more open again ... this openness is part of me, but it still takes practice". They enjoyed being confronted with challenges and found that they were more confident, and that the dance sessions shifted boundaries within them. Schärli and Guss-West (2025, p. 6) suggest that participants' willingness to take new risks indicates possible increases in movement variability and that "dance might increase the functionality of the motor system and thus contribute to an enhanced adaptability to new situations".

Beyond its benefits as a physical activity, dance is a medium for experiencing and expressing a wide range of emotions and fosters growth by prompting participants to challenge boundaries. As one participant states, "there is no pressure, but it is demanding. This mixture of no pressure and yet demands, I often think that it should have started earlier" (Mataj, 2023, p. 25).

Dance for health participants' experiences are documented in abundant qualitative research evidencing the transformative power of dance and the physical, mental, emotional and social well-being benefits (Bearss & DeSouza, 2021; Brook & Booth, 2022; Carapellotti et al., 2023; DeFarias et al., in press; Jola et al., 2022; McRae et al., 2018). These narratives reveal how dance supports not only physical but also emotional adaptability, resilience, and social connection. For individuals facing health challenges, dance offers a space to reclaim agency, explore and redefine their relationship with their bodies, frequently renewing a sense of joy and life purpose. Participants share inspirational observations such as, "life [is easier for me because of dance]. ... It lifts your spirits ... there are things that you wouldn't normally do in life ... it pushes you to your limits. So that you go beyond them" (Mataj, 2023, p. 21). This phenomenon is also identified by Carel (2007), who proposes that serious illness can foster a deep appreciation for the present moment and often leads to a unique, creative perspective.

Participants report that this renewed sense of joy and purpose transcends the boundaries of the dance session to permeate life's challenging situations (Andreasson et al., 2024). They shared emotional examples of how dance enabled them to transfer their experiences: "I did that in the hospital too. I imagined myself dancing" (Mataj, 2023, p. 19).

Practical collaborative learning strategies

Dance for health teaching artists play a central role in fostering this multidimensional recovery and growth through dance. They create an environment where participants feel safe to explore, to try new challenges, and connect with their artistic selves, by emphasising non-judgmental learning approaches that promote individual agency.

Dance offers a framework to reshape narratives about what is achievable. Jeffrey connected dance to possibilities: "it's having the opportunity to practice possibility – in order to be able to see possibilities or a different life journey" (personal communication, December 11, 2024). Using non-body-focused instructions, teaching artists guide participants' focus strategically to artistic components such as movement quality, imagery and musicality. This focus on artistic dance elements facilitates motor control and learning (Chua et al., 2021) and allows participants to immerse themselves in the process and enjoyment of dancing, in the moment. Together with autonomy supportive strategies, this focus reinforces a cycle of increased motivation, enhanced mental and emotional well-being, and, potentially, dopamine release (Guss-West & Leventhal, 2024; Wulf & Lewthwaite, 2016).

These are transformative focus of attention strategies (Guss-West, 2021; Guss-West & Leventhal, 2024) that transfer beyond the dancing space to provide tools for day-to-day challenges. Shifting perspectives renders dance a kind of physical meditation that has the capacity to promote profound physiological and emotional change witnessed in dance practice.

Across multiple contexts, participants describe the transformative experience of rediscovering beauty and joy in their movement, an antidote to the perception of their bodies as 'problems' to be managed (Bek et al., 2022; Houston, 2019). The teaching artist and dance context enable participants to be immersed in the creative process (Dingle et al., 2021). "Permission to be in the 'present' moment is a powerful tool for healing and transformation", suggested Guss-West; it relieves, for that moment, pressure to focus on limitation and control of symptoms (personal communication, February 13, 2025). The authors witness that the process of facilitating dance can also be a deeply transformative experience for the teaching artists themselves, reigniting a sense of meaning and passion for dance and redefining their continuing role within the art form.

Conclusions and recommendations for practice

Exploring the intersection of dance, health, and recovery, the multidimensional physical, social, and creative elements of dance are seen to contribute to well-being. By emphasising creativity, connection, and artistic expression, dance redefines what it means to recover in the context of degenerative conditions and the challenges of ageing. This perspective expands conventional narratives of loss of functionality and quality of life, offering options of flourishing, courage, agency and transformation.

The potential of dance as a vital modality for recovery in all its dimensions – biomedical, personal, and social – warrants further investigation and innovation. By incorporating perspectives from teaching artists, participants, and interdisciplinary researchers, the field can continue to expand its application in health and well-being. Grounded in embodied dimensions, dance serves as a lifeline, reinforcing the intricate connection between mind and body while offering a dynamic, nuanced and creative pathway to healing, resilience, and personal transformation.

Note

1 The unpublished, research study and thesis of Arbëri Mataj, Bern University, Institute for Sport Science (2023) "Tanz für die Gesundheit: Wie ältere Frauen von regelmässigem Tanz profitieren" (Dance for Health: How Older Women benefit from regular dance), Institut für Sportwissenschaft, Universität Bern, supervisor Dr Andrea Schärli. The bachelor study captured qualitative feedback on the physical, mental, and social impact of participation in 'Seniorstars', creative dance programme, Bern Ballet led by Clare Guss-West. It was part of a larger research "Dance Interventions for different population groups" with ethics approval and the basis for the Schärli and Guss-West (2024) publication.

References

Albrecht, G. L., & Devlieger, P. J. (1999). The disability paradox: High quality of life against all odds. *Social Science & Medicine*, *48*(8), 977–988.

Andonian, C. S., Freilinger, S., Achenbach, S., Ewert, P., Gundlach, U., Hoerer, J., Kaemmerer, H., Pieper, L., Weyand, M., Neidenbach, R. C., & Beckmann, J. (2021). 'Well-being paradox' revisited: A cross-sectional study of quality of life in over 4000 adults with congenital heart disease. *BMJ Open*, *11*(6), e049531. https://doi.org/10.1136/bmjopen-2021-049531

Andreasson, I., Ann, B., Sofi, F., Paula, B., Katarzyna, F., Ida-Klara, J., & Santos Tavares Silva, I. (2024). Dance for Parkinson, multifaceted experiences of persons living with Parkinson's Disease. *Scandinavian Journal of Occupational Therapy*, *31*(1), 2411206. https://doi.org/10.1080/11038128.2024.2411206

Bearss, K. A., & DeSouza, J. F. X. (2021). Parkinson's disease motor symptom progression slowed with multisensory dance learning over 3-years: A preliminary longitudinal investigation. *Brain Sciences*, *11*(7), 895. https://doi.org/10.3390/brainsci11070895

Beckmann, J., Kellmann, M., & Jakowski, S. (2023). Recovery is more than just healing: Advocating a broader perspective on recovery in physical and mental health. In M. Kellmann, S. Jakowski, & J. Beckmann (Eds.), *The importance of recovery for physical and mental health: Negotiating the effects of underrecovery* (pp. 266–270). Routledge.

Bek, J., Arakaki, A. I., Derbyshire-Fox, F., Ganapathy, G., Sullivan, M., & Poliakoff, E. (2022). More than movement: Exploring motor simulation, creativity, and function in co-developed dance for Parkinson's. *Frontiers in Psychology*, *13*, 731264. https://doi.org/10.3389/fpsyg.2022.731264

Blevins, P., Erskine, S., Hopper, L., & Moyle, G. M. (2020). Finding your balance. *Journal of Dance Education*, *20*(1), 12–22.

Booth, E. (2003). Seeking definition: What is a teaching artist? *Teaching Artist Journal*, *1*(1), 5–12.

Brook, J., & Booth, A. (2022). May I have this dance: Examining a community based dance program for people living with Parkinson's disease. *Research in Dance Education*, *23*(4), 470–484.

Bruyneel, A. V. (2019). Effects of dance activities on patients with chronic pathologies: Scoping review. *Heliyon*, *5*(7), e02104. https://doi.org/10.1016/j.heliyon.2019.e02104

Campbell, J. (1990). *The hero's journey*. Harper & Row.

Carapellotti, A. M., Meijerink, H., Gravemaker-Scott, C., Thielman, L., Kool, R., Lewin, N., & Abma, T. A. (2023). Escape, expand, embrace: The transformational lived experience of rediscovering the self and the other while dancing with Parkinson's or Multiple Sclerosis. *International Journal of Qualitative Studies on Health and Well-being*, *18*(1), 2143611. https://doi.org/10.1080/17482631.2022.2143611

Carel, H. (2007). Can I be ill and happy? *Philosophia*, *35*(2), 95–110.

Chappell, K., Redding, E., Crickmay, U., Stancliffe, R., Jobbins, V., & Smith, S. (2021). The aesthetic, artistic and creative contributions of dance for health and wellbeing across the lifecourse: A systematic review. *International Journal of Qualitative Studies on Health and Well-Being*, *16*(1), 1950891. https://doi.org/10.1080/17482631.2021.1950891

Chua, L. K., Jimenez-Diaz, J., Lewthwaite, R., Kim, T., & Wulf, G. (2021). Superiority of external attentional focus for motor performance and learning: Systematic reviews and meta-analyses. *Psychological Bulletin*, *147*(6), 618–645.

Clifford, A. M., Joanne, S., Jennifer, M., Triona, C., Aoife, O. N., Marie, O. G., Quinette, L., & Ní Bhriain, O. (2023). The effect of dance on physical health and cognition in community dwelling older adults: A systematic review and meta-analysis. *Arts & Health*, *15*(2), 200–228.

Cross, L., Turgeon, M., & Atherton, G. (2019). How moving together binds us together: The social consequences of interpersonal entrainment and group processes. *Open Psychology*, *1*, 273–302.

DeFarias, E. G. A., DeJesus, B. M., DeSantana, J. M., & Teixeira-Machado, L. (in press). Dancing through Parkinson's: Impacts on quality of life and socioemotional experiences. *Journal of Dance Medicine & Science*. https://doi.org/10.1177/1089313X251330753

De Wet, J. S., Africa, E., & Venter, R. (2022). Recovery-stress states of professional ballet dancers during different phases of a ballet season. *Journal of Dance Medicine & Science*, *26*(1), 8–15.

Dingle, G. A., Sharman, L. S., Bauer, Z., Beckman, E., Broughton, M., Bunzli, E., Davidson, R., Draper, G., Fairley, S., Farrell, C., Flynn, L. M., Gomersall, S., Hong, M., Larwood, J., Lee, C., Lee, J., Nitschinsk, L., Peluso, N., Reedman, S. E., … Wright, O. R. L. (2021). How do music activities affect health and well-being? A scoping review of studies examining psychosocial mechanisms. *Frontiers in Psychology*, *12*, 713818. https://doi.org/10.3389/fpsyg.2021.713818

Fellinghauer, B., Reinhardt, J. D., Stucki, G., & Bickenbach, J. (2012). Explaining the disability paradox: A cross-sectional analysis of the Swiss general population. *BMC Public Health*, *12*(1), 655. https://doi.org/10.1186/1471-2458-12-655

Fong Yan, A., Nicholson, L. L., Ward, R. E., Hiller, C. E., Dovey, K., Parker, H. M., Low, L. F., Moyle, G., & Chan, C. (2024). The effectiveness of dance interventions on psychological and cognitive health outcomes compared with other forms of physical activity: A systematic review with meta-analysis. *Sports Medicine*, *54*(5), 1179–1205.

Fortin, S., Lucie, B., Raymond, C., Duval, H., Patricia, M., Sylvie, T., Guylaine, V., & Swaine, B. (2023). All dancing bodies matter: Six facilitators aiming for inclusion and wellbeing for people with special needs. *Research in Dance Education*, *24*(4), 392–409.

Frank, A. W. (1995). *The wounded storyteller: Body, illness, and ethics*. University of Chicago Press.

Friedman, Y. (2021). On recovery: Re-directing the concept by differentiation of its meanings. *Medicine, Health Care and Philosophy*, *24*(3), 389–399.

Guss-West, C. (2021). *Attention and focus in dance: Enhancing, power, precision, and artistry*. Human Kinetics.

Guss-West, C., & Leventhal, D. (2024). *Attention and focus strategies for dance educators*. Human Kinetics.

Haputhanthirige, N. K. H., Sullivan, K., Moyle, G. M., Brauer, S., Jeffrey, E. R., & Kerr, G. (2023). Effects of dance on gait and dual-task gait in Parkinson's disease. *PloS ONE*, *18*(1), e0280635. https://doi.org/10.1371/journal.pone.0280635

Hernandez, K.-A. C., Chang, H., & Ngunjiri, F. W. (2017). Collaborative autoethnography as multivocal, relational, and democratic research: Opportunities, challenges, and aspirations. *a/b: Auto/Biography Studies*, *32*(2), 251–254.

Houston, S. (2019). *Dancing with Parkinson's*. Intellect Books.

Huber, M., Knottnerus, J. A., Green, L., van der Horst, H., Jadad, A. R., Kromhout, D., Leonard, B., Lorig, K., Loureiro, M. I., van der Meer, J. W., Schnabel, P., Smith, R., van Weel, C., & Smid, H. (2011). How should we define health? *BMJ*, *343*, d4163. https://doi.org/10.1136/bmj.d4163

Iezzoni, L. I., Rao, S. R., Ressalam, J., Bolcic-Jankovic, D., Agaronnik, N. D., Donelan, K., Lagu, T., & Campbell, E. G. (2021). Physicians' perceptions of people with disability and their health care. *Health Affairs*, *40*(2), 297–306.

Jola, C., Sundström, M., & McLeod, J. (2022). Benefits of dance for Parkinson's: The music, the moves, and the company. *PloS ONE*, *17*(11), e0265921. https://doi.org/10.1371/journal.pone.0265921

Kallus, K. W. (2016). Stress and recovery: An overview. In K. W. Kallus & M. Kellmann (Eds.), *The Recovery-Stress Questionnaires: User manual* (pp. 27–48). Pearson Assessment.

Kalyani, H. H. N., Sullivan, K., Moyle, G. M., Brauer, S., Jeffrey, E. R., & Kerr, G. (2019). Impacts of dance on cognition, psychological symptoms and quality of life in Parkinson's disease. *NeuroRehabilitation*, *45*(2), 273–283.

Kalyani, H. H., Sullivan, K. A., Moyle, G. M., Brauer, S. G., Jeffrey, E. R., & Kerr, G. K. (2020). Dance improves symptoms, functional mobility and fine manual dexterity in people with Parkinson disease: A quasi-experimental controlled efficacy study. *European Journal of Physical and Rehabilitation Medicine*, *56*(5), 563–574.

Kellmann, M., & Kallus, K. W. (2001). *The Recovery-Stress Questionnaire for Athletes; manual*. Human Kinetics.

Kellmann, M., & Kallus, K. W. (Eds.). (2025). *The Recovery-Stress Questionnaires: A user manual*. Routledge.

Lapadat, J. C. (2017). Ethics in autoethnography and collaborative autoethnography. *Qualitative Inquiry*, *23*(8), 589–603.

Malorni, A., Diaz, A., Spencer, M. S., & Jones, T. (2023). Collaborative autoethnography as a tool for research–practice partnerships: Facilitating self and school transformation. *Qualitative Social Work*, *22*(4), 643–662.

Mataj, A. (2023). *Tanz für die Gesundheit: Wie ältere Frauen von regelmässigem Tanz profitieren* [Dance for health: How older women benefit from regular dancing]. Bern University.

McRae, C., Leventhal, D., Westheimer, O., Mastin, T., Utley, J., & Russell, D. (2018). Long-term effects of dance for PD® on self-efficacy among persons with Parkinson's disease. *Arts & Health*, *10*(1), 85–96.

Podolski, O. S., Whitfield, T., Schaaf, L., Cornaro, C., Köbe, T., Koch, S., & Wirth, M. (2023). The impact of dance movement interventions on psychological health in older adults without dementia: A systematic review and meta-analysis. *Brain Sciences*, *13*(7), 981. https://doi.org/10.3390/brainsci13070981

Rehfeld, K., Lüders, A., Hökelmann, A., Lessmann, V., Kaufmann, J., Brigadski, T., Müller, P., & Müller, N. G. (2018). Dance training is superior to repetitive physical exercise in inducing brain plasticity in the elderly. *PLoS ONE*, *13*(7), e0196636. https://doi.org/10.1371/journal.pone.0196636

Schärli, A., & Guss-West, C. (2025). Exploring the essence of a creative dance programme for older adults: Programme overview and research insights. *Geriatric Nursing*, *62*(Pt A), 254–261.

Waugh, M., Youdan, G., Jr., Casale, C., Balaban, R., Cross, E. S., & Merom, D. (2024). The use of dance to improve the health and wellbeing of older adults: A global scoping review of research trials. *PLoS ONE*, *19*(10), e0311889. https://doi.org/10.1371/journal.pone.0311889

Westheimer, O. (2008). Why dance for Parkinson's disease. *Topics in Geriatric Rehabilitation*, *24*(2), 127–140.

Wulf, G., & Lewthwaite, R. (2016). Optimizing performance through intrinsic motivation and attention for learning: The optimal theory of motor learning. *Psychonomic Bulletin & Review*, *23*(5), 1382–1414.

16

THE REPARATIVE ARTIST

CoActive therapeutic theatre in service of recovery

Dave Mowers and Laura L. Wood

Introductory framework: Drama therapy and therapeutic theatre

Stress and lack of or inadequate recovery are major problems for artists in the performing arts, but also for society as a whole. One-dimensional approaches to recovery are inadequate. Drama therapy appears to be an excellent way to achieve individualised, comprehensive recovery. Drama therapy is defined as the intentional use of drama and theatre techniques for therapeutic purposes (Landy, 1994) and positions the practitioner as both a clinician and an artist, balancing mental health expertise with creative expression. This dual focus allows the field and practice of drama therapy to be applied across diverse settings and to address a wide range of diagnoses as well as community-oriented work. On the clinical side, drama therapy may be used to treat formal diagnoses such as anxiety, depression, or post-traumatic stress disorder (PTSD). Regarding community-based work drama therapy may be delivered in places such as after-school programmes, religious organisations, community centres, or summer camps and focus on topics such as character development, skill development, or bullying. In both settings, successful drama therapy interventions have demonstrated their capacity to foster psychological resilience, advance personal growth, and support the development of healthy relationships (Johnson & Emunah, 2020). Drama therapy is practised globally in a wide range of clinical and community settings.

Mowers, D., & Wood, L. L. (2026). The reparative artist: CoActive therapeutic theatre in service of recovery. In E. Altenmüller, M. Kellmann, J. Beckmann, & G. M. Moyle (Eds.), *Recovery and well-being in the performing arts* (pp. 267–283). Routledge.

DOI: 10.4324/9781003566885-20

Drama therapy approaches are as varied as the artists, researchers, and clinicians who practice them, reflecting the diversity of theoretical foundations within the field. As a profession, drama therapists receive training in a wide range of frameworks, including *Developmental Transformations* (Johnson, 2009), *Role Theory and Method* (Landy, 1994), and the *Five-Phase Model* (Emunah, 2019). Additionally, they gain skills in psychodrama (Moreno, 1987), explore playback theatre (Fox, 2004), and examine the therapeutic applications of performance (Pendzik et al., 2017). Despite these varied approaches, a set of core processes unites the field. These core processes, first articulated by Jones (2007), serve as the foundation for effective drama therapy. Frydman et al. (2022) formalised these core processes in drama therapy in North America by conducting a Delphi study, which gave North American drama therapists a shared definition of these processes. These include: dramatic reality, dramatic play, multidimensional relationship, active witnessing, distancing, dramatic projection, and embodiment. Additionally, De Witte et al. (2021) examined the therapeutic factors and mechanisms of change in creative arts therapies, identifying how various artistic modalities contribute to psychological and emotional healing, further advancing the field's understanding of its efficacy and adaptability across diverse contexts.

These core processes lay the groundwork for more specialised approaches within the field, such as therapeutic theatre. Therapeutic theatre involves the intentional use of performance to address psychological, social, and physical concerns while promoting health and well-being (Snow et al., 2003). At its essence, therapeutic theatre asserts that performance is healing as a way to explore oneself, a presenting problem, or a set of relationships. In a recent film on therapeutic theatre, Israeli drama therapist Susana Pendzik noted that "therapeutic theater" can include many types of material, including 'plays that a group thinks are interesting to them for some reason' (Sajnani, 2022, w. p.). The presence of an audience is considered a helpful adjunct to personal goals. In therapeutic theatre an audience may be closed, invited, or public.

There is extensive writing on the use of therapeutic theatre for readers who would like a comprehensive overview (Emunah, 2019; Hodermarska, 2013; Pendzik et al., 2017). However, the primary research on therapeutic theatre has been qualitative, with criticism from larger psychological disciplines struggling to replicate the process to drive empirical data (Addis et al., 2006). Thus, Wood and Mowers (2019, 2024) have worked to manualise a model that also occupies a distinctive space by offering structured guidelines for integrating performance into recovery-oriented practices called The CoActive Therapeutic Theatre (CoATT) model. CoATT, situated at the intersection of drama therapy and community theatre, involves creating and performing an original play for a public audience in support of mental health recovery.

The CoActive therapeutic theatre model: A structured approach to recovery through performance

The CoATT model occupies a distinct place within what Wood and Mowers (2024, p. 13) have termed the "quilt of therapeutic theater" as the only manualised model of its kind. Unlike broader therapeutic theatre approaches, which often operate without a set framework, CoATT provides structured guidelines for practitioners to engage participants in play-making and performance as part of the recovery process.

At its core, CoATT is designed to support individuals in transition, whether they are moving between levels of care, reintegrating into daily life after intensive treatment, or navigating the complexities of sustained recovery. The model recognises that this transitional phase is often marked by uncertainty and a sense of disconnection, and it seeks to bridge this gap by fostering connection, agency, and creative exploration. Unlike models that frame recovery as an endpoint, CoATT understands recovery as an active, evolving process, in which participants reclaim their narratives and re-engage with their communities.

CoATT productions are guided by six key principles, each of which reinforces the model's commitment to intentionality, collaboration, and narrative transformation:

1 CoATT productions answer a question. Each production begins with a central inquiry: *What is a theme of recovery you want to explore and share with an audience in service of strengthening your recovery?* This question acts as a guiding framework, ensuring that the creative process remains anchored in the participants' lived experiences while maintaining aesthetic distance.
2 Participants must identify as being in active recovery. CoATT defines active recovery as "an action-oriented process of engagement, driven by the new narrative one constructs for themselves beyond treatment" (p. 14). This definition bridges medical models of recovery – such as those outlined by the DSM – with socially constructed approaches that centre lived experience and personal agency.
3 CoATT is co-active in all elements of creation, performance, and interdisciplinary collaboration. The model is fundamentally collaborative, integrating participants, facilitators, and audience members into a shared creative process. This co-active approach ensures that power is distributed rather than hierarchical, reinforcing the idea that recovery is a communal effort rather than an isolated experience.
4 CoATT is not autobiographical. As Butler notes in the foreword to *Recovery and Drama Therapy: The CoActive Therapeutic Theatre Model*, CoATT "uses therapeutic theatre to focus on the active experience of recovery"

through a "co-constructed fictional narrative" (Wood & Mowers, 2024, p. xi). This use of metaphor and aesthetic distance allows participants to engage deeply with their experiences without becoming retraumatised or overly exposed. By crafting fictional narratives, participants can explore multiple facets of their identity, including the selves they hope to become.

5 CoATT requires a public presentation. The final performance is not merely a showcase but a ritual of reintegration, in which participants step into the role of both performer and storyteller, reclaiming their agency in a public space. Unlike traditional theatre, where an audience passively observes, CoATT positions the audience as witnesses, co-creating an interactive and communal experience that reinforces recovery as a shared, social process.

6 CoATT is manualised and offered at a specific point in the treatment continuum. Unlike less structured therapeutic theatre approaches, CoATT is designed to be introduced at a specific moment in a person's recovery journey, when they are ready to take ownership of their story and engage in an active, creative process. This structure ensures that participants can safely and effectively navigate the complexities of recovery while benefiting from the model's emphasis on autonomy and self-expression.

Once participants in recovery are identified, the principles are delivered across seven movements, which are typically delivered over 12–18 weeks. The seven movements facilitated by a team of two CoATT practitioners are: recruitment, discovery, generation, performance intensive, rehearsal, public performance and launch. In recruitment participants recovering from a similar ailment are identified, screened, and contracted for inclusion. In the discovery movement, the group organises itself around themes common to their recovery and answers the CoATT question. In generation, participants are generating material towards the creation of a script, such as scenes and monologues. The generation is driven by the manualised drama therapy exercises. In the performance-intensive shifts the focus of the group towards making and presenting a play with a focus on acting skills and story development. In rehearsal the play is being staged and rehearsed while participants are reflecting on how does the play mirror the recovery process. In movement six the CoATT model culminates in a performance for a public, open audience. The launch movement allows the group to reflect on the experience, solidify new relationship and recovery skills, and terminate with the CoATT practitioners (Figure 16.1).

CoATT research indicates that growth in recovery happens against the process of producing a play. By working together as a group, exploring new roles through metaphor, and practising recovery through the life-drama connection participants use public performance as a successful re-connection with the community at large.

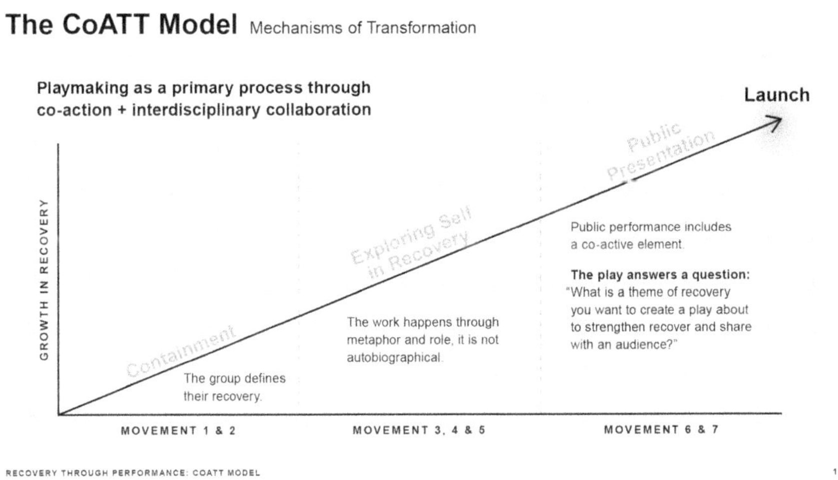

FIGURE 16.1 The CoATT model.

Through its structured yet flexible approach, CoATT reframes recovery as a creative and communal journey, rather than a solitary or clinical process. By using story, role, and performance, CoATT helps participants explore their identities, reconnect with their communities, and engage in a meaning-making process that extends beyond treatment and into their lived experience (Wood & Mowers, 2024).

Recovery in mental health

Recovery in mental health encompasses a range of definitions and frameworks, each reflecting distinct perspectives on how individuals regain a sense of wellness and functionality and aligning with the theoretical underpinnings of a view of human nature (Beckmann et al., 2023). That 'extension of perspective' on recovery describes the landscape in which CoATT came into practice. A central focus of the CoATT Model is for participants to operationalise a concept of recovery that serves their individual needs and reflects their values. This conception revolves around understanding how recovery works and what actions or support are needed to maintain the state of recovery. In North America, this awareness may begin in treatment centres but is often developed outside of formal treatment.

Medical and psychiatric models define recovery as the absence of criteria listed in classification manuals such as the DSM-5-TR (American Psychiatric Association, 2013). For instance, an individual with an eating disorder is considered 'recovered' when binge-purge or restrictive behaviours cease; someone with a substance-use disorder meets recovery criteria when substances are no longer consumed; and a client with

PTSD is deemed in recovery when intrusive flashbacks and hypervigilance subside. These diagnostic boxes are easy to track, yet they often miss the subtle truths of comprehensive recovery. For example, medical models will say recovery from an eating disorder is purely an absence of symptoms, whereas true recovery from an eating disorder often requires a deep renegotiation with the body, primary relationships that the ED had replaced, and movement (Noordenbos, 2011a, 2011b). These less tangible components to recovery have been overlooked in the medical and psychiatric models but are increasingly being understood as necessary for long-lasting, meaningful recovery.

CoATT recognising the limitations of medical models aligns with Altenmüller et al. (this volume, Chapter 1) view which state that recovery is more than simply 'getting back to normal' (or as we might equate in a mental health framework, more than just the absence of symptoms). Building on Kellmann and Kallus's multilevel model (2001, 2025), in CoATT we define recovery as an ongoing psychological, physiological, and social process that restores, and ideally expands, one's recovery beyond the medical baseline. In our work, the rehearsal space becomes a microcosm for this process, offering individuals the opportunity to practice new roles and rehearse emerging scripts of identity and agency, including being re-introduced to stressful situations in recovery. We rehearse this through metaphor in our theatrical process and see this view as resonating with Antonovsky's (1987) salutogenic model, in which recovery functions as a resource that strengthens resistance and preparation for future stress.

Social constructivist models offer a more expansive view of recovery, recognising it as a highly individualised and collective process that honours multiple truths in defining recovery (Cottone, 2017). In these models, individuals and communities co-create pathways towards recovery by identifying and adopting behaviours that support meaningful and fulfilling lives post-crisis. For example, harm-reduction approaches work with each individual to assess their own goals, meeting the client where they are in the recovery process with a focus on agency and community engagement. This perspective aligns recovery with ongoing personal growth and social reintegration, rather than an endpoint (Marlatt, 1996).

Populations using new recovery frameworks, including those living with chronic or serious and persistent mental illness (SPMI), find that wellness recovery models may offer a more sustainable approach to treatment. These models adapt the action-oriented strategies of other recovery paradigms but apply them within the context of conditions that may never fully resolve. By centring the lived experiences of individuals with SPMI, wellness recovery models challenge the medical model's reliance on expert knowledge and its implicit assumptions about normalcy and functionality (Cheung et al., 2022).

Biopsychosocial models of stress and recovery

Biopsychosocial models of stress and recovery begin with an understanding of stress as a fundamental physiological and psychological process. Within these frameworks, recovery is conceptualised as the return to an optimal state of performance readiness or a balanced psychobiological equilibrium (Kellmann & Kallus, 2025). These models extend beyond a simple stress-response cycle by identifying stress as the internal and external conditions that push an individual's body and mind beyond its normal range of functioning. Recovery, then, is the critical process by which both the mind and body regain their equilibrium after peak performance, ensuring resilience and continued performance.

Established definitions in psychological and ergonomic research create a conceptual framework distinguishing stress and recovery, while emphasising their interrelated nature. Stress is defined as a state beyond normal functioning, while recovery is a broader concept. Such a framework supports a nuanced assessment of individual responses to stressors and recovery processes.

The Recovery-Stress Questionnaire (Kellmann & Kallus, 2001, 2025) integrates findings from various fields, including psychology and biology, to assess stress and recovery. The assessment tool is based on a biopsychosocial model that connects stress with health and illness through physiological and psychological pathways. This model emphasises the importance of recovery processes in maintaining health.

The recovery-stress balance model integrates cognitive stress concepts with action-oriented approaches, highlighting the importance of recovery in managing stress. Recovery is essential for restoring resources depleted during stress. Recovery is a complex, multilevel process that encompasses various physiological and psychological components. It can be categorised into passive, active, and proactive recovery methods.

Given the challenge for empirical measurement in mental health care settings, these qualitative methodologies may offer a more nuanced understanding of strain, capturing its subjective and individualised nature in ways that quantitative measures alone may not (Strauss & Corbin, 1990).

Understanding stress, strain, and recovery within biopsychosocial models is essential for developing effective interventions, particularly in high-performance domains. By recognising the delicate balance between exertion and recuperation, practitioners can better support individuals in maintaining long-term well-being and peak performance.

Stress and strain in the CoATT model

Participants in the CoATT model frequently report both stress and strain in their recovery journeys. Many addictions impose significant physical tolls on the body, and survivors of medical trauma may face ongoing challenges as they attempt to reintegrate into a world not always accommodating of their new abilities. The tension between external stressors and internal strain is as apparent in mental health recovery as it is in sports performance, further highlighting the need for individualised and context-sensitive approaches.

Recovery beyond 'before and after'

In traditional conceptions of recovery, there is an implied 'before and after' in the lived experience of individuals struggling with mental health challenges. These models often assume a trajectory in which a person moves from illness to wellness, from dysfunction to function. This linear notion of recovery is insufficient for those living with SPMI or chronic physical conditions as they require a model that acknowledges that their condition may not change or resolve in a traditional sense.

This is where wellness recovery models emerge. Unlike conventional recovery frameworks that emphasise a return to a prior state of health, wellness recovery integrates action-oriented approaches while recognising that recovery may mean adapting, growing, and finding equilibrium within an ongoing condition. Using a post-modern lens, wellness recovery remains grounded in the lived experience of those with serious and persistent challenges.

CoATT and the space between

The CoATT model is introduced at a specific moment in the treatment continuum – a point that exists between the 'before' and 'after' of conventional recovery. This undefined space is often a time of vulnerability, where individuals may have stabilised but are still grappling with what comes next. A helpful starting point for understanding this space comes from psychologists Kuhl and Beckmann (1994), who explore alienation. They described alienation as a state of powerlessness, social isolation, and estrangement from shared cultural beliefs. Drawing on Karl Marx's concept of labour alienation, they suggest that alienation can arise when an individual engages in an activity that is no longer intrinsically rewarding (Bottomore, 1963). This perspective provides a compelling lens through which to understand the experiences of many CoATT participants.

Medical models offer structured interventions that address immediate mental health crises. Once those crises have passed, patients may find themselves disconnected from a sense of engagement or incentive. The routines of structured care may leave them feeling like passive recipients rather than active participants in their recovery. This loss of autonomy, what Kuhl and Beckmann (1994) describe as a volitional impairment, can create a cycle in which individuals struggle to perceive their own emotional needs and preferences, feeling trapped between external expectations and an internal disconnection from self.

CoATT as an antidote to alienation

This exploration of alienation is central to the discovery and generation movements within the CoATT model, corresponding to the treatment phase of "exploring self in recovery" (p. 33). CoATT practitioners view this exploration not just as an exercise in role-play but as an essential component of growth in recovery. Through play-making, individuals engage with their sense of self in a way that restores autonomy, fosters creative agency, and reconnects them with intrinsic motivation.

The work of Landy (1994) on aesthetic distancing further illuminates this process. Drawing from Bertolt Brecht's concept of the alienation effect, who was both a theatre-maker and a clinician, argued that theatrical techniques could create a necessary distance between an individual and their emotions, allowing for deeper reflection and transformation, putting cognition and affect in harmony. In CoATT, this principle is at play as participants collaboratively construct narratives that externalise and examine their experiences. Through the shared act of play-making, they are able to step outside of feelings of alienation and move toward a re-engagement with their own agency and self-perception.

As participants approach the final phase of CoATT – the moment of performance – they are not simply stepping into a role but launching into a newly constructed reality, one that they have actively shaped. This process embodies the very heart of wellness recovery: not a return to a previous state, but the creation of new possibilities for meaning, connection, and self-determination.

The role of the reparative artist

CoATT plays allow participants (and audience members) to explore the power of the artist. Beckmann et al. (2023) posited that a multidimensional recovery would include strengthening an individual's personal understanding of meaning and purpose to foster resilience. Recalling that 'role' is a projective object that is central to the core processes of dramatherapy, *Landy's Role Taxonomy* described the function of the Artist as "asserting the creative principle, envisioning new forms, and transforming old ones" (Landy, 1996, p. 241). The inclusion of an *artist* in the story, or choosing to portray an *artist,* is an implicit statement that transformation is vital to recovery. Such roles may appear as sub-types such as *the poet, the dreamer*, or *the performer.* Stevens (2023) acknowledged the many forms that role may take in his Black American Role Taxonomy, expanding the repertoire of roles with awareness of cultural specificity and lived experience. CoATT practitioners view the artist figure as a conduit to intuition, coping tools, and the ability to reconnect to deeper truths. It should be no surprise that this role is needed when stepping into a new narrative after overcoming a serious challenge in life. CoATT sees the artist as reparative.

Outcomes of CoATT productions are measured against our participants' goals. These goals rarely include 'creating and presenting a play', focusing instead on how they hope their lives will improve through active recovery. CoATT addresses treatment goals on both individual and group levels. Therefore, engaging with the model is best achieved in a cohort facing a shared health challenge.

CoATT productions are not intended to be didactic, nor educational about diseases or conditions, but rather to tell good stories that engage an audience. Participants stay close to their personal experience but expand the idea to be relevant to others. CoATT practitioners leverage the future audience in each movement of the play by asking, 'is this what an audience needs to see or understand?' The core process of life-drama connection is invoked with the question, 'How is this moment in our play/rehearsal like recovery?' to underline the parallels in play-making and growth in recovery.

Later, groups build a 'co-active element' in each performance, inviting the audience to participate in the play-making process and facilitating an opportunity to reconnect to one's community. A co-active element can be any activity that helps to level the power dynamics between audience and performers, those in recovery and those in community, those who are the 'sick ones' and those who are 'not sick ones'. Destroying the binary, locked dynamic is key to reconnection with the world outside of treatment, a meaningful step in recovery.

What is the power of the artist in recovery?

CoATT plays offer many examples of the *artist* role invoked to assist in recovery. When the *artist* appears as a *performer*, or shows another form of art such as *painter*, or *entertainer*, the role may empower the physical transformation of recovery, especially salient in CoATT plays with participants living with Aphasia.

In *Aphasia Park*, a participant with treatment goals of expanding her spoken vocabulary to pronounce one two-syllable word played a *painter*. In addition to speaking the word, she was actively painting a canvas on the stage. For a person recovering from a stroke, the demonstration of fine muscle control, sustained effort, and dual mental processes of performing a task and speaking on cue is a marked transformation. In *The Gift*, another participant with aphasia was insistent on playing the piano as part of the performance. In this instance, the participant identified himself as a performer and wanted to offer his musical gift as a demonstration of love. The ability to create demonstrates recovery.

CoATT play-making in recovery

The CoATT Model positions 'active recovery' as "engagement in regular activity, reflection, and relationships that reinforce (my own) definition of recovery beyond treatment" (Wood & Mowers, 2024, p. 22). The model operates in concert with conceptions of recovery put forward by Kellmann (2002).

Recovery is a process in time and is dependent on the type and duration of stress

The CoATT process is time-bound and manualised, therefore offered at a specific time trajectory in the treatment continuum. A public performance focuses the participants around a 'planned crisis' when presenting their work to an open audience, marking a new beginning and an end of formal treatment. The presentation itself is an inflexion of stress into the process, as most participants do not perform or act in public during their everyday lives. Type and duration of stress are key in planning the performance.

Recovery depends on a reduction of stress, a change of stress, or a break from stress

CoATT productions offer a change in stress by presenting participants in roles that differ from their everyday lives. Participants who are known by their families to be 'the sick one' or 'the problem one' or 'a liar' step onto the stage as Artists, and portray roles including hero, helper, and friend. The transformation allows for a different relationship to emerge.

Recovery is individually specific and depends on individual appraisals

Participants begin by defining recovery in ways that are meaningful to the group. CoATT practitioners test these appraisals of recovery throughout the process by asking "how is this moment like recovery?".

Recovery can be passive, active, and pro-active

While CoATT prefers action and self-direction, it straddles medical definitions of recovery. In practice, this may mean that some participants agree that recovery is simply an absence of a particular behaviour, abstinence from substance use, or the cessation of symptoms. Yet, CoATT is designed as a group treatment protocol facilitating shared knowledge and strategies, a framework for reflection, and ongoing support; these elements may be pro-active efforts to prevent or delay relapse.

Recovery is closely tied to situational conditions

Flexibility is key to the CoATT Model conception of recovery. Definitions are individually driven and socially constructed and therefore reflect the changing conditions in which an individual operates. In practice, participants and practitioners accept each other in the immediate state and work towards a healthy balance in future states.

Recovery is not merely regeneration or healing. It is an inter- and intra-individual multilevel (e.g., psychological, physiological, social) process in time for the re-establishment of personal resources and their full functional capacity.

The manualised CoATT model assumes that participants have reached a point in their treatment where they have considered the impact of illness, trauma, or addiction on their mental state, physical health, and social situation. Most participants will have been labelled 'sick' or 'patient' and can discuss how this impacts their view of themselves and the people around them. They must have the ability and desire to identify a definition of active recovery.

CoATT model recovery for professional performing artists

In short, CoATT endows non-professional performers with the status of artist in a search for growth in recovery. How might professional Artists view a similar process?

In private practice we experience that professional performing artists conceptualise the drain on personal resources in a career in the arts as injurious. The business structures of the professional performing arts in North America, including the rejection and denial that accompany auditions (for theatre, dance, and music), strict and subjective criteria for advancing through conservatory training, exclusion from opportunities for training and advancement that require financial investment unavailable to many people of the working class perpetually deplete personal resilience. CoATT may help develop a wellness recovery model for individuals working in a system that is unlikely to change and may never have actually been a healthy endpoint state.

Career inflexion points may be particularly distressing for performers as these moments can be abrupt or at the whim of the marketplace (Middelton & Middelton, 2017). Imagine a touring soloist dropped by a booking agent and unable to make a living or a recognised master of a form that falls out of favour and is denied a venue for work. The external threat to well-being causes fear that meets the definition of trauma.

Professional performers are also subject to public scrutiny and criticism that can be the equivalent of bullying or hazing (Quigg, 2016). Nemiro (1997) noted that social influences, such as evaluation, can undermine an actor's creativity. Therefore, we surmise that creation is personal, and violent language or reaction can be felt as violence toward the self. For performing arts workers, alienation from self is intimately tied to alienation from their work.

Burnout has a psychological, physiological, and social component (Mainwaring & Mor, 2019). Performers may over-identify with their role, bound by their skillset. Without it, some believe they would have no self. Elite performers rely on the physical body to deliver peak performance as well as emotional resilience. Both resources may diminish through over-extension, age, and illness (Edel, 1985).

In our clinical practise we often hear stories of when artists' reward for the work of creativity is withheld, or arbitrary, the result is an inability to meet basic needs for security and self-esteem. CoATT productions address the social aspect of recovery through group work. Participants build supportive relationships that form a safety net for performers who work alone or cannot work unless accepted by a professional organisation.

The work of play-making can involve externalising both the nature of burnout and a desired state, allowing for reflection and action-planning. CoATT refocuses the meaning of (art)work towards connections (or re-connection) between artist and self, artist and group, and artist and audience. CoATT is therefore an intervention against alienation.

Conclusion and recommendations for practice

CoATT is conceived as an intervention for people who identify as living in 'active recovery'. CoATT plays support well-being, but are not intended to replace commercial theatre or the professional performing arts. As such, CoATT may or may not have strong relevance to the world of professional performers.

Nonetheless, the model may provide a safety net or release valve for the societal and systemic pressures of the performing arts. Artists who choose to work outside of their professional realm, either by taking creative risks or shielding the work from commercial purposes, may experience a renewed sense of self-determination. Overuse of the artist's instrument can be detrimental, though. This may disqualify CoATT as a treatment of choice for some artists suffering from burnout or fatigue.

Our participants often begin with the complaint that discussing the problem again, even in a new way, seems unappealing and unlikely to provide a new lens on recovery. Professional artists who experience role constriction, or over-identification with their work, may not respond to expressive therapy that feels too close to work.

Practitioners considering CoATT with artist populations should assess readiness for creative re-engagement. For artists in acute burnout, too much expressive work too soon may exacerbate symptoms. A pacing plan or use of unfamiliar art forms (e.g., a dancer writing or a musician drawing) may lower internalised expectations and shift the goal from mastery to exploration.

While the full expression of the model may not be a fit, some exercises derived from the CoATT model may offer a meaningful reflection for artists to use as component of their recovery, therefore, we suggest:

1 **Define your recovery:** In the CoATT model participants derive great benefit from defining their active recovery. We suggest that artists could define their own active recovery as a part of the process. By articulating

a personal definition of active recovery, artists can create a concrete and intentional framework for healing, ensuring that their recovery aligns with their own needs, values, and artistic identity.

2 **Externalise through a new medium:** CoATT relies on the power of metaphor to help groups express and externalise their recovery journeys. We suggest that artists may benefit from choosing an artistic medium different from their primary discipline to externalise their experiences. Engaging in unfamiliar forms of artistic expression can transform burnout into something visible and workable – offering fresh perspectives and new pathways for renewal.

3 **Reconnect to community:** The CoATT model draws on Herman's (1992) foundational assertion that reconnection to community is a vital stage in trauma recovery. Herman outlines a three-phase model – establishing safety, remembrance and mourning, and reconnection – emphasising that healing is incomplete without the restoration of meaningful relationships and social roles. In the context of burnout, which is often rooted in secondary or vicarious trauma (Shoji et al., 2015), isolation becomes both a symptom and a barrier to recovery. Artists experiencing burnout may withdraw from peers, audiences, and collaborative networks. Actively seeking opportunities for reconnection can serve as a powerful corrective – restoring a sense of belonging, reinforcing resilience, and reigniting creative purpose.

4 **Rehearse new roles in a safe space:** CoATT helps participants expand their sense of identity by trying on roles they may not yet feel ready to live out in everyday life. For artists in recovery, this principle could be beneficial. Burnout often comes with role exhaustion, feeling trapped in identities like 'the performer', or 'the perfectionist'. In response, artists may feel the urge to abandon the role entirely. Instead, recovery can invite rehearsal. What does it feel like to be 'the artist who rests', 'the collaborator who says no', or 'the person who makes art just for themselves'? Exploring these new roles in a low-stakes environment, whether through journaling, improvisation, collage, or movement, can potentially help soften rigid patterns and introduce a wider, more sustainable range of self-expression.

By integrating these strategies, artists can move toward a more sustainable and self-determined creative life, navigating the demands of their profession while maintaining their well-being. Furthermore, when this work is shared with other artists who may be similarly struggling, the benefits of group process may enhance our suggestions.

In 2024, a group of emerging professional theatre-makers in Akron, Ohio, USA, employed the CoATT model to explore healing from the traumatic experiences that result from working in the arts as Queer individuals. This is the first group of artists to come together and identify (a) a shared experience from which to recover and (b) an interest in defining recovery from those experiences. Outstanding questions for this group included: Does this deplete the artist further, especially in the realm of physical recovery? How is recovery defined when the behaviour in question may continue?

Emerging anecdotal feedback from the group suggests that using a play-making process to address harms incurred by other play-making processes was a successful intervention. Participants appreciated the ability to set boundaries on their time and the opportunity to develop new group norms for emotional demand and physical contact. Through experiencing these new norms, a reparative model for ongoing professional work began to emerge. Among the most powerful elements of CoATT practice was the focus on the *launch movement*. Leaders and practitioners welcomed structured reflection on the experience of working as an artist, particularly as differentiated from an evaluation of the production itself. For this group, the CoATT process did indeed provide a space for community connection as an antidote to alienation.

References

Addis, M. E., Cardemil, E. V., Duncan, B. L., & Miller, S. D. (2006). Does manualization improve therapy outcomes? In J. C. Norcross, L. E. Beutler, & R. F. Levant (Eds.), *Evidence-based practices in mental health: Debate and dialogue on the fundamental questions* (pp. 131–160). American Psychological Association.

American Psychiatric Association. (2013). *Diagnostic and statistical manual of mental disorders* (5th ed.). American Psychiatric Publishing.

Antonovsky, A. (1987). *Unraveling the mystery of health*. Jossey-Bass.

Beckmann, J., Kellmann, M., & Jakowski, S. (2023). Recovery is more than just healing: Advocating a broader perspective on recovery in physical and mental health. In M. Kellmann, S. Jakowski, & J. Beckmann (Eds.), *The importance of recovery for physical and mental health: Negotiating the effects of underrecovery* (pp. 266–270). Routledge.

Bottomore, T. B. (Ed.). (1963). *Karl Marx: Early writings*. McGraw Hill.

Cheung, A., Agwu, V., Stojcevski, M., Wood, L., & Fan, X. (2022). A pilot remote drama therapy program using the CoActive therapeutic theater model in people with serious mental illness. *Community Mental Health Journal*, *58*(8), 1613–1620.

Cottone, R. R. (2017). In defense of radical social constructivism. *Journal of Counseling & Development*, *95*(4), 465–471.

De Witte, M., Orkibi, H., Zarate, R., Karkou, V., Sajnani, N., Malhotra, B., & Koch, S. C. (2021). From therapeutic factors to mechanisms of change in the creative arts therapies: A scoping review. *Frontiers in Psychology*, *12*, 678397. https://doi.org/10.3389/fpsyg.2021.678397

Edel, L. (1985). The artist in old age. *Hastings Center Report*, *15*(4), 38–44.

Emunah, R. (2019). *Acting for real: Drama therapy process, technique, and performance*. Routledge.

Fox, J. (2004). *Playback theatre compared to psychodrama and theatre of the oppressed*. Centre for Playback Theatre.

Frydman, J. S., Cook, A., Armstrong, C. R., Rowe, C., & Kern, C. (2022). The drama therapy core processes: A Delphi study establishing a North American perspective. *The Arts in Psychotherapy*, *80*, 101939. https://doi.org/10.1016/j.aip.2022.101939

Herman, J. L. (1992). *Trauma and recovery: The aftermath of violence—from domestic abuse to political terror*. Basic Books.

Hodermarska, M. (2013). Autism as performance. *Dramatherapy*, *35*(1), 64–76.

Johnson, D. R. (2009). Developmental transformations: Towards the body as presence. *Current Approaches in Drama Therapy*, 2, 65–88.

Johnson, D. R., & Emunah, R. (Eds.). (2020). *Current approaches in drama therapy* (3rd ed.). Charles C Thomas Publisher.

Jones, P. (2007). *Drama as therapy: Theory, practice and research*. Routledge.

Kellmann, M. (2002). Current status and directions of recovery research. In M. Kellmann (Ed.), *Enhancing recovery: Preventing underperformance in athletes* (pp. 301–311). Human Kinetics.

Kellmann, M., & Kallus, K. W. (2001). *The Recovery-Stress Questionnaire for Athletes; manual*. Human Kinetics.

Kellmann, M., & Kallus, K. W. (Eds.). (2025). *The Recovery-Stress Questionnaires: A user manual*. Routledge.

Kuhl, J., & Beckmann, J. (1994). Alienation: Ignoring one's preferences. In J. Kuhl & J. Beckmann (Eds.), *Volition and personality: Action and state orientation* (pp. 375–390). Hogrefe & Huber.

Landy, R. J. (1994). *Drama therapy: Concepts, theories, and practices*. Charles C. Thomas Publisher.

Landy, R. J. (1996). *Persona and performance: The meaning of role in drama, therapy, and everyday life*. Guilford Press.

Mainwaring, L., & Mor, S. (2019). Managing psychological disturbances in performing artists. In L. Carder (Ed.), *Performing arts medicine* (pp. 151–162). Springer.

Marlatt, G. A. (1996). Harm reduction: Come as you are. *Addictive Behaviors*, *21*(6), 779–788.

Middleton, J. C., & Middleton, J. A. (2017). Review of literature on the career transitions of performing artists pursuing career development. *International Journal for Educational and Vocational Guidance*, *17*, 211–232.

Moreno, J. L. (1987). *The essential Moreno: Writings on psychodrama, group method, and spontaneity*. Springer.

Nemiro, J. (1997). Interpretive artists: A qualitative exploration of the creative process of actors. *Creativity Research Journal*, *10*(2–3), 229–239.

Noordenbos, G. (2011a). When have eating disordered patients recovered and what do the DSM-IV criteria tell about recovery? *Eating Disorders*, *19*(3), 234–245.

Noordenbos, G. (2011b). *Recovery from eating disorders: A guide for clinicians and their clients*. Wiley-Blackwell.

Pendzik, S., Emunah, R., & Johnson, D. R. (2017). *Self in performance*. Palgrave Macmillan.

Quigg, A. M. (2016). *Bullying in the arts: Vocation, exploitation and abuse of power*. Routledge.

Sajnani, N. (2022). *Autobiographical therapeutic performance* [Video]. YouTube. Retrieved June 30, 2025 from https://www.youtube.com/watch?v=KOH6mRbl66k

Snow, S., D'Amico, M., & Tanguay, D. (2003). Therapeutic theatre and well-being. *The Arts in Psychotherapy*, *30*(2), 73–82.

Shoji, K., Lesnierowska, M., Smoktunowicz, E., Bock, J., Luszczynska, A., Benight, C. C., & Cieslak, R. (2015). What comes first, job burnout or secondary traumatic stress? Findings from two longitudinal studies from the US and Poland. *PloS ONE*, *10*(8), e0136730. https://doi.org/10.1371/journal.pone.0136730
Stevens, A. D. F. (2023). BART, the Black American Role Taxonomy: A culturally expansive approach to role theory and method. *Drama Therapy Review*, *9*(1), 81–99.
Strauss, A., & Corbin, J. (1990). *Basics of qualitative research*. Sage.
Wood, L. L., & Mowers, D. (2019). The Co-Active therapeutic theatre model: A manualized approach to creating therapeutic theatre with persons in recovery. *Drama Therapy Review*, *5*(2), 217–234.
Wood, L. L., & Mowers, D. (2024). *Dramatherapy and recovery: The CoActive therapeutic theatre model and manual*. Taylor & Francis.

17

MUSIC AS A RESOURCE FOR HEALTH AND WELL-BEING

Epidemiological and big data studies

J. Matt McCrary and Christina Davies

Introduction

An increasing body of evidence supports broad associations between engaging in the arts (in a non-professional context) and a range of positive health and well-being outcomes in clinical and healthy populations, including benefits at the individual and population levels (Davies & Pescud, 2020; Fancourt & Finn, 2019; McCrary et al., 2021). Extending beyond the performing arts, 'arts engagement' encompasses the various ways in which people actively and receptively take part in the arts (e.g., listening to music, playing a musical instrument, singing, dancing, reading novels, photography, painting, sewing, concert attendance, and art class participation) as part of their everyday life for enjoyment, entertainment, socially or as a hobby (Davies & Clift, 2022). The emerging relationship between arts engagement and health, well-being and recovery has inspired investment and attention from prominent health organisations – for example, the World Health Organization (Sajnani & Fietje, 2023) and the US National Institutes of Health (Collins & Fleming, 2017) – aiming to inspire research, policy and practice that can ultimately operationalise this presently broad evidence into tangible health outcomes. Additionally, the presumed economic efficiency of the arts provides further impetus at a time of globally stretched health resources (Frontier Economics, 2024).

McCrary, J. M., & Davies, C. (2026). Music as a resource for health and well-being: Epidemiological and big data studies. In E. Altenmüller, M. Kellmann, J. Beckmann, & G. M. Moyle (Eds.), *Recovery and well-being in the performing arts* (pp. 284–298). Routledge.

DOI: 10.4324/9781003566885-21

A wide range of theories related to physiological, psychological, social, and behavioural mechanisms of arts effects has been proposed (Fancourt et al., 2021; McCrary & Altenmüller, 2021), with most focused on the ability of arts engagement to support recovery from various life stressors (i.e., recreational arts engagement as a promoter of better recovery-stress balance). Driven by this emerging evidence, references to health and well-being are increasingly included in arts policies at a national, state, and local government level; however, the arts are only sparsely included in corresponding public health policies, indicating that further rigorous research is still required to support broad implementation (Davies et al., 2015; Dow et al., 2023; Kaasgaard et al., 2024). In particular, consistent and specific dose-response relationships between arts engagement and population health (i.e., mental, physical, social) are lacking, as is convincing evidence supporting a physiological rationale underpinning such dose-response relationships. Together, consistency, specificity, a 'biological gradient' (i.e., dose-response relationship), and 'biological plausibility' (i.e., physiological rationale) are cornerstones of the Bradford Hill criteria for distinguishing causal relationships in epidemiologic research (Hill, 1965), with continued relevance to the modern scientific context (Fedak et al., 2015). Establishing causality is of critical importance in justifying and facilitating the application and efficient use of scarce health resources, and the possibility/probability of cross-government departmental collaboration (e.g., government health departments with arts departments).

Music is globally the most popular form of arts engagement, with estimates from the USA, Australia, and European Union indicating that > 70% of adults regularly listen to music (Australia Council for the Arts, 2017; Eurostat, 2019; National Endowment for the Arts, 2019). Music is also the most widely studied artform in a health and experimental physiological context (Collins & Fleming, 2017). Accordingly, music engagement (i.e., defined in this chapter as 'all' the ways you can take part in music including singing, playing a musical instrument, listening to music, etc.) is an excellent use case for the development of new epidemiologic research approaches which can address knowledge and evidence gaps relevant to arts engagement and population health more broadly, while also providing valuable insights into the direct impact of music on health (McCrary & Altenmüller, 2021).

Mirroring the broader arts and health evidence base, the literature specific to music supports general associations between music engagement interventions and improved physical and mental health in healthy and clinical populations (Finn & Fancourt, 2018; McCrary et al., 2021). Further, key proposed mechanisms of action specific to music similarly relate to the promotion of better recovery-stress balance (McCrary & Altenmüller, 2021). At the population level, the evidence is varied, with prior epidemiologic studies finding both positive links and no significant relationships between music engagement

TABLE 17.1 Prior epidemiologic studies of the impact of music engagement on population health outcomes.

Study	*Type of engagement*	*Outcome(s)*	*Music effects*
Konlaan et al. (2000)	Music-making	All-cause mortality	Positive
Story et al. (2021)	Music-making & listening	All-cause mortality	Positive
Verghese et al. (2003)	Music-making	Dementia	Positive
Balbag et al. (2014)	Music-making	Dementia	Positive
Bygren et al. (1996)	Music-making	All-cause mortality	No effect
Løkken et al. (2018)	Music-making	All-cause mortality	No effect
Ekholm and Bonde (2018)	Music-making	Self-reported NCDs	No effect
Hughes et al. (2010)	Music-making	Dementia	No effect

Note: NCD = Non-communicable disease.

and all-cause mortality and dementia incidence (Table 17.1). To date, no epidemiologic studies have investigated the links between music engagement as a stand-alone variable – i.e., analysed as an independent activity, rather than as part of a group of broader arts activities – and physical and mental well-being outcomes (e.g., health-related quality of life, happiness). However, high-quality evidence supports positive effects of music engagement interventions on self-reported health and well-being in healthy populations, suggesting that population-level links may also exist (McCrary et al., 2021).

Inadequate capture of music engagement – A key driver of conflicting epidemiologic results

Conflicting epidemiologic results suggest that one or both of the following methodological inadequacies confound the 'true' relationship between music and health and well-being outcomes: (1) incomplete and/or inconsistent capture of the music engagement 'signal'; (2) insufficient and/or inconsistent filtering of the 'noise' of co-variates. We propose that current inadequacies in capturing the music engagement 'signal' are far more significant than those related to co-variate 'noise'. This hypothesis is based on variation in individual responses to music engagement appearing even in intervention studies, which suggests systemic inadequacies in measuring the music engagement signal also within more controlled settings. For example, a meta-analysis of 26 studies (McCrary, Altenmüller et al., 2022) found that music interventions were associated, on average, with a clinically significant three-point improvement in mental health-related quality of life, as quantified by the Short Form-36 (SF-36) and Short Form-12 (SF-12) questionnaires (Ware Jr, 2000). However, 95% confidence intervals of these effects within individual studies ranged from 5 to 67 points, indicating that it is still difficult to precisely predict music's health impact on a given individual even in controlled intervention settings. This interindividual variability is only likely to be further magnified in uncontrolled, observational epidemiologic studies.

Assessments of music engagement in prior epidemiologic studies have focused on 'practical characteristics' surrounding music engagement: the frequency of engagement (i.e., how often an individual plays an instrument, sings, or listens to music); the duration of engagement (i.e., how long an individual plays an instrument, sings, or listens to music daily/weekly/monthly); and the type of music engagement (e.g., playing an instrument, singing, listening). However, assessing only practical characteristics treats all music engagement as being equivalent, when we know that significant variation in responses to music exists – playing or listening to the exact same piece of music can elicit a strong emotional and related physiological response in one individual, but a minimal or completely different response in another individual, or even the same individual at different time points (Grewe et al., 2007; McCrary et al., 2021; Nakahara et al., 2009; Salimpoor et al., 2009). We propose that this individual variation in responses to music underpins differential longer-term impacts of music engagement on recovery-stress balance and, by extension, disease and well-being outcomes; this differential impact is particularly driven by autonomic nervous system (ANS) components of varied individual responses to music engagement.

Autonomic nervous system variation – Implications for epidemiologic studies and population health

The ANS is a division of the peripheral nervous system that controls, mostly involuntarily, the major peripheral organs/organ systems (e.g., cardiovascular, digestive, endocrine, reproductive, respiratory, visual). The ANS is divided into two branches, a sympathetic branch associated with 'fight-or-flight' responses (i.e., energy mobilisation, increased heart rate, blood pressure, stress hormone release), and a parasympathetic response associated with 'rest and digest' or 'recovery' responses (i.e., vegetative and restorative functions; decreased heart rate and blood pressure; McCorry, 2007).

ANS responses to music engagement are, as noted previously, highly individual, reflecting emotional experiences and, when making music, also physical and cognitive demands (McCrary & Altenmüller, 2021). Engaging with music for pleasure and enjoyment, the most common motivation in the general population (Sanfilippo et al., 2020), induces a characteristic ANS 'relaxation/recovery response': increased sympathetic activation during engagement, followed by increased parasympathetic activation after the music stops (Bernardi et al., 2006; Grape et al., 2002; Grewe et al., 2007; Lynar et al., 2017; Nakahara et al., 2009; Salimpoor et al., 2009). A similar

ANS relaxation/recovery response is also associated with exercise engagement (Curtis & O'Keefe Jr, 2002; Fu & Levine, 2013), with more pleasurable music engagement and more intense exercise both associated with greater sympathetic response magnitudes (Fu & Levine, 2013; Grewe et al., 2007; Lynar et al., 2017; Salimpoor et al., 2009).

In exercise, the cumulative weekly magnitude of sympathetic responses – i.e., the product of weekly duration * average intensity – are correlated, in a dose-response fashion, with an improved feeling of physical and mental well-being and a reduced risk of all-cause mortality and 20+ NCDs including cancers, cardiovascular diseases, and mental illnesses (Arem et al., 2015; Rhodes et al., 2017). These effects on health and disease are largely driven by the impact of repeated exercise on the 'autonomic tone', the balance point of baseline sympathetic and parasympathetic activity and a physiological indicator of recovery-stress balance (Curtis & O'Keefe Jr, 2002; Fu & Levine, 2013; Thayer et al., 2010). In healthy individuals, the ANS responds dynamically to daily situations by activating the sympathetic/parasympathetic branches before returning to the autonomic tone, a point of relative stability and minimal energy use. Poor autonomic tone or baseline autonomic *im*balance, generally sympathetic overactivation (i.e., chronic stress state), can be resolved over time through activities which improve the 'elasticity' of acute ANS responses; for example, regular exercise, which increases the efficiency of parasympathetic responses in returning ANS activity to baseline following sympathetic activation (Fu & Levine, 2013). Music engagement is hypothesised to be another activity which promotes such ANS elasticity, and, accordingly, can support broad benefits to population health and well-being through improved recovery-stress balance (McCrary & Altenmüller, 2021). Similar physiological mechanisms can also be inferred for other modes of arts engagement, albeit without the support of a comparable body of experimental evidence.

Capturing variable ANS responses to music engagement: The 'FITT' approach

In the exercise and physical activity domain, capturing and translating individual ANS responses into public health impact has been achieved using the 'FITT' model – evaluation of the Frequency, Intensity, Timing (i.e., duration), and Type of exercise (Barisic et al., 2011). In just four criteria, FITT captures the individual ANS response (Intensity), dose parameters [Frequency and Timing (i.e., duration)], and practical information informing the replication of the dose (Type). These FITT data have been effectively captured both using questionnaires (e.g., International Physical Activity Questionnaire; Hagströmer et al., 2006) and wearable devices (e.g., Apple and Garmin smart watches) in epidemiologic and intervention studies. Further, FITT is also used as a framework for 'prescribing' exercise in both clinical and public health scenarios, facilitating direct translation of research insights into practice. For example, the World Health Organization (2010) global physical activity recommendations are prescribed according to FITT criteria: 150 minutes (Timing) of weekly (Frequency) moderate to vigorous (Intensity) aerobic activity (Type).

An adaptation of FITT also presents potential utility for epidemiologic studies of music engagement. Frequency, Timing, and Type information are already captured to some extent in epidemiologic studies of music engagement, albeit using unvalidated self-report questions which introduce confounding variability (Warren et al., 2010) and also fail to quantify the specificity of engagement needed to support causal inferences (i.e., number of minutes of music engagement per week). The Intensity of music engagement, i.e., ANS responses and their emotional correlates, has yet to be captured or considered as a moderator of music's effects in both intervention and epidemiologic studies. Conceptually, the same broad approaches to capturing Intensity in exercise can be applied to assess music engagement Intensity: wearable heart rate data and questionnaires. Wrist-worn and chest-strap heart rate data can be used to capture ANS responses to music, as demonstrated in numerous experimental settings (Lynar et al., 2017; Nakahara et al., 2009; Salimpoor et al., 2009). These data have, however, yet to be captured during music engagement in non-experimental settings, nor as part of an epidemiologic approach. Similarly, the physical, cognitive, and emotional Intensity of music engagement have been previously captured using self-report measures in experimental settings (McCrary et al., 2016; Nagel et al., 2007; Robinson, 2001; Senn et al., 2020); however, a single validated questionnaire assessment tool combining all Intensity domains with rigorous, specific assessment of Frequency, Timing, and Type criteria does not presently exist.

Applied FITT approaches to capturing music's population health impact: The role of 'big data'

In the context of established lifestyle factors (e.g., smoking, physical activity), the impact of music engagement on population-level health and well-being is likely to be small but significant. The meta-analysis introduced above (McCrary, Altenmüller et al., 2022) demonstrated that music interventions (listening, singing, playing a musical instrument; no significant differences between Types) have approximately half the impact of exercise interventions on health-related quality of life, with both measured using the same SF-36/SF-12 questionnaires (Ware Jr, 2000). Extrapolating this relative effect size to the global population, music engagement could prevent 800,000 annual premature NCD deaths, 3–4% of global mortality, 17 million annual years lost to ill health (disability adjusted life years), and save up to $40 billion in annual global healthcare expenditure and $10 billion in annual productivity (Danaei et al., 2009; Ding et al., 2016; Forouzanfar et al., 2016; World Health Organization, 2010).

The consequence of this hypothesised small but significant effect of music is that sample sizes and/or data volumes collected in epidemiologic cohort studies will need to be large to observe clear and reliable effects. However, prior study underscores the need for collected data to be large *and* targeted, using appropriately specific and sensitive measures to assess music engagement. A study of over 103 million United States residents analysing the links between performing arts engagement, estimated using a financial modelling approach, and 13 health outcomes produced equivocal results (McCrary, Großbach et al., 2022). Integrating new, validated self-report music engagement FITT assessments into national population cohort studies presents a promising means of linking specific music engagement data founded upon a plausible physiological rationale (improved recovery-stress balance) to longitudinally collected health outcomes. Additionally, the increasing prevalence of commercial wearables (e.g., Apple Watch, Garmin Watch, etc.) presents a new means of directly capturing extremely large quantities of 'objective' music engagement FITT data remotely, automatically, and non-invasively. These wearable FITT data can then be linked to epidemiologic and other health record data and analysed both cross-sectionally and longitudinally.

This 'big data' commercial wearables approach to capturing music engagement FITT data is currently in development in a joint project (ALLEVIATE) between Hannover Medical School and the Institute of Music Physiology and Musicians' Medicine at the Hannover University of Music, Drama and Media in Germany. In brief, a new app will enable commercial wearables to be used as 'musical engagement trackers', similar to their established use as physical activity trackers. Heart rate data (i.e., ANS response Intensity) will be captured whenever music engagement occurs, as detected either through an onboard music player (e.g., Spotify, Apple Music) or in the external environment using the microphone and a lightweight artificial intelligence classification system. Through this process, Frequency, Timing, and Type data will also be captured with minute accuracy. Data related to physical activity occurring during music engagement and responses to push notifications asking individuals to confirm active music-making will be used to control for and/or integrate the additive impact of physical activity on the Intensity signal.

Translation case study: Good Arts, Good Mental Health®

The *Good Arts, Good Mental Health®* (GAGMH) initiative and media campaign is an Australian research translation success story that provides an applied example of how epidemiologic evidence supporting a dose-response relationship (Davies et al., 2015) can be mobilised into public health action and cross-government departmental collaboration.

Arts-mental well-being study

The GAGMH initiative is based on a landmark study which established a two-hour per week dose-response relationship between recreational arts engagement (definition above – including, but not limited to music) and mental well-being for adults in the general population (Davies et al., 2015). The 'arts-mental health dose' was calculated by: (1) defining arts engagement for population based research (Type of activities and their average engagement Intensity; Davies et al., 2012), (2) measuring respondent engagement for each arts activity (Type) on a continuous, numeric scale (days/hours/minutes; Timing), (3) controlling for eleven confounding and effect modifying variables to the arts-mental health relationship, and (4) measuring the dependent variable of mental well-being via the validated Warwick-Edinburgh Mental Well-being Scale (Davies et al., 2015). The dose-response evidence from this study was fundamental in building the case to support translation. However, mobilising this evidence into a public health initiative/campaign also required substantial time, advocacy, collaboration, financial investment, networks to stakeholders/structures/facilitators, and knowledge of relevant government policy and policy cycles (Davies et al., 2024).

GAGMH initiative

The GAGMH initiative is based at the University of Western Australia, in partnership with six other universities, the community, and 31 industry, philanthropic and government (health, mental health, arts departments) partners. The focus of GAGMH was a media campaign, but also demonstration programmes and learning opportunities to support the campaign. Overall, GAGMH aims to communicate the arts-mental well-being relationship and dose – i.e., arts' ability to promote, maintain and improve mental health and well-being, including recovery-stress balance – to Western Australian general population adults (18–64 years, all genders, metropolitan and regional areas). For further details see Davies et al. (2025).

GAGMH media campaign

The creative components of the GAGMH campaign were guided by the literature, arts-mental health dose and co-designed through a rigorous co-design research process (surveys, focus groups, interviews) with project partners, i.e., 3,560 community members, industry, philanthropy, a consumer reference

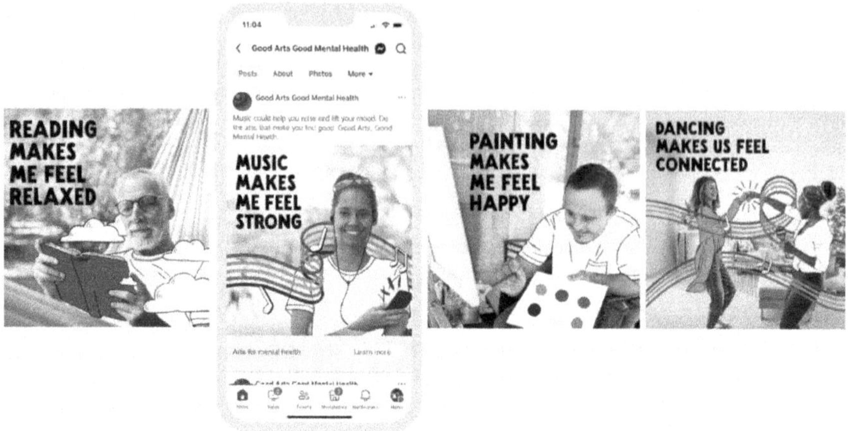

FIGURE 17.1 GAGMH Meta ads/tiles.

group and cross-government departmental reference group (health, mental health, arts departments). From this process, the **tagline** *Good Arts, Good Mental Health®* was established, along with the following campaign **manifesto:**

> You don't have to be good at art for the arts to be good for you. Do the art that makes YOU feel GOOD. TRY for two hours per week. It could make a difference to your mental health. Good Arts, Good Mental Health.
> *(Davies et al., 2025, p. 4)*

Guided by theories of social psychology and social epidemiology (psychosocial, eco-social; Ajzen, 1991; Krieger, 2001; Nutbeam & Harris, 2002), the specific objectives of the campaign were to increase brand *awareness*, *comprehension,* and *acceptance* of the tagline *Good Arts, Good Mental Health®* and encourage community members to form an *intention* to engage in the arts for their mental health and well-being (including improved recovery-stress balance). Overall, the media campaign cost AUD $198,965 and was delivered through a variety of distribution channels including radio, Meta (Instagram, Facebook; see Figure 17.1 for music, reading, painting, and dance ads/tiles), Spotify (Figure 17.2 for the Spotify ad), editorials, signage, and free/organic media e.g., media releases and interviews (TV, radio, print), newsletters, unpaid social media posts via GAGMH, project partner, and community accounts (e.g., Instagram, Facebook, Linked-In, Twitter, YouTube).

GAGMH campaign evaluation

A process evaluation and (short-term) outcome evaluation were conducted by sourcing online analytics and conducting an online, general population

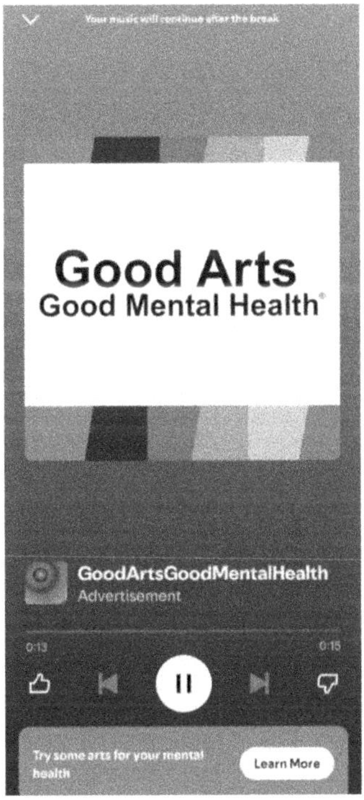

FIGURE 17.2 Spotify ad.

survey, which ran for 14 days, starting the day the campaign ended. Post-campaign, engagement with the GAGMH website substantially increased (pre-campaign = 7,505 events, one month post-campaign = 53,810 events).

In terms of outcomes, when measured as a proportion of the total survey sample (n = 661), one in four respondents were aware of the tagline *Good Arts, Good Mental Health®*. This is comparatively high for a new tagline without TV advertising (goal 4–30%). Overall, comprehension of the message was found to be satisfactory (49%), while agreement (89%; goal = 40%) and intention to act on the message (42%; goal 16%) were found to be higher than other Western Australian health promotion campaigns. As this was the first time the GAGMH campaign was run, collecting data on behavioural action over time (resulting from reported intentions) would have been premature. However, for extrapolation and comparison purposes, established Western Australian messages related to exercise with intention scores between 35% and 43% have been linked to behavioural actions scores between 10% and 11% (Mills et al., 2007). Theoretically, increased arts engagement behaviour could lead to enhanced well-being via mechanisms including improved recovery-stress balance. Future waves of the GAGMH campaign will aim to reinforce the campaign message, dose, and extend the evaluation to interrogate theoretically plausible biological and behavioural effects, via established and innovative approaches including those described above i.e., wearables to capture arts engagement FITT data.

Conclusions and recommendations for practice

The success of the GAGMH campaign indicates a general population, cross-government, philanthropic and industry receptiveness for evidence-based, epidemiological, dose-response approaches to utilising the arts to improve mental health. The epidemiologic research on which GAGMH was based provides specific, dose-response evidence, along with implicit biological plausibility – self-selected arts activities are most likely to elicit stronger emotional and ANS responses (i.e., higher Intensity), with hypothesised links to greater impacts on recovery-stress balance and long-term health (McCrary & Altenmüller, 2021). However, returning to the Hill (1965) criteria for inferring causality from epidemiologic studies, a key unfulfilled criterion across both music and broader arts and health epidemiologic research remains consistency. To enable uptake of music engagement-based strategies into public health practice, new approaches are still needed. FITT presents a promising approach, enabling specific, dose-response music data with clear biological plausibility (improved ANS recovery-stress balance) to be captured using both self-report and 'big data' methods. Accordingly, key methodological confounds can be removed, facilitating more precise epidemiologic research into the 'true' relationship between music/arts and health, which further supports future arts-public health policy and practice.

References

Ajzen, I. (1991). The theory of planned behavior. *Organizational Behavior and Human Decision Processes*, *50*(2), 179–211.

Arem, H., Moore, S. C., Patel, A., Hartge, P., De Gonzalez, A. B., Visvanathan, K., Campbell, P. T., Freedman, M., Weiderpass, E., & Adami, H. O. (2015). Leisure time physical activity and mortality: A detailed pooled analysis of the dose-response relationship. *Journal of the American Medical Association Internal Medicine*, *175*(6), 959–967.

Australia Council for the Arts. (2017). *Connecting Australians: Results of the National Arts Participation Survey*. Retrieved February 25, 2025 from https://www.australiacouncil.gov.au/workspace/uploads/files/connecting-australians-natio-59520692c614a.pdf

Balbag, M. A., Pedersen, N. L., & Gatz, M. (2014). Playing a musical instrument as a protective factor against dementia and cognitive impairment: A population-based twin study. *International Journal of Alzheimer's Disease*, *2014*, 836748. https://doi.org/10.1155/2014/836748

Barisic, A., Leatherdale, S. T., & Kreiger, N. (2011). Importance of frequency, intensity, time and type (FITT) in physical activity assessment for epidemiological research. *Canadian Journal of Public Health*, *102*(3), 174–175.

Bernardi, L., Porta, C., & Sleight, P. (2006). Cardiovascular, cerebrovascular, and respiratory changes induced by different types of music in musicians and non-musicians: The importance of silence. *Heart*, *92*(4), 445–452.

Bygren, L. O., Konlaan, B. B., & Johansson, S.-E. (1996). Attendance at cultural events, reading books or periodicals, and making music or singing in a choir as determinants for survival: Swedish interview survey of living conditions. *British Medical Journal*, *313*(7072), 1577–1580.

Collins, F. S., & Fleming, R. (2017). Sound health: An NIH-Kennedy center initiative to explore music and the mind. *Journal of the American Medical Association*, *317*(24), 2470–2471.

Curtis, B. M., & O'Keefe Jr, J. H. (2002). Autonomic tone as a cardiovascular risk factor: The dangers of chronic fight or flight. *Mayo Clinic Proceedings*, *77*(1), 45–54.

Danaei, G., Ding, E. L., Mozaffarian, D., Taylor, B., Rehm, J., Murray, C. J., & Ezzati, M. (2009). The preventable causes of death in the United States: Comparative risk assessment of dietary, lifestyle, and metabolic risk factors. *PLoS Medicine*, *6*(4), e1000058. https://doi.org/10.1371/journal.pmed.1000058

Davies, C. R., & Clift, S. (2022). Arts and health glossary - A summary of definitions for use in research, policy and practice. *Frontiers in Psychology*, *13*, 949685. https://doi.org/10.3389/fpsyg.2022.949685

Davies, C. R., Knuiman, M., & Rosenberg, M. (2015). The art of being mentally healthy: A study to quantify the relationship between recreational arts engagement and mental well-being in the general population. *BMC Public Health*, *16*, 15. https://doi.org/10.1186/s12889-015-2672-7

Davies, C. R., & Pescud, M. (2020). *The arts, creative industries and health: An evidence check rapid review brokered by the Sax Institute for The Victorian Health Promotion Foundation Sax Institute, New South Wale*s. Retrieved February 25, 2025 from https://www.saxinstitute.org.au/wp-content/uploads/20.12_Evidence-Check_arts-and-health-promotion.pdf

Davies, C. R., Pescud, M., Clifford, R., McGrath, R., Thomson, A., Jeffrey, M., Stoneham, M., Pikora, T., Wright, P., Gridler, S., Baldassar, L., & Clift, S. (2025). Good Arts, Good Mental Health ®: The effectiveness of an Australian health promotion media campaign in promoting community mental wellbeing via the arts. *Frontiers in Public Health*, *13*, 1594846. https://doi.org/10.3389/fpubh.2025.1594846

Davies, C. R., Pescud, M., Maury, S., & Sullivan, D. (2024). A new perspective to an old problem – Mobilizing research into policy and practice using an arts and health case study. *Frontiers in Public Health*, *12*, 1392146. https://doi.org/10.3389/fpubh.2024.1392146

Davies, C. R., Rosenberg, M., Knuiman, M., Ferguson, R., Pikora, T., & Slatter, N. (2012). Defining arts engagement for population-based health research: Art forms, activities and level of engagement. *Arts & Health*, *4*(3), 203–216.

Ding, D., Lawson, K. D., Kolbe-Alexander, T. L., Finkelstein, E. A., Katzmarzyk, P. T., Van Mechelen, W., & Pratt, M. (2016). The economic burden of physical inactivity: A global analysis of major non-communicable diseases. *The Lancet*, *388*(10051), 1311–1324.

Dow, R., Warran, K., Letrondo, P., & Fancourt, D. (2023). The arts in public health policy: Progress and opportunities. *The Lancet Public Health*, *8*(2), e155–e160.

Ekholm, O., & Bonde, L. O. (2018). Music and health in everyday life in Denmark: Associations between the use of music and health-related outcomes in adult danes. In L. O. Bonde & T. Theorell (Eds.), *Music and public health: A Nordic perspective* (pp. 15–31). Springer.

Eurostat. (2019). *Culture statistics*. Retrieved February 25, 2025 from https://ec.europa.eu/eurostat/documents/3217494/10177894/KS-01-19-712-EN-N.pdf/915f828b-daae-1cca-ba54-a87e90d6b68b?t=1571393532000

Fancourt, D., Aughterson, H., Finn, S., Walker, E., & Steptoe, A. (2021). How leisure activities affect health: A narrative review and multi-level theoretical framework of mechanisms of action. *The Lancet Psychiatry*, *8*(4), 329–339.

Fancourt, D., & Finn, S. (2019). *What is the evidence on the role of the arts in improving health and well-being? A scoping review*. Retrieved February 25, 2025 from https://www.ncbi.nlm.nih.gov/books/NBK553773/

Fedak, K. M., Bernal, A., Capshaw, Z. A., & Gross, S. (2015). Applying the Bradford Hill criteria in the 21st century: How data integration has changed causal inference in molecular epidemiology. *Emerging Themes in Epidemiology*, *12*, 14. https://doi.org/10.1186/s12982-015-0037-4

Finn, S., & Fancourt, D. (2018). The biological impact of listening to music in clinical and nonclinical settings: A systematic review. *Progress in Brain Research*, *237*, 173–200.

Forouzanfar, M. H., Afshin, A., Alexander, L. T., Anderson, H. R., Bhutta, Z. A., Biryukov, S., Brauer, M., Burnett, R., Cercy, K., & Charlson, F. J. (2016). Global, regional, and national comparative risk assessment of 79 behavioural, environmental and occupational, and metabolic risks or clusters of risks, 1990–2015: A systematic analysis for the Global Burden of Disease Study 2015. *The Lancet*, *388*(10053), 1659–1724.

Frontier Economics. (2024). *Culture and heritage capital: Monetising the impact of culture and heritage on health and wellbeing*. Department for Culture, Media and Sport (UK). Retrieved February 25, 2025 from https://assets.publishing.service.gov.uk/media/678e2ecf432c55fe2988f615/rpt_-_Frontier_Health_and_Wellbeing_Final_Report_09_12_24_accessible_final.pdf

Fu, Q., & Levine, B. D. (2013). Exercise and the autonomic nervous system. *Handbook of Clinical Neurology*, *117*, 147–160.

Grape, C., Sandgren, M., Hansson, L.-O., Ericson, M., & Theorell, T. (2002). Does singing promote well-being? An empirical study of professional and amateur singers during a singing lesson. *Integrative Physiological & Behavioral Science*, *38*(1), 65–74.

Grewe, O., Nagel, F., Kopiez, R., & Altenmüller, E. (2007). Emotions over time: Synchronicity and development of subjective, physiological, and facial affective reactions to music. *Emotion*, 7(4), 774. https://doi.org/10.1037/1528-3542.7.4.774

Hagströmer, M., Oja, P., & Sjöström, M. (2006). The International Physical Activity Questionnaire (IPAQ): A study of concurrent and construct validity. *Public Health Nutrition*, *9*(6), 755–762.

Hill, A. B. (1965). The environment and disease: Association or causation? *Journal of the Royal Society of Medicine*, *58*(5), 295.

Hughes, T. F., Chang, C.-C. H., Vander Bilt, J., & Ganguli, M. (2010). Engagement in reading and hobbies and risk of incident dementia: The MoVIES project. *American Journal of Alzheimer's Disease & Other Dementias*, *25*(5), 432–438.

Kaasgaard, M., Grebosz-Haring, K., Davies, C., Musgrave, G., Shriraam, J., McCrary, J. M., & Clift, S. (2024). Is it premature to formulate recommendations for policy and practice, based on culture and health research? A robust critique of the CultureForHealth (2022) report. *Frontiers in Public Health*, *12*, 1414070. https://doi.org/10.3389/fpubh.2024.1414070

Konlaan, B. B., Bygren, L. O., & Johansson, S.-E. (2000). Visiting the cinema, concerts, museums or art exhibitions as determinant of survival: A Swedish fourteen-year cohort follow-up. *Scandinavian Journal of Public Health*, *28*(3), 174–178.

Krieger, N. (2001). Theories for social epidemiology in the 21st century: An ecosocial perspective. *International Journal of Epidemiology*, *30*(4), 668–677.

Løkken, B. I., Rangul, V., Merom, D., Ekholm, O., Krokstad, S., & Sund, E. R. (2018). Are playing instruments, singing or participating in theatre good for population health? Associations with self-rated health and all-cause mortality in the HUNT3 study (2006–2008), Norway. In L. O. Bonde & T. Theorell (Eds.), *Music and public health: A Nordic perspective* (pp. 33–54). Springer.

Lynar, E., Cvejic, E., Schubert, E., & Vollmer-Conna, U. (2017). The joy of heartfelt music: An examination of emotional and physiological responses. *International Journal of Psychophysiology*, *120*, 118–125.

McCorry, L. K. (2007). Physiology of the autonomic nervous system. *American Journal of Pharmaceutical Education*, *71*(4), 78. https://doi.org/10.5688/aj710478

McCrary, J. M., & Altenmüller, E. (2021). Mechanisms of music impact: Autonomic tone and the physical activity roadmap to advancing understanding and evidence-based policy. *Frontiers in Psychology*, *12*, 727231. https://doi.org/10.3389/fpsyg.2021.727231

McCrary, J. M., Altenmüller, E., Kretschmer, C., & Scholz, D. S. (2022). Association of music interventions with health-related quality of life: A systematic review and meta-analysis. *Journal of the American Medical Association Network Open*, *5*(3), e223236. https://doi.org/10.1001/jamanetworkopen.2022.3236

McCrary, J. M., Großbach, M., & Altenmüller, E. (2022). Are culturally vibrant communities healthier? Relationships between performing arts activity and health outcomes in the 500 largest US cities. *Perspectives in Public Health*, *142*(2), 94–101.

McCrary, J. M., Halaki, M., Sorkin, E., & Ackermann, B. J. (2016). Acute warm-up effects in submaximal athletes: An EMG study of skilled violinists. *Medicine and Science in Sports and Exercise*, *48*(2), 307–315.

McCrary, J. M., Redding, E., & Altenmüller, E. (2021). Performing arts as a health resource? An umbrella review of the health impacts of music and dance participation. *PLoS ONE*, *16*(6), e0252956. https://doi.org/10.1371/journal.pone.0252956

Mills, C., Rosenberg, M., Mitchell, J., & Wood, L. (2007). *Sponsorship monitor evaluation results 2006/2007*. The University of Western Australia.

Nagel, F., Kopiez, R., Grewe, O., & Altenmüller, E. (2007). EMuJoy: Software for continuous measurement of perceived emotions in music. *Behavior Research Methods*, *39*(2), 283–290.

Nakahara, H., Furuya, S., Obata, S., Masuko, T., & Kinoshita, H. (2009). Emotion-related changes in heart rate and its variability during performance and perception of music. *Annals of the New York Academy of Sciences*, *1169*(1), 359–362.

National Endowment for the Arts. (2019). *U.S. Patterns of Arts Participation: A full report from the 2017 survey of public participation in the arts*. Retrieved February 25, 2025 from https://www.arts.gov/impact/research/publications/us-patterns-arts-participation-full-report-2017-survey-public-participation-arts

Nutbeam, D., & Harris, E. (2002). *Theory in a nutshell: A guide to health promotion theory*. McGraw-Hill.

Rhodes, R. E., Janssen, I., Bredin, S. S., Warburton, D. E., & Bauman, A. (2017). Physical activity: Health impact, prevalence, correlates and interventions. *Psychology & Health*, *32*(8), 942–975.

Robinson, P. (2001). Task complexity, task difficulty, and task production: Exploring interactions in a componential framework. *Applied Linguistics*, *22*(1), 27–57.

Sajnani, N., & Fietje, N. (2023). The Jameel Arts & Health Lab in collaboration with the WHO–Lancet global series on the health benefits of the arts. *The Lancet*, *402*(10414), 1732–1734.

Salimpoor, V. N., Benovoy, M., Longo, G., Cooperstock, J. R., & Zatorre, R. J. (2009). The rewarding aspects of music listening are related to degree of emotional arousal. *PLoS ONE*, *4*(10), e7487. https://doi.org/10.1371/journal.pone.0007487

Sanfilippo, K. R. M., Spiro, N., Molina-Solana, M., & Lamont, A. (2020). Do the shuffle: Exploring reasons for music listening through shuffled play. *PLoS ONE*, *15*(2), e0228457. https://doi.org/journal.pone.0228457

Senn, O., Bechtold, T., Rose, D., Câmara, G. S., Düvel, N., Jerjen, R., Kilchenmann, L., Hoesl, F., Baldassarre, A., & Alessandri, E. (2020). Experience of Groove Questionnaire: Instrument development and initial validation. *Music Perception: An Interdisciplinary Journal*, *38*(1), 46–65.

Story, K. M., Yang, Z., & Bravata, D. M. (2021). Active and receptive arts participation and their association with mortality among adults in the United States: A longitudinal cohort study. *Public Health*, *196*, 211–216.

Thayer, J. F., Yamamoto, S. S., & Brosschot, J. F. (2010). The relationship of autonomic imbalance, heart rate variability and cardiovascular disease risk factors. *International Journal of Cardiology*, *141*(2), 122–131.

Verghese, J., Lipton, R. B., Katz, M. J., Hall, C. B., Derby, C. A., Kuslansky, G., Ambrose, A. F., Sliwinski, M., & Buschke, H. (2003). Leisure activities and the risk of dementia in the elderly. *New England Journal of Medicine*, *348*(25), 2508–2516.

Ware Jr, J. E. (2000). SF-36 health survey update. *Spine*, *25*(24), 3130–3139.

Warren, J. M., Ekelund, U., Besson, H., Mezzani, A., Geladas, N., & Vanhees, L. (2010). Assessment of physical activity – A review of methodologies with reference to epidemiological research: A report of the exercise physiology section of the European Association of Cardiovascular Prevention and Rehabilitation. *European Journal of Preventive Cardiology*, *17*(2), 127–139.

World Health Organization. (2010). *Global recommendations on physical activity for health*. Retrieved February 25, 2025 from https://www.who.int/publications/i/item/9789241599979

18

TOWARDS IMPLEMENTING SCIENTIFICALLY BASED RECOVERY STRATEGIES IN THE PERFORMING ARTS

Eckart Altenmüller and Gene M. Moyle

Why do performing artists need specific recovery strategies?

This volume provides an overview of the unique challenges, working conditions, and needs of performing artists. It highlights the importance of recovery for performance quality, well-being, health, and career longevity. Performing arts include theatre/drama (acting, playwriting, stagecraft), dance (ballet, contemporary, ballroom, commercial, hip hop, jazz, tap, musical theatre, traditional dance), music (instrumental, vocal, opera, musical theatre, jazz, rock, pop), circus arts, and physical theatre (acrobatics, mime, clowning, puppetry). These disciplines share specific demands and requirements, which we summarise below. Challenges include:

- Performance delivered publicly before an audience
- High degree of controllability exercised by both performers and audience members
- Requirement for specialised skills that must be developed over many years and maintained through continuous practice
- Sustained work at mental and physical limits for extended periods
- Prevalence of an 'error culture' linked to an uncompromising societal reward or failure system
- Emotional engagement closely tied to the performer's personality and identity

Altenmüller, E., & Moyle, G. M. (2026). Towards implementing scientifically based recovery strategies in the performing arts. In E. Altenmüller, M. Kellmann, J. Beckmann, & G. M. Moyle (Eds.), *Recovery and well-being in the performing arts* (pp. 299–310). Routledge.

DOI: 10.4324/9781003566885-22

- Mastering of expressive movements, facial expressions, gestures, and postures and in some performing arts voice timbre (i.e., singing, acting)
- Vocational orientation towards the professional pursuit, profession as a 'way to live'
- Frequently unstable financial conditions, short-term contracts, and freelance employment

To face all the above-mentioned challenges, recovery has emerged as a central determinant of performance, health, and career sustainability in the performing arts. However, unlike sports science, where recovery has long been studied, its role in music, dance, acting, and circus performance has gained little attention. For this reason, we invited experts from all fields of performing arts to contribute to this volume. As already explained in the introductory chapter (Altenmüller et al., this volume, Chapter 1), in this volume recovery is understood as a multilevel biopsychosocial process that balances stress exposure with resource replenishment (Beckmann, 2023; Kellmann & Kallus, 2001). This model emphasises recovery not just as 'returning to baseline' but as a resource that builds resilience and buffers against future stress. Failure to maintain this balance leads to underrecovery, non-functional overreaching, and in severe cases, overtraining syndromes and functional breakdowns (Lobinger et al., 2014; Meeusen et al., 2013).

Performers face highly demanding conditions: early specialisation beginning in childhood shapes self-identity, limits leisure, and heightens vulnerability to overuse and musculoskeletal disorders (Kogan, 2002). Emotional attachment and intrinsic motivation often mask fatigue and delay recovery. This is particularly evident in flow, a mental state of complete absorption and focus on an activity where time feels distorted, and the activity itself becomes intrinsically rewarding (Csikszentmihalyi, 1990). Performing artists frequently report these flow experiences and enjoy their energising potential; however, they tend to ignore signs of exhaustion in this state (Moral-Bofill et al., 2022; Storm, 2006).

In the performing arts, physical and cognitive limits are constantly tested, with illness, infections, and hormonal fluctuations affecting the reliability of the performance (Ackermann & Steiner, this volume, Chapter 2). Ergonomic challenges are widespread; for instance, musical instruments such as violins and trombones or traditional 'classical' ballet postures were developed without consideration of modern ergonomic guidelines, which can increase the risk of chronic pain and injury (Boyette, 2005; Zamorano et al., 2023). Additionally, societal and organisational factors such as audience expectations, hierarchical structures in orchestras and dance companies, and globalised schedules in artists who are active on an international level may contribute to elevated stress, to anxieties, repetitive thoughts, and perfectionistic tendencies (Alpheis & Altenmüller, 2024).

Drawing from sports science, monitoring systems are increasingly applied to the performing arts (Jeffries & Coutts, this volume, Chapter 3). Tools measuring training load, fitness, fatigue, and recovery status help predict injury risk and optimise schedules. However, data-driven approaches remain underutilised in dance, music, and theatre due to cultural and financial barriers. Dance studies reveal that long rehearsals, overlapping productions, and poorly planned schedules create overuse injuries (Brown-Appenzeller et al., this volume, Chapter 4). Recovery planning at both the individual and company level is essential; however requires a cultural shift in management.

While physical recovery has long dominated discourse, psychological recovery is now recognised as equally vital. Mindfulness interventions have been shown to mitigate mental fatigue, stress, and performance anxiety (Blevins et al., this volume, Chapter 5). Barriers include scepticism within conservatories and training institutions and a lack of time in rehearsal schedules. Systemic adoption of mindfulness practices could transform resilience in dancers and actors.

Discipline-specific insights concerning the need for recovery

Musicians are often likened to 'peak-performance athletes of small muscles' (Steinhausen, 1907). Therefore, musicians need systemic prevention strategies and recovery protocols to address musculoskeletal and psychological issues (Schuppert & Altenmüller, this volume, Chapter 6). Retraining programmes and regulated reintegration (e.g., Hamburg model in Germany) are seemingly effective but need to be further developed (Altenmüller, this volume, Chapter 10). In dancers, injuries are common and underreported. Psychological consequences of injuries, such as a fear of being stigmatised as unable to cope, are common. In this 'Darwinist' climate, isolation, and maladaptive coping are often overlooked. Here, recovery requires addressing both the physical and psychosocial dimensions (Mainwaring, this volume, Chapter 7; Wirdnam et al., this volume, Chapter 11). Singers have their instrument, the voice, internalised. Even small impairments, such as a simple cold or lack of sleep, directly affect performance. Therefore, the quality of the voice is a constant source of concern. Recovery is strongly tied to vocal hygiene, career planning, and stage ergonomics (Richter, this volume, Chapter 8). Actors frequently face precarious employment, rejection, and emotional immersion. Recovery strategies such as de-rolling, resilience-building, and institutional intimacy consent practices are increasingly important. Circus artists blend artistry and athleticism under extreme physical demands. Holistic frameworks for recovery include sleep hygiene, nutrition, physical preparation, stress management, and social support (Richard et al., this volume, Chapter 12; Stuckey et al., this volume, Chapter 9).

Beyond self-management: Recovery concepts for improved ageing, rehabilitation, and arts interventions

In this volume we extend the recovery concepts into the effects of performing arts itself on health, well-being, and cognition. These beneficial effects are mediated by several brain networks, including the limbic systems and neuro-hormones involved in positive emotions, such as dopamine, related to reward, and endogenous opioids, related to pleasure (Salimpoor et al., 2013). Furthermore, music and dance can reduce stress and decrease blood levels of cortisol (Dimitriadis et al., 2024; Hankir et al., 2017; Karkou et al., 2019; Rodríguez-Jiménez et al., 2022; Sreepetch et al., 2025; West et al., 2004). These stress responses are 'programmed' by the autonomic nervous system and are primarily regulated by the hypothalamic-pituitary-adrenal axis. Under stress, the hypothalamus releases corticotropin-releasing hormone, which leads to the release of cortisol via the pituitary gland. Music and other performing arts can modulate this process: studies, including those conducted in domestic settings and not just under laboratory conditions, show that music perceived as calming by the individual lowers cortisol levels, slows the heart rate, and reduces blood pressure (Linnemann et al., 2017). This physiological reduction in stress has a calming effect in the short term. But it also improves resilience in the long term (Wong et al., 2021).

In addition to dampening negative emotions, performing arts also produce positive emotions. Listening to music increases the release of dopamine in the nucleus accumbens of the limbic system (Salimpoor et al., 2013), which improves emotional balance. Anxiety and stress are not only reduced but replaced by joy and relaxation. In certain circumstances, watching performances or listening to music can lead to intense feelings of happiness, known as 'chill-experiences'. 'Chills' are accompanied by brain activation in the reward centres of the limbic system including areas of the midbrain and the above-mentioned nucleus accumbens, as well as the lower front part of the orbitofrontal cortex and the superior temporal gyrus (Blood & Zatorre, 2001); in contrast, the activity of the amygdala is inhibited (Sescousse et al., 2013). The dopaminergic activation described above regulates and increases attention, supports motivation, and aids memory formation in episodic and procedural memory (Blum et al., 2017). These effects may also contribute to the general popularity and importance of the arts in all societies.

Linked to these powerful effects on emotions, motivation, and the autonomic nervous system, music and arts engagement foster cognitive resilience, delay neurocognitive decline, and promote social well-being (Moisseinen & Särkämö, this volume, Chapter 13). For example, a one-year music intervention in 156 seniors, which included randomised either weekly piano lessons or weekly intensive listening to music slowed brain ageing, improved executive functions, memory, speech-in-noise hearing and general quality of life (Worschech et al., 2021, 2024, 2025). These changes were accompanied by neuroplastic adaptations of the brain with increased neural connectivity in auditory-motor circuits and in the hippocampal-prefrontal circuits (Jünemann et al., 2023).

Not only music making and music listening, but also dance supports motor control, emotional health, and social connectedness, especially in neurodegenerative conditions (Jeffrey et al., this volume, Chapter 15). These findings align with broader neuroscience evidence for arts-induced neuroplasticity as a protective factor across the lifespan. The performing arts can be considered as an important resource which can support recovery in many domains. Finally, the potential of performing arts for healing needs to be emphasised. Music therapy and dance interventions leverage both neurobiological and psychosocial mechanisms to promote healing in clinical populations. Music therapy has been established in neurological rehabilitation (Särkämö et al., 2008; Schneider et al., 2007), in pain medicine, oncology, addiction and mental health (Stegemann & Silvermann, this volume, Chapter 14). Dance interventions have proven to be enormously effective in Parkinson's Disease, improving mobility, stride length, cadence, and quality of life (Jeffrey et al., this volume, Chapter 15; Liu et al., 2025). Also, dance interventions are helpful in many psychiatric conditions (Li et al., 2025). Theatre interventions, such as the 'CoActive Therapeutic Theater' provide therapeutic pathways through creative, co-produced performances, especially for populations experiencing alienation (Mowers & Wood, this volume, Chapter 16).

Future directions: Towards evidence-based recovery strategies in the performing arts

This volume underscores that recovery is not optional but central to the sustainability of performing arts careers. By integrating physiological, psychological, organisational, and societal perspectives, performers can flourish while avoiding long-term health impacts. Across the chapters, four unifying hypotheses emerged:

1 **Early recovery education** builds resilience and prevents high dropout and injury rates in young performers.
2 **Performing arts medicine** can humanise a profession often dominated by external control and perfectionism.
3 **Knowledge cultures** within institutions can transform training into a holistic, health-supportive practice.
4 **Recovery research** offers insights not only into human performance but also into mechanisms of failure, informing prevention, rehabilitation, and broader public health strategies.

Implementation of recovery strategies according to our understanding of recovery as a holistic (neuro)biological, psycho-mental, socio-cultural requirement needs a change in education, working conditions, and performance culture. To follow, we will outline what is needed across the domains of music, dance, theatre, and circus to reach such a goal in interdisciplinary research, in education, in the health literacy of performing artists and in institutions across the different performing arts domains.

When assembling the articles for this volume, it became apparent that recovery science in the performing arts is still nascent. There is a clear lack of studies, although some facets of recovery have been studied in classical musicians (McCrary & Davis, this volume, Chapter 17; McCrary et al., 2022; Norris, 1996) and dancers (Hrubes & Janowski, 2021). Unfortunately, these studies mostly cover either monitoring of physical load or recovery from injury in the sense of healing, clearly concepts that do not cover our holistic approach.

What is urgently needed are longitudinal controlled prospective randomised intervention studies with large cohorts, well-defined target parameters and covering as many aspects as possible of our enlarged recovery concept. This is difficult to organise, as funding for such research in performing arts is still scarce. If RCTs are not feasible, scientifically sound evaluations for programmes covering aspects of recovery are required. For example, at the Music University in Hannover (Germany), a longitudinal study of physical and mental health-related attitudes among music students was conducted (Rosset et al., 2022). Factors such as health status, health-related attitudes, behaviours, knowledge, skills, and coping strategies of students were assessed at the beginning of their education at a music university, and at the end of their second semester. Interestingly, music students are already in demand when they enter a music university, practising on average almost three hours daily. Compared to other body regions, pain in shoulders/back is most prevalent in first-year students, especially in those playing string instruments. Performance majors reported better knowledge about health risks and recovery measures for musicians, better coping abilities, and practised more than music education majors. First-year students assessed their overall and mental health status at the beginning of their first semester as mainly good, but found a decrease in mental health status at the end of the second semester. After two semesters, students attending courses on musicians' health showed increased knowledge and skills regarding different aspects of musicians' health, prevention and recovery (Rosset et al., 2022).

Similarly, Junge et al. (2024) found in their longitudinal study of 57 professional ballet dancers over 44 weeks that their ability to dance at full potential was affected due to health problems (i.e., musculoskeletal injuries, illness or mental health issues) every second week, or at least on 29.1% of the days documented in the weekly reports. Depression, low mood, and generalised anxiety were the most frequently reported mental health symptoms, while

95.6% of dancers reported sustaining at least one injury, and 64.9% an illness (i.e., respiratory). With regards to injuries, dancers reported the primary causes due to issues such as too much workload, tiredness/exhaustion, and stress/overload/insufficient regeneration. Junge et al. (2024) noted that preventative interventions and evaluations of these were urgently required, and even more so for dance students who presented with higher levels of mental health challenges.

These studies highlight the need for **education for recovery**, accompanying students already from the beginning of training in the respective performing art form. This way, routines and habits for recovery strategies are formed before overload and injury are pending (Gillison et al., 2014). At present, there is no scientific literature available concerning evaluation or implementation of a respective recovery-literacy programme.

Beyond education, changes in institutional culture are essential for effective recovery. As discussed by Altenmüller et al. (this volume, Chapter 1), recovery means not only restoring individual resources but also building stress buffers or resilience (Kellmann & Kallus, 2001). Achieving a balance between recovery and stress involves more than simply recovering from stress. It includes developing and maintaining resources that support overall well-being (World Health Organization, 2019). Here, time is needed, and employers, orchestra directors or company managers need to consider this when choosing repertoire, choreographic, or concept programmes. This applies to the planning of tours or whole seasons, where recovery time must be included in the individual schedule of each employee. 'Client-tailored' recovery plans should be available, since recovery is highly individuum-specific. Coaches or trained 'recovery experts' will be needed to accomplish this complex task. Besides financial constraints, time pressures, linked among others to concert-seasons, dance festivals or touring programmes need to be taken into account, and best compromises between necessary (and frequently voluntarily chosen), stressors, and recovery-time need to be negotiated. Since we regard recovery as a multifaceted restorative process in time, the above-mentioned external conditions, leading to heavy workload in an unyielding competitive societal system, such as an orchestra or a ballet company, need to be addressed. Here, a general 'humanising process' of the performing arts seems appropriate.

Requirements for recovery on an individual level

Individual recovery involves physiological, psychological, and social factors. Insufficient recovery, whether from mental, muscular, or general fatigue caused by exertion, disrupts balance. Effective recovery restores both physiological and psychological resources, helping to regain psycho-mental equilibrium. Ideally, the following requirements for individual recovery need to be met:

1 **Long-term preparation:**

   a Participation (at least partly and where possible) in choice of repertoire (Wulf & Lewthwaite, 2016)
   b Training plans, avoiding overtraining, and loss of motivation (Daley et al., 2023)
   c Psychological support enhancing self-confidence, focus, and reducing performance anxiety (Spahn, 2015)
   d Bodily preparation specific for performance including endurance training, strength training, mobility training, stretching, Pilates, and yoga.
   e Among others, regular post-training stretches, warm relaxation baths, cold-water immersion, and rest to reduce muscular fatigue and muscular micro-lesions (Gabbett & Oetter, 2025)
   f Mental imagery and mental training to reduce bodily overload (Bernardi et al., 2013)

2 **Short-term preparation:**

   a Sufficient sleep and time to recover from travel and jetlag (Decker et al., 2019)
   b Individualised pre-performance nutrition and routines
   c Opportunity to withdraw before the performance (e.g., use of 'green rooms')

3 **Performance venues:**

   a Optimised temperature, ventilation, lighting, and acoustics
   b According to performance domain: ergonomic sprung dance floor, security net, etc.

4 **Post-performance recovery, depending on performance domain:**
   Individualised regeneration approaches are needed. Depending on stressors, post-performance stretching or mobilisation might be helpful (Järvinen et al., 2007). Mental fatigue and cognitive exhaustion following extended performances may be managed through cognitive self-regulation, resource activation, psychological relaxation techniques, and sleep (Rattray et al., 2015). Kellmann (2002) categorises recovery approaches as passive, active, or pro-active. Passive methods include external treatments such as massage or periods of rest with minimal activity. Active recovery involves physical activities like cooldown exercises or jogging that address metabolic responses to physical fatigue. Pro-active recovery, such as participation in social activities, involves selecting activities tailored to individual needs and preferences. Recovery strategies should be adjusted based on specific requirements and the types of performance stressors encountered.

Outlook

The holistic recovery concept for performing artists presented in this volume has the potential to induce a major change in the world of performers. On an individual level, life quality, professional satisfaction, well-being, creativity, and performance quality will be enhanced. On a systemic level, societal justice, recognition, respect, and valuation of performing artists will increase. The importance of performing arts for our society is growing. Performing arts are a language of emotion, a catalyst for reflection and change, a source of meaning and healing. Art is a mirror of humanity, and not merely an ornament of civilisation; it is one of its foundations. It connects reason and emotion, the individual and the collective, the past and the future. Through art, we remember who we are, imagine who we might become, and find meaning in the in-between. To sustain a healthy society, we must therefore not only tolerate but actively cultivate art and artists – in our schools, cities, and everyday lives. For in the end, it is through art that humanity learns to feel, to reflect, and to hope.

References

Alpheis, S., & Altenmüller, E. (2024). Comparison of perfectionism between music and medical students and its association with anxiety. *Medical Problems of Performing Artists*, *39*(2), 82–92.

Beckmann, J. (2023). Self-regulation of recovery. In M. Kellmann, S. Jakowski, & J. Beckmann (Eds.), *The importance of recovery for physical and mental health: Negotiating the effects of underrecovery* (pp. 53–69). Routledge.

Bernardi, N. F., Schories, A., Jabusch, H.-C., Colombo, B., & Altenmüller, E. (2013). Mental practice in music memorization: An ecological-empirical study. *Music Perception*, *30*(3), 275–290.

Blood, A. J., & Zatorre, R. J. (2001). Intensely pleasurable responses to music correlate with activity in brain regions implicated in reward and emotion. *Proceedings of the National Academy of Sciences USA*, *98*(20), 11818–11823.

Blum, K., Simpatico, T., Febo, M., Rodriquez, C., Dushaj, K., Li, M., Braverman, E. R, Demetrovics, Z., Oscar-Berman, M., & Badgaiyan, R. D. (2017). Hypothesizing music intervention enhances brain functional connectivity involving dopaminergic recruitment: Common neuro-correlates to abusable drugs. *Molecular Neurobiology*, *54*(5), 3753–3758.

Boyette, J. (2005). Splinting for adaptation of musical instruments. *Work*, *25*(2), 99–106.

Csikszentmihalyi, M. (1990). *Flow: The psychology of optimal experience*. Harper and Row.

Daley, M. M., Shoop, J., & Christino, M. A. (2023). Mental health in the specialized athlete. *Current Reviews in Musculoskeletal Medicine*, *16*(9), 410–418.

Decker, A., Aubertin, P., & Kriellaars, D. (2019). Sleep and fatigue of elite circus student-artists during one year of training. *Medical Problems of Performing Artists*, *34*(3), 125–131.

Dimitriadis, T., Della Porta, D., Perschl, J., Evers, A. W. M., Magee, W. L., & Schaefer, R. S. (2024). Motivation and music interventions in adults: A systematic review. *Neuropsychological Rehabilitation*, *34*(5), 649–678.

Gabbett, T. J., & Oetter, E. (2025). From tissue to system: What constitutes an appropriate response to loading? *Sports Medicine*, *55*(1), 17–35.
Gillison, F., Standage, M., & Verplanken, B. (2014). A cluster randomised controlled trial of an intervention to promote healthy lifestyle habits to school leavers: Study rationale, design, and methods. *BMC Public Health*, *4*(1), 221. https://doi.org/10.1186/1471-2458-14-221
Hankir, A., Kirkcaldy, B., Carrick, F. R., Sadiq, A., & Zaman, R. (2017). The performing arts and psychological well-being. *Psychiatria Danubina*, *29*(Suppl. 3), 196–202.
Hrubes, M., & Janowski, J. (2021). Rehabilitation of the dancer. *Physical Medicine and Rehabilitation Clinics of North America*, *32*(1), 1–20.
Järvinen, T. A., Järvinen, T. L., Kääriäinen, M., Äärimaa, V., Vaittinen, S., Kalimo, H., & Järvinen, M. (2007). Muscle injuries: Optimising recovery. *Best Practice & Research: Clinical Rheumatolology*, *21*(2), 317–331.
Jünemann, K., Engels, A., Marie, D., Worschech, F., Scholz, D. S., Grouiller, F., Kliegel, M., Van De Ville, D., Altenmüller, E., Krüger, T. H. C., James, C. E., & Sinke, C. (2023). Increased functional connectivity in the right dorsal auditory stream after a full year of piano training in healthy older adults. *Science Reports*, *13*(1), 19993. https://doi.org/10.1038/s41598-023-46513-1
Junge, A., Hauschild, A., Stubbe, J. H., & van Rijn, R. M. (2024). Health problems of professional ballet dancers: An analysis of 1627 weekly self-reports on injuries, illnesses and mental health problems during one season. *Sports Medicine – Open*, *10*, 79. doi.org/10.1186/s40798-024-00753-1
Karkou, V., Aithal, S., Zubala, A., & Meekums, B. (2019). Effectiveness of dance movement therapy in the treatment of adults with depression: A systematic review with meta-analyses. *Frontiers in Psychology*, *10*, 936. https://doi.org 10.3389/fpsyg.2019.00936
Kellmann, M. (2002). Underrecovery and overtraining: Different concepts – Similar impact? In M. Kellmann (Ed.), *Enhancing recovery: Preventing underperformance in athletes* (pp. 3–24). Human Kinetics.
Kellmann, M., & Kallus, K. W. (2001). *The Recovery-Stress Questionnaire for Athletes: User manual.* Human Kinetics.
Kogan, N. (2002). Careers in the performing arts: A psychological perspective. *Creativity Research Journal*, *14*(1), 1–16. https://doi.org/10.1207/S15326934CRJ1401_1
Li, G., He, H., Gao, K., Yu, Y., Liu, Y., Li, T., Xi, P., Pollick, F., Lu, J., Yin, L., Yao, D., Duan, M., Mi, L., & Luo, C. (2025). The effects of dance intervention on clinical symptoms and cognitive deficits in hospitalized patients with chronic schizophrenia: A randomized controlled trial. *PeerJ*, *13*, e19840. https://doi.org/10.7717/peerj.19840
Linnemann, A., Strahler, J., & Nater, U. M. (2017). Assessing the effects of music listening on psychobiological stress in daily life. *Journal of Visualized Experiments*, *2*(120), 54920. https://doi.org.10.3791/54920
Liu, Z., Hui, C., Liu, S., Chen, Y., Zhang, Y., & Ye, W. (2025). The effectiveness of art therapy on motor function in Parkinson's disease: A systematic review and meta-analysis. *Frontiers in Psychology*, *16*, 1542405. https://doi.org/10.3389/fpsyg.2025.1542405
Lobinger, B., Klämpfl, M., & Altenmüller, E. (2014). We are able, we intend, we act - but we do not succeed: A theoretical framework for a better understanding of paradoxical performance in sports. *Journal of Clinical Sport Psychology*, *8*(4), 357–377.

McCrary, J. M., Ascenso, S., Savvidou, P., Schraft, S., McAllister, L., Redding, E., Bastepe-Gray, S., & Altenmüller, E. (2022). Load and fatigue monitoring in musicians using an online app: A pilot study. *Frontiers in Psychology*, *13*, 1056892. https://doi.org/10.3389/fpsyg.2022.1056892

Meeusen, R., Duclos, M., Foster, C., Fry, A., Gleeson, M., Nieman, D., Raglin, J., Rietjens, G., Steinacker, J., Urhausen, A., European College of Sport Science, & American College of Sports Medicine (2013). Prevention, diagnosis, and treatment of the overtraining syndrome: Joint consensus statement of the European College of Sport Science and the American College of Sports Medicine. *Medicine and Science in Sports and Exercise*, *45*(1), 186–205.

Moral-Bofill, L., López de la Llave, A., Pérez-Llantada, M. C., & Holgado-Tello, F. P. (2022). Development of flow state self-regulation skills and coping with musical performance anxiety: Design and evaluation of an electronically implemented psychological program. *Frontiers in Psychology*, *13*, 899621. https://doi.org/10.3389/fpsyg.2022.899621

Norris, R. N. (1996). Return to play after injury: Strategies to support a musician's recovery. *Work*, *7*(2), 89–93.

Rattray, B., Argus, C., Martin, K., Northey, J., & Driller, M. (2015). Is it time to turn our attention toward central mechanisms for post-exertional recovery strategies and performance? *Frontiers in Physiology*, 6, 79. https://doi.org/10.3389/fphys.2015.00079

Rodríguez-Jiménez, R. M., Carmona, M., García-Merino, S., Díaz-Rivas, B., & Thuissard-Vasallo, I. J. (2022). Stress, subjective wellbeing and self-knowledge in higher education teachers: A pilot study through bodyfulness approaches. *PLoS ONE*, *17*(12), e0278372. https://doi.org/10.1371/journal.pone.0278372

Rosset, M., Baumann, E., & Altenmüller, E. (2022). A longitudinal study of physical and mental health and health-related attitudes among music students: Potentials and challenges for university health promotion programs. *Frontiers in Psychology*, *13*, 885739. https://doi.org/10.3389/fpsyg.2022.885739

Salimpoor, V. N., van den Bosch, I., Kovacevic, N., McIntosh, A. R., Dagher, A., & Zatorre, R. J. (2013). Interactions between the nucleus accumbens and auditory cortices predict music reward value. *Science*, *340*(6129), 216–219.

Särkämö, T., Tervaniemi, M., Laitinen, S., Forsblom, A., Soinila, S., Mikkonen, M., Autti, T., Silvennoinen, H. M., Erkkilä, J., Laine, M., Peretz, I., & Hietanen, M. (2008). Music listening enhances cognitive recovery and mood after middle cerebral artery stroke. *Brain*, *131*, 866–876.

Schneider, S., Schönle, P. W., Altenmüller, E., & Münte, T. F. (2007). Using musical instruments to improve motor skill recovery following a stroke. *Journal of Neurology*, *254*(10), 1339–1346.

Sescousse, G., Caldú, X., Segura, B., & Dreher, J. C. (2013). Processing of primary and secondary rewards: A quantitative meta-analysis and review of human functional neuroimaging studies. *Neuroscience and Biobehavioral Reviews*, *37*(4), 681–696.

Spahn, C. (2015). Treatment and prevention of music performance anxiety. *Progress in Brain Research*, *217*, 129–140.

Sreepetch, S., Ramyarangsi, P., Mukda, S., Siripornpanich, V., & Ajjimaporn, A. (2025). Recovery effects of slow-tempo preferred music on brain activity, physiological and psychological responses following high-intensity interval exercise in healthy male adults. *Acta Psychologica*, *259*, 105456. https://doi.org 10.1016/j.actpsy.2025.105456

Steinhausen, F. A. (1907). *Die Physiologie der Bogenführung auf den Streich-Instrumenten* [The physiology of bowing on string instruments]. Breitkopf & Härtel.

Storm, S. A. (2006). Assessing the instrumentalist interface: Modifications, ergonomics and maintenance of play. *Physical Medicine and Rehabilitation Clinics of North America*, *17*(4), 893–903.

West, J., Otte, C., Geher, K., Johnson, J., & Mohr, D. C. (2004). Effects of hatha yoga and African dance on perceived stress, affect, and salivary cortisol. *Annals of Behavioural Medicine*, *28*(2), 114–118.

Wong, M. M., Tahir, T., Wong, M. M., Baron, A., & Finnerty, R. (2021). Biomarkers of stress in music interventions: A systematic review. *Journal of Music Therapy*, 58(3), 241–277.

World Health Organization. (2019). *Recovery practices for mental health and well-being: WHO Quality rights core training: Mental health and social services: Course guide*. Retrieved October 11, 2025 from https://apps.who.int/iris/handle/10665/329602

Worschech, F., Marie, D., Jünemann, K., Sinke, C., Krüger, T. H. C., Großbach, M., Scholz, D. S., Abdili, L., Kliegel, M., James, C. E., & Altenmüller, E. (2021). Improved speech in noise perception in the elderly after 6 months of musical instruction. *Frontiers in Neuroscience*, *15*, 696240. https://doi.org/10.3389/fnins.2021.696240

Worschech, F., Marie, D., Sinke, C., Kliegel, M., Jünemann, K., Scholz, D. S., Krüger, T. H., James, C. E., & Altenmüller, E. (2025). Quality of life in older adults is enhanced by piano practice: Results from a randomized controlled trial. *Annals of the New York Academy of Sciences*, *1550*(1), 239–254.

Worschech, F., Passarotto, E., Losch, H., Oku, T., Lee, A., & Altenmüller, E. (2024). What does it take to play the piano? Cognito-motor functions underlying motor learning in older adults. *Brain Sciences*, *14*(4), 405. https://doi.org/10.3390/brainsci14040405

Wulf, G., & Lewthwaite, R. (2016). Optimizing performance through intrinsic motivation and attention for learning: The OPTIMAL theory of motor learning. *Psychonomic Bulletin and Review*, *23*(5), 1382–1414.

Zamorano, A. M., Kleber, B., Arguissain, F., Vuust, P., Flor, H., & Graven-Nielsen, T. (2023). Extensive sensorimotor training enhances nociceptive cortical responses in healthy individuals. *European Journal of Pain*, *27*(2), 257–277.

INDEX

For Product Safety Concerns and Information please contact our EU representative GPSR@taylorandfrancis.com
Taylor & Francis Verlag GmbH, Kaufingerstraße 24, 80331 München, Germany

www.ingramcontent.com/pod-product-compliance
Ingram Content Group UK Ltd.
Pitfield, Milton Keynes, MK11 3LW, UK
UKHW020153200926
475702UK00016B/2694
* 9 7 8 1 0 3 2 9 3 6 3 6 9 *